HORMONAL MANIPULATION OF CANCER

Peptides, Growth Factors, and New (Anti) Steroidal Agents

Monograph Series of the European
Organization for Research on Treatment of Cancer
Volume 18

MONOGRAPH SERIES OF THE EUROPEAN ORGANIZATION FOR RESEARCH ON TREATMENT OF CANCER

The Monograph Series of the EORTC deals with selected topics related to cancer treatment. Volumes are usually, but not necessarily, based on the proceedings of an EORTC symposium. The responsibility of the Editorial Advisory Board is to approve the subject of each monograph; the Board does not review individual manuscripts.

Hormonal Manipulation of Cancer

PEPTIDES, GROWTH FACTORS, AND NEW (ANTI) STEROIDAL AGENTS

Monograph Series of the European Organization for Research on Treatment of Cancer
Volume 18

Editor

Jan G. M. Klijn, M.D.

Head, Department of Endocrine Oncology
(Clinical Endocrinology and Biochemistry)
The Dr. Daniel den Hoed Cancer Center
Rotterdam, The Netherlands

Co-Editors

Robert Paridaens, M.D.

Assistant Director of Clinical Affairs
EORTC Data Center
and Department of Medicine
Institute Jules Bordet
Brussels, Belgium

John A. Foekens, Ph.D.

Head, Department of Biochemistry
The Dr. Daniel den Hoed Cancer Center
Rotterdam, The Netherlands

Raven Press New York

Raven Press, 1185 Avenue of the Americas, New York, New York 10036

Made in the United States of America

Library of Congress Cataloging-in-Publication Data

Hormonal manipulation of cancer.

(Monograph series of the European Organization for Research on Treatment of Cancer ; v. 18)
Based on the International Symposium on "Hormonal Manipulation of Cancer: Peptides, Growth Factors and New (Anti)steroidal Agents" held in Rotterdam, the Netherlands from 4–6 June 1986; organized by the Rotterdam Dr. Daniel den Hoed Cancer Center in cooperation with the European Organization for Research on Treatment of Cancer (EORTC).
Includes index.
1. Cancer—Chemotherapy—Congresses. 2. Steroid hormones—Antagonists—Therapeutic use—Congresses. 3. Peptide hormones—Therapeutic use—Congresses. 4. Growth promoting substances—Therapeutic use— Congresses. 5. Cancer—Endocrine aspects—Congresses. I. Klijn, Jan G. M. II. Paridaens, Robert. III. Foekens, John A. IV. International Symposium On "Hormonal Manipulation of Cancer: Peptides, Growth Factors and New (Anti)steroidal Agents" (1986 : Rotterdam, Netherlands) V. Dr. Daniël den Hoed Kliniek (Rotterdam, Netherlands) VI. European Organization for Research on Treatment of Cancer. VII. Series. [DNLM: 1. Hormones—congresses. 2. Neoplasms—drug therapy—congresses. W1 M0559U v.18 / QZ 267 H8122 1986] RC271.H55H67   1987   616.99'4061   86-42601 ISBN 0-88167-301-3

Preface

Developments in the hormonal treatment of cancer have progressed rapidly. The number of new hormonal agents and treatment modalities has expanded enormously in the past five to ten years and is still doing so. A number of new agents are already in an advanced phase of preclinical research and will become available in the near future for use in treatment of cancer patients; however, not only is the number of treatment modalities for the classical endocrine-related tumors increasing, but the number of clinical indications for hormonal treatment of other tumor types is increasing simultaneously. With the accumulating insight into the endocrine, paracrine, and autocrine functions of hormones and growth factors, we may expect that in the future, apart from the classical forms of endocrine-related cancers (i.e., breast and prostate cancer), new forms of hormonal therapy or therapy based on growth factors and their receptors will be employed in the treatment of patients with cerebral, pancreatic, gastrointestinal, gynecologic, urologic, lung, and skin tumors. In addition, hormonal treatment of cancer is of increasing importance because side effects are in general negligible or less serious compared to those of cytostatic chemotherapy.

The introduction of recombinant DNA techniques make possible the production of (analogs of) peptide hormones on a large scale, and, moreover, the application of monoclonal antibodies and the detection of growth factors (receptors) have opened wide fields for preclinical and clinical research. In the areas of endocrinology and oncology especially these developments are very exciting and offer new possibilities for treatment.

Having observed these developments and having participated for five years in (pre)clinical research in the field of endocrine oncology, the Editor judged the time appropriate to bring together a large number of experts in the field of laboratory and clinical research to review newly acquired knowledge, especially with respect to new modes of treatment.

We trust that this volume will contribute to an exchange of new ideas and will stimulate people in setting up new studies that will ultimately benefit our present and future patients.

JAN G. M. KLIJN
ROBERT PARIDAENS
JOHN A. FOEKENS

Contents

New Antisteroidal Agents, Enzyme Inhibitors, and New Treatment Modalities

Luteinizing Hormone Releasing Hormone
Analogs in Cancer Treatment

PROSTATE CANCER

BREAST AND OVARIAN CANCER

DIRECT EFFECTS OF LHRH ANALOGS

Growth Factors

Somatostatin Analogs and Cancer

Hormones as Stimulatory Agents of Tumor Cell Growth in the Treatment of Cancer

Contributors

HORMONAL MANIPULATION OF CANCER

Peptides, Growth Factors, and New (Anti) Steroidal Agents

Monograph Series of the European
Organization for Research on Treatment of Cancer
Volume 18

Hormonal Manipulation of Cancer: Peptides, Growth Factors, and New (Anti) Steroidal Agents, edited by Jan G. M. Klijn et al. Raven Press, New York © 1987.

10 YEARS OF TAMOXIFEN IN BREAST CANCER

A REVIEW

J. S. Patterson

Clinical Research Department,
I.C.I. Pharmaceuticals Division,
Alderley Park, Macclesfield Cheshire England

Tamoxifen (Nolvadex *, ICI 46474) has been widely available for more than 10 years for the treatment of breast cancer. Its pharmacology (3, 7, 9, 10), toxicology (8), human safety (4, 5, 6) and antineoplastic efficacy (1, 2, 4, 6) have been subject to a number of large and exhaustive reviews. The drug has become widely accepted in the palliative treatment of metastatic breast cancer and as an agent capable of improving survival in the adjuvant situation (1, 2). It can be conservatively estimated that over one million women have been treated with tamoxifen worldwide.

It is surprising that such a successful drug is the only non steroidal anti-oestrogen available in the market place 17 years after the first clinical studies were commenced and 28 years after the discovery of MER-25. This review examines the clinical profile of tamoxifen in relation to its animal and human pharmacology and attempts to explain the present lack of newer improved agents, in contrast to many other therapeutic areas such as the β-blockers, where more than 20 variants are available, and the new ACE inhibitors where already 2 drugs are available and more than 30 are in the wings.

It is clear that any further antioestrogens will have to exhibit "real" pharmacological advantages to justify being brought to the market place, as the average development time before a new drug is marketed is in the region of 11 years, from a patent life of 16-20 years

* Nolvadex is a trade mark property of Imperial Chemical Industries PLC.

1

at a cost of more than £ 40 million. They will also be in a direct price competition with generic tamoxifens. While these factors may inhibit future developments, the underlying reasons for a lack of new anti-oestrogens today lie with the difficulty in defining a relevant clinical advantage which can be successfully modelled in the laboratory. The current safety, endocrine and efficacy profiles of Nolvadex will be used to illustrate the problems in this quest.

Prediction of Human Tolerability from Animals

Tamoxifen was designed to circumvent two problems seen with clomiphene in animals; namely a build up of a cholesterol precursor-desmosterol - with associated cataract formation and removal of the oestrogenic component by isomer separation. The former appears to have been successful while the latter is only partly so, due to the interspecies variability of endocrine target organ responses.

The human tolerability picture is built up from publications in both adjuvant and advanced disease together with case reports and company files. The data on a marketed drug are of necessity incomplete and with the advent of multiple tamoxifens in the market place, will become even more fragmented. The second problem of interpretation of the data lies with the lack of controlled studies especially in advanced breast cancer, in a group of already severely ill patients. Placebo studies do not exist here and thus a genuine background incidence of spontaneously occuring events is unavailable. Even against this background, Nolvadex has been well tolerated with a low withdrawal rate due to intolerance and the major side effects such as nausea, hot flushes occurring in around 10% of women (4, 6). Thus, a significant improvement in tolerability for a new agent would be unlikely and is notoriously difficult to model with preclinical studies. This problem has already manifest itself with 2 other members of this class of compound, nafoxidine and MER-25 which have shown unpredicted phototoxicity and CNS problems respectively, in man.

Prediction of Human Endocrine Effects from Animals

When the human data are examined it is hard to decide whether Nolvadex can genuinely be called an antioestrogen, defined as an agent which blocks the response of an oestrogen sensitive cell to oestrogenic stimulation. It is certainly not a pure anti-oestrogen as both the vaginal cornification index rise and gonadotrophin fall in postmenopausal women testify. However, the majority of its effects can be construed as anti-oestrogenic with some partial agonism. It is also clear that different cells and organs can respond quite differently to the agent. An illustration lies with the premenopausal woman who has a marked elevation of circulating oestradiol (E2) in the presence of a fall in karyopyknotic index (K.P.I.) and antioestrogenic side effects and antineoplastic effects while continuing to menstruate.

All laboratory models show differing responses to tamoxifen and other anti-oestrogens and the menstruating primate (m.nemestrina) shows the drug to be a pure anti-oestrogen with an opposite effect on circulating E2 than in the premenopausal woman (3). Thus, the search for an endocrinologically better anti-oestrogen begs the question of what is better and what is a relevant test species. There is no doubt, however, that an agent which showed no partial agonism in the rat uterus and did not elevate E2 in young women, would be extremely interesting.

Prediction of Human Efficacy from the Laboratory

The complete or partial response rate in 68 published studies involving 4,000 patients treated with Nolvadex has remained unchanged from the earliest publications and remarkably consistant at 33% (5). A further 20% of patients show disease stabilization. These response rates are very similar to those achieved with other endocrine modalities such as the oestrogens, androgens, progestins or aminoglutethimide that have been compared with tamoxifen. As the primary mode of action of tamoxifen is thought to be through the cytoplasmic oestrogen receptor (ER) selection of patients with receptor rich

tumours was predicted to improve the effect.
This appears so, especially in advanced disease
although even so, only 55% of these patients are
seen to respond. It is known that tamoxifen is a
relatively weak binder to the ER and it has been
postulated that compounds with a higher binding
affinity would improve the tumour response rate.
This approach, too, has run into problems as the
effects would appear to depend on binding which
is temperature dependant and the kinetics of the
binding. Thus some very tightly bound compounds
appear to be rapidly displaced and produce less
anti tumour effects in DMBA tumours than tamoxifen. Further, tamoxifen has, at high but pharmacologically realistic concentrations, an inhibitory effect on some ER negative tumours. It also
has other pharmaceutical effects, as do other
members of the class, such as prostaglandin
synthetase inhibitor activity. These effects may
be relevant to the human anti tumour activity
and need to be considered when new compounds are
assessed although it is not known exactly how to
do so. Finally, attempts to obtain additive
endocrine effects by giving several endocrine
modalities with different mechnisms of action
have been tried with little success, suggesting
that all the effects of these agents may run
down a final common pathway, as yet undefined.

In the adjuvant situation, the work of Jordan
and his coworkers has shown that in the DMBA
tumour model in rats, prolonged adjuvant therapy
has led to a greater disease free interval and
survival than a short tamoxifen course. It is
difficult to know how long term therapy in the
rat life should be translated to man. However,
the significant improvements in DFI and survival
seen with a 2 year Nolvadex adjuvant course have
led to work now in progress to assess much
longer term therapy and to attempts to find markers that would allow earlier intervention in
preventing recurrent breast cancer.

Conclusion

This review has sought to clarify the reason why
tamoxifen stands alone as the single commercially available anti-oestrogen for breast cancer
therapy after so many years. It is salutory to
quote the words of the discoverer of tamoxifen,

Dr. Arthur Walpole, at the first meeting on the effect of Nolvadex in breast cancer in 1974.

He said "The action of Nolvadex is extremely complex. It has quite definite oestrogenic properties but it is also a true anti-oestrogen in certain circumstances and in certain species."

The intervening years have done nothing to clarify this situation - if anything the discoveries have had the opposite effect.

My grateful thanks to my colleagues Dr. Alan Wakeling, Dr. Ian Jealson, Dr. Barry Furr and Dr. Jo Diver for their help in preparing this paper and Frau C. Schell for typing the manuscript.

References

1. Baum, M., Brinkley, D.M., Dossett, J.A., McPherson, K., Patterson, J.S., Rubens, R.D., Smiddy, F.G., Stoll, B.A., Wilson, A., Richards, D. and Ellis, H. (1985): Lancet, 1:836-840.
2. Consensus Conference on Adjuvant Breast Cancer Chemotherapy (1985): JAMA 254:3461-3463.
3. Furr, B.J., Jordan, V.C. (1984): In: Pharmac. Ther. Vol 25, edited by J.H. Clark and B.M. Markaverich, pp. 127-205, Pergamon Press, Oxford.
4. Heel, R.C., Brogden, R.N. and Speight, J.M. (1978): Drugs, 16:1. Adis Press.
5. ICI Data on file.
6. Patterson, J.S., Edwards, D.G. and Battersby, L. (1981): Japan. Journal of Cancer Clinics Suppl. (Nov.) 157.
7. Sutherland, R. and Jordan, V.C., editors (1981): Non-Steroidal Anti Oestrogens. Molecular Pharmacology and Anti Tumour Activity. Academic Press, Sydney.
8. Tucker, M.J., Adam, H.K. and Patterson, J.S. (1984): In: Safety Testing of New Drugs, edited by D. R. Lawrence, A.E.M. McLean and M. Weatherall, pp. 125-163. Academic Press, London.
9. Wakeling, A.E. (1985): In: Antioestrogens in Oncology, Past, Present and Prospects, edited by F.Pannuti, pp. 43-54. Excerpta Medica, Amsterdam.

10. Wakeling, A.E. In: Pharmacology and Clinical Uses of Inhibitors of Hormone Action and Secretion, edited by A.E. Wakeling and B.J. Furr (in press). Holt Saunders.
11. Wakeling, A.E., Valcaccia, B., Newboult E. and Green, L.R. (1984): J. Steroid Biochem. Vol. 20. 1:111-120.

Hormonal Manipulation of Cancer: Peptides, Growth Factors, and New (Anti) Steroidal Agents, edited by Jan G. M. Klijn et al.
Raven Press, New York © 1987.

ADRENAL STEROIDS EXERT POTENT ESTROGENIC ACTION IN BOTH NORMAL AND CANCER TISSUE

F. Labrie, R. Poulin, J. Simard, J.-F. Hubert,
P. Spinola and B. Marchetti

MRC Group in Molecular Endocrinology
Laval University Medical Center, Quebec G1V 4G2, Canada

SUMMARY

Human adrenals are unique in having a high secretion rate of steroids which are converted into estrogens and androgens in peripheral tissues. In order to obtain further information about the potential role of these steroids as estrogens in target tissues, we have studied the activity of dehydroepiandrosterone-sulfate (DHEA-S), dehydroepiandrosterone (DHEA) and androst-5-ene-3β,17β-diol (Δ^5-diol) in normal and cancer tissues. Following incubation with normal rat anterior pituitary cells in culture, Δ^5-diol, DHEA and DHEA-S cause a 3- to 8-fold maximal increase in prolactin cell content, the effect being reversed by the antiestrogen LY156758. Similarly, the stimulatory effect of the three steroids on LH, FSH and GH release is blocked competitively by the antiestrogen. The effect of Δ^5-diol was next studied in the human mammary carcinoma cell line ZR-75-1. In this tissue, it caused a strong mitogenic effect on cell growth. Since the half-maximal concentration of Δ^5-diol required to stimulate cell growth is 2.5 nM, a concentration which is within the range of normal serum levels of the adrenal steroid in women, the present data clearly indicate the potential role of Δ^5-diol in breast cancer growth and development in women. We have also found a potent stimulatory effect of Δ^5-diol and DHEA on the growth of the DMBA-induced mammary tumor in the rat. The present data indicate that the adrenal steroids, either in the form of Δ^5-diol, or of its precursors, DHEA-S and DHEA, should be taken into consideration for the efficient control of estrogen-sensitive cancer. Drugs able to more efficiently block adrenal steroid secretion and pure antiestrogenic compounds able to neutralize the action of estrogens of various sources should become a priority in the field of research on estrogen-sensitive cancer, especially breast cancer.

INTRODUCTION

Man is unique among species in having a high secretion rate
of adrenal steroids other than glucocorticoids (17). Despite the
fact that dehydroepiandrosterone sulfate (DHEAS), their main
secretion product, is present in human serum at far higher concentrations than any other steroid, the biological functions of
this so-called adrenal "androgen" remain almost entirely unknown.
Delay in this field is partly due to the fact that all the animal
models used do not secrete appreciable amounts of adrenal precursor steroids, thus focusing all attention to the testes and
ovaries as exclusive sources of sex steroids for target tissue
growth and function.

However, recent data clearly indicate that the adrenal steroids dehydroepiandrosterone-sulfate (DHEAS), DHEA, androst-5-
ene-3β,17β-diol (Δ^5-diol) and androstenedione (Δ^4-dione) can be
converted into active estrogens (and androgens) in peripheral
tissues, especially the breast (13, 21). Moreover, Δ^5-diol, a
metabolite of DHEAS and DHEA has been shown to induce classical
estrogenic responses in target tissues (4, 5, 26). These data
pertain to the stimulatory effect of Δ^5-diol on estrogen-sensitive parameters in cultured human mammary carcinoma MCF-7 (4, 26)
and ZR-75-1 (25) cell lines. In addition, Δ^5-diol exerts typical
estrogenic activity at physiological concentrations on the growth
of the uterus of immature rats (27).

Since the effects of C_{19}-Δ^5 adrenal steroids on tumor growth
had not been reported, we have investigated, as a first approach,
their potential effect on the growth of the human breast carcinoma cell line ZR-75-1 in vitro as well as on the growth of the
dimethylbenz(a)anthracene (DMBA)-induced mammary tumor in the
rat. In addition, we have studied the effect of the same adrenal
steroids in normal rat anterior pituitary cells in culture on the
release of LH, FSH, growth hormone and prolactin. The present
data indicate that C_{19}-Δ^5-adrenal steroids, especially Δ^5-diol,
may well be the main estrogen in breast cancer.

RESULTS AND DISCUSSION

As illustrated in Fig. 1, an 8-day incubation with maximal
concentrations of estradiol increases ZR-75-1 cell number by
about 3.5-fold. The concentration of estradiol required to induce
half-maximal stimulation of cell proliferation is approximately 5
pM. It can be seen that Δ^5-diol has a strong mitogenic effect on
ZR-75-1 cells, this steroid leading to a maximal increase in cell
number 2.8-fold above control values, the half-maximal effect
being observed at approximately 2.5 nM Δ^5-diol. It should be
mentioned that this concentration lies within the range of normal
serum levels of Δ^5-diol in women (1-3 nM) (16, 24).

On the other hand, DHEA and DHEAS have a much less potent
action on cell proliferation, both steroids increasing cell
number up to about 75% above control at the maximal concentration

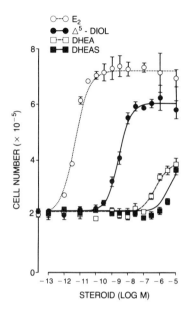

FIG. 1. Effect of increasing concentrations of estradiol and C_{19}-Δ^5-steroids on the proliferation of ZR-75-1 cells in culture. Cells were plated at an initial density of 2.0×10^4 cells/well in 24-well culture plates in RPM1 1640-5% DCC-treated FBS. After 48h, estradiol, Δ^5-diol, DHEA or DHEAS were added with fresh medium at the indicated concentrations. Cell number was measured after 8 days in the presence of the steroids. Values represent means ± SEM of triplicate determinations from a representative experiment.

used (10 µM). DHEA was more potent than its 3β-sulfate ester, a significant increase in cell number being observed at concentrations greater than 100 nM, while DHEAS did not have a significant effect on the growth of ZR-75-1 cells at concentrations lower than 3000 nM. It should however be mentioned that the normal serum concentration of DHEAS in adult women lies within the range of concentrations having a stimulatory effect on cell growth.

The potent antiestrogen LY156758, a benzothiophene derivative having minimal agonistic activity in vivo (10) and behaving as a pure estrogen antagonist in rat pituitary gonadotrophs (28), was next used to assess the estrogenic nature of C_{19}-Δ^5-steroid action. The antiestrogen alone exerted a 50% inhibition of cell growth, this inhibitory effect remaining maximal up to 0.3 nM estradiol and 0.3 µM Δ^5-diol (data not shown). That the effect of LY156758 was not cytotoxic is indicated by the finding that 100 nM estradiol could completely reverse the effect of the antiestrogen. The inhibitory effect of the antiestrogen was thus of a competitive nature for both estradiol and Δ^5-diol, the calculated (9) K_D value of LY156758 action being 0.54 nM. Growth stimulation by the less potent DHEA and DHEAS was completely abolished by LY156758 at all steroid concentrations used.

The expression of the progesterone receptor is known to be under specific estrogenic control in human breast cancer cells (14). We have thus measured the level of progesterone-specific binding sites after incubation of the ZR-75-1 cells for 4 days in the presence of estradiol and of the C_{19}-Δ^5-steroids. The specific uptake of ^{3}H-labeled R5020 was increased up to 5-fold in

ZR-75-1 cells incubated with estradiol (data not shown). When present up to 10 µM, Δ^5-diol, DHEA and DHEAS maximally increased the number of high-affinity R5020 binding sites by 3.7-, 3.2- and 2.0-fold, respectively. A half-maximal stimulatory effect was obtained at 0.025, 13 and 200 nM with estradiol, Δ^5-diol and DHEA, respectively. Therefore, the relative potency of the C_{19}-Δ^5-steroids in increasing the number of specific progesterone binding sites is parallel to their ability to stimulate cell proliferation.

The estrogen-like effects of Δ^5-diol, DHEA and DHEAS could have been mediated through metabolism including an endogenous aromatase with the subsequent formation of the known estrogenic compounds estrone and/or estradiol (1, 19, 23).

However, considering its action at low concentrations, it is likely that Δ^5-diol acts at physiological concentrations as a genuine estrogen on the ZR-75-1 cells through its direct interaction with the estrogen receptor (ER) (16). In order to better define the pathways through which C_{19}-Δ^5-steroids exert their estrogenic effects, ZR-75-1 cells were incubated with [^{3}H] DHEA for various time periods. As shown in Fig. 2, DHEA can be conver-

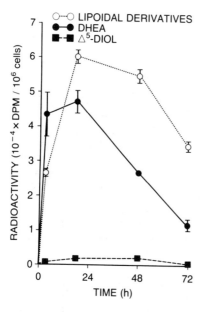

FIG. 2. Metabolism of [1,2-^{3}H]DHEA in ZR-75-1 human breast cancer cells in monolayer culture. Sub-confluent cultures of ZR-75-1 cells maintained in RPMI 1640 medium supplemented with 5% DCC-coated FBS were incubated for the indicated time periods with 51 nM [1,2-^{3}H]DHEA (60 Ci/mmol). Cells were then washed with Hank's Balanced Salt Solution, trypsiniz-ed, and extracted twice with die-thyl ether. Extracts were then submitted to Sephadex LH-20 liquid chromatography, and the various fractions thus obtained were ace-tylated overnight with acetic anhydride: pyridine (2:3, v/v), and analyzed by silica gel thin-layer chromatography. Areas of the chromatograms containing radioac-tivity were located with a Ber-thold thin-layer scanner, scraped, and eluted with 10 ml diethyl ether. Radioactivity was then measured by scintillation spectro-metry. Values are expressed as mean ± SEM of triplicate measu-rements.

ted into Δ^5-diol in this cell line. Though the maximal yield of conversion of [^{3}H] Δ^5-diol was 2.4 ± 0.1% of total incorporation after 48h, it corresponds to an intracellular Δ^5-diol concentration equal to approximately 1.5 nM. No significant formation of androstenedione, testosterone, estrone or estradiol could be detected at any sampling time. In fact, the only other products of [^{3}H]DHEA metabolism detected were highly hydrophobic derivatives ("lipoidal derivatives"), the identity of which is currently under investigation, but do not correspond to non-polar esters of estradiol (20). Moreover, increasing DHEA concentrations up to 1 µM in the incubation medium led to further accumulation of Δ^5-diol, thus reaching intracellular levels equivalent to approximately 9 nM (results not shown). In experiments not shown here, the only radiolabelled products found in ZR-75-1 cells incubated with [^{3}H] Δ^5-diol for up to 72 h were [^{3}H]DHEA as well as the corresponding tritiated non-polar derivatives.

From these data, it is most likely that Δ^5-diol exerts its estrogenic effect directly, i.e. without the involvement of the aromatase pathway, which has been reported to be virtually absent in the ZR-75-1 cell line (22). Moreover, the present experiments also suggest that DHEA must first be metabolized into Δ^5-diol in order to have estrogenic activity.

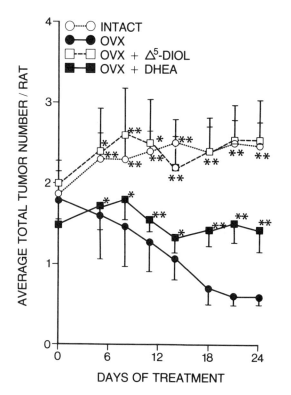

FIG. 3 Effect of ovariectomy (OVX) or of 24-day treatment of OVX animals with the C_{19}-Δ^5-steroids Δ^5-diol or DHEA (2 mg, twice daily) on the total number of DMBA-induced mammary tumors in the rat.

   Dimethylbenz(a)anthracene (DMBA)-induced mammary carcinoma in the rat is a widely accepted model of hormone-dependent breast cancer in the human (6, 7, 15). The development and growth of this tumor are particularly sensitive to the stimulatory action of estrogens and prolactin (6, 7). We have thus studied the effect of Δ^5-diol and DHEA on the growth of this tumor in the rat.

   Figure 3 illustrates the changes in total tumor number under the influence of the various treatments. It can be seen that there is a steady increase in the total number of tumors in the intact animals from 1.87 ± 0.27 to 2.47 ± 0.29 during the 24 days of observation. In the OVX animals, the tumor number shows a marked reduction from 1.80 ± 0.26 to 0.60 ± 0.19 per rat (p < 0.01). More importantly, it can be seen that treatment of OVX rats with Δ^5-diol or DHEA completely prevents the decrease found after OVX. In fact, the total number of tumors in these two groups increased to 2.54 ± 0.50 after Δ^5-diol treatment (p < 0.01 vs OVX) while it remained constant in the group of OVX rats treated with DHEA with values going from 1.50 ± 0.23 to 1.42 ± 0.26 tumors/rat for the same 24-day period. Both Δ^5-diol and DHEA treatments caused a highly significant (p < 0.01) increase in total tumor number as compared to OVX animals who received the vehicle only.

   Figure 4 illustrates the effect of the same treatments on average tumor area (cm^2) in each group of animals. It can be seen that while average tumor area is dramatically reduced to 0.75 ± 0.27 cm^2 (p < 0.01) after OVX, treatment of OVX animals with Δ^5-diol and DHEA increases tumor area to 9.79 ± 2.25 and 3.93 ± 0.86 cm^2, respectively (p < 0.01). In intact animals, tumor area is measured at 4.70 ± 0.95 cm^2 at the end of the experiment.

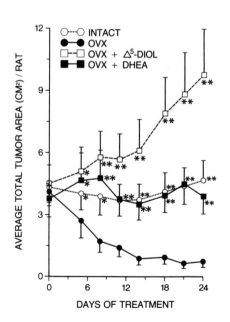

FIG. 4 Effect of ovariectomy (OVX) or of 24-day treatment of OVX animals with the C_{19}-Δ^5-steroids Δ^5-diol or DHEA (2 mg, twice daily) on the average total area (cm^2) of DMBA-induced mammary tumors in the rat.

Estrogens are known to exert a specific stimulatory effect on LHRH-induced LH release in rat anterior pituitary cells in primary culture (11, 12) while androgens and progestins act as inhibitors and glucocorticoids have no effect. We have thus taken advantage of the specificity, sensitivity and reliability of rat adenohypophysial cells in culture to investigate the activity of Δ^5-diol and DHEA at the pituitary level.

Pretreatment with 17β-estradiol (E_2), Δ^5-diol or DHEA induces a 2.4-, 2.7- and 4.2-fold stimulation of LH release induced by 0.3 nM LHRH, the effect being exerted at respective 50% maximally effective concentrations (ED_{50} values) of 0.015, 45 and 110 nM for the respective steroids. On the other hand, the sensitivities of the LH and FSH responses to LHRH as assessed by ED_{50} values of LHRH action are increased by about 4.5- to 7-fold. As further proof of the estrogenic nature of the effect of Δ^5-diol and DHEA, the effects of E_2, Δ^5-diol and DHEA are inhibited competitively by simultaneous incubation with the antiestrogen LY156758 (Keoxifene). Δ^5-diol and DHEA also exert a potent stimulatory effect on growth hormone and PRL secretion as well as on PRL cell content (3- to 8-fold stimulation) (results not shown).

In direct binding studies, Δ^5-diol and DHEA have approximately 85- and > 10,000 lower affinities than E_2, respectively, for the estrogen receptor in rat anterior pituitary homogenate and human breast carcinoma cytosols. The present data clearly show that Δ^5-diol and DHEA can exert full estrogenic activity on LHRH-induced LH and FSH release in rat adenohypophysial cells, thus supporting the potential estrogenic role of these C_{19} adrenal steroids in estrogen-dependent diseases.

The above-described data show that physiological concentrations of Δ^5-diol can exert a marked stimulatory effect on the proliferation of ZR-75-1 cells. Since the half-maximal stimulation of cancer cell growth was observed at 2.5 nM and the serum levels of Δ^5-diol in adult women are 1 to 3 nM (16, 24), the present data clearly indicate the potential role of Δ^5-diol in breast cancer growth and development in women.

The implications of the present findings for breast cancer are important. As mentioned above, the average plasma concentration of Δ^5-diol in women (1-3 nM) is sufficient to cause a sustained estrogenic stimulus in responsive breast tumor cells, the serum level of Δ^5-diol being maintained by continuous peripheral conversion from DHEAS and DHEA (3, 4). Moreover, the cytosolic concentrations of Δ^5-diol and DHEA in breast tissue are 2- to 5-fold higher than in plasma (3, 8) and breast cancer tissue homogenates are known to convert DHEA into Δ^5-diol (2, 18).

The present demonstration that C_{19}-Δ^5-steroids can stimulate breast cancer cell growth indicates that adrenal estrogens, either in the form of Δ^5-diol or of its precursors, should be taken into consideration for the efficient control of estrogen-sensitive breast cancer. Thus, medical or surgical oophorectomy offers no more than a partial blockade of estrogens in premenopausal women. Neutralization by a pure antiestrogen of the continuous action of C_{19}-Δ^5 steroids should therefore become an essential part of the endocrine treatment of breast cancer.

REFERENCES

1. Abul-Hajj, Y.J. (1975): Metabolism of dehydroepiandrosterone by hormone-dependent and hormone-independent human breast carcinoma. Steroids, 26:488-500.
2. Adams, J.B., and Wang, M.S.F. (1968): Paraendocrine behaviour of human breast carcinoma. In vitro transformation of steroids to physiologically active hormones. J. Endocrinol., 41:41-52.
3. Adams, J.B., Archibald, L., and Seymour-Munn, K. (1980): Dehydroepiandrosterone and androst-5-ene-3β,17β-diol on human mammary cancer cytosolic and nuclear compartments and their relationship to estrogen receptor. Cancer Res., 40:3815-3820.
4. Adams, J.B., Garcia, M., and Rochefort, H. (1981). Estrogenic effects of physiological concentrations of 5-androstene-3β,17β-diol and its metabolism in MCF-7 human breast cancer cells. Cancer Res., 41: 4720-4726.
5. Adams, J.B. (1985): Control of secretion and the function of C_{19}-Δ^5-steroids of the human adrenal gland. Mol. Cell. Endocrinol., 41:1-17.
6. Asselin, J., Kelly, P.A., Caron, M.G. and Labrie, F. (1977): Control of hormone receptor levels and growth of 7,12-dimethylbenz(a)anthracene-induced mammary tumors by estrogens, progesterone and prolactin. Endocrinology, 101: 666-671.
7. Asselin, J., and Labrie, F. (1977): Effects of estradiol and prolactin on steroid receptor levels in 7,12-dimethylbenz-(a)anthracene-induced mammary tumors and uterus in the rat. J. Steroid Biochem., 9:1079-1082.
8. Bonney, R.C., Scanlon, M.J., Reed, M.J., Jones, D.L., Beranek, P.A., and James, V.H.T. (1984): Adrenal androgen concentrations in breast tumours and in normal breast tissue. The relationship to oestradiol metabolism. J. Steroid Biochem., 20:501-504.
9. Cheng, Y., and Prusoff, W.H. (1973): Relationship between the inhibition constant (Ki) and the concentration of inhibitor which causes 50% inhibition (IC_{50}) of an enzymatic reaction. Biochem. Pharmacol., 22:3099-3108.
10. Clemens, J.A., Bennett, D.R., Black, L.J., and Jones, C.D. (1983): Effects of a new antiestrogen, keoxifene (LY156758), on growth of carcinogen-induced mammary tumors and on LH and prolactin levels. Life Sci., 32:2869-2875.
11. Drouin, J., and Labrie, F. (1976): Selective effect of androgens on LH and FSH release in anterior pituitary cells in culture. Endocrinology, 98: 1528-1534.
12. Drouin, J., Lagacé, L., and Labrie, F. (1976): Estradiol-induced increase of the LH responsiveness to LHRH in anterior pituitary cells in culture. Endocrinology, 99: 1477-1481.

13.Griffiths, K., Jones, D., Cameron, E.H.D., Gleave, E.N., and Forrest, A.P.M. (1972): Transformation of steroids by mammary cancer tissue. In: Estrogen target tissues and neoplasia, edited by T.L. Dao, pp. 151-162, University of Chicago Press, Chicago.

14.Horwitz, K.B., and McGuire, W.L. (1978): Estrogen control of progesterone receptors in human breast cancer. J. Biol. Chem., 253:2223-2228.

15.Huggins, C., Grand, L.C., and Brillantes, F.P. (1961): Mammary cancer induced by a single feeding of polynuclear hydrocarbons, and its suppression. Nature, 189: 204-247.

16.Kreitmann, B. and Bayard, F. (1979): Androgen interaction with the oestrogen receptor in human tissues. J. Steroid Biochem., 11:1589-1595.

17.Labrie, F., Dupont, A. and Bélanger, A. (1985). Complete androgen blockade for the treatment of prostate cancer. In: Important Advances in Oncology, edited by V.T. De Vita, S. Hellman and S.A. Rosenberg, pp. 193-217. J.B. Lippincott, Philadelphia.

18.Li, K., Foo, T. and Adams, J.B. (1978). Products of dehydro-epiandrosterone metabolism by human mammary tumors and their influence on estradiol receptor binding. Steroids, 31:113-127.

19.McIndoe, J.H. (1979): Estradiol formation from testosterone by continuously cultured human breast cancer cells. J. Clin. Endocrinol. Metab., 49: 272-277.

20.Mellon-Nussbaum, S.H., Ponticorvo, L., Schatz, F., and Hochberg, R.B. (1982). Estradiol fatty acid esters. The isolation and identification of the lipoidal derivatives of estradiol synthesized in the bovine uterus. J. Biol. Chem., 257: 5678-5684.

21.Miller, W.R., and Forrest, A.P.M. (1976). Oestradiol synthesis from C19 steroids by human breast cancers. Brit. J. Cancer, 33:116-118.

22.Perel, E., Daniilescu, D., Kharlip, L., Blackstein, M.E. and Killinger, D.W. (1985). The relationship between growth and androstenedione metabolism in four cell lines of human breast carcinoma cells in culture. Mol. Cell. Endocrinol., 41: 197-203.

23.Perel, E., Wilkins, D., and Killinger, D.W. (1980): The conversion of androstenedione to estrone, estradiol and testosterone in breast tissue. J. Steroid Biochem., 13:89-94.

24.Poortman, J., Prenen, J.A.C., Schwarz, F., and Thijssen, J.H.H. (1975): Interaction of Δ^5-androstene-3β,17β-diol with estradiol and dihydrotestosterone receptors in human myometrial and mammary cancer tissue. J. Clin. Endocrinol. Metab., 40:133-143.

25.Poulin, R., and Labrie, F. (1985): Stimulation of cell growth by C19 steroids of adrenal origin in a human breast cancer cell line. Clin. Invest. Med., 8:A162.

26.Rochefort, H., and Garcia, M. (1984): The estrogenic and antiestrogenic activities of androgens in female target tissues. Pharmacol. Ther., 23: 193-216.

27.Seymour-Munn, K., and Adams, J.B. (1983): Estrogenic effects of 5-androstene-3β,17β-diol at physiological concentrations and its possible implication in the etiology of breast cancer. Endocrinology, 112: 486-491.

28.Simard, J., and Labrie, F. (1985): Keoxifene shows pure antiestrogenic activity in pituitary gonadotrophs. Mol. Cell. Endocrinol., 39:141-144.

Hormonal Manipulation of Cancer: Peptides, Growth Factors, and New (Anti) Steroidal Agents, edited by Jan G. M. Klijn et al. Raven Press, New York © 1987.

TOTAL ANDROGEN BLOCKADE vs ORCHIECTOMY

IN STAGE D   PROSTATE CANCER

Preliminary results of a multicentre French trial*

J.M. Brisset, C. Bertagna, J. Fiet, A. de Géry, M. Hucher, J.M. Husson, D. Tremblay and J.P. Raynaud.

Centre Médico-Chirurgical de la Porte de Choisy, 75634 Paris Cedex 13 (JMB) ; Hôpital St-Louis, 75010 Paris (JF) ; Roussel-Uclaf, 75007 Paris (CB, AG, MH, JMH, DT, JPR), France.

Total androgen blockade, i.e., the elimination of all sources of androgen influence on prostate cancer growth, is not an entirely new concept. Several studies in the past have investigated the effect of bilateral adrenalectomy or of adrenal biosynthesis inhibitors in patients who have relapsed after castration [1,3, 28,30(review),36] or of a steroid antiandrogen in orchiectomized or estrogen-treated patients [5,6,10-13,18]. The rationale of these treatments is the elimination of the source or action of both testicular and adrenal androgens. However, these treatments have been criticized for a variety of reasons : both adrenalectomy and the use of biosynthesis inhibitors necessitate replacement

---

* Clinical study centres : J-M. Brisset, L. Boccon-Gibod, H. Botto, M. Camey, G. Cariou, J-M. Duclos, F. Duval, D. Gontiès, R. Jorest, L. Lamy, A. Le Duc, A. Mouton, M. Petit, A. Prawerman, F. Richard, I. Savatovsky, G. Vallancien.

Centre Médico-Chirurgical de la Porte de Choisy, Paris (J-M.B., G.V.), Hôpital Saint-Joseph, Paris (J-M.B., J-M.D.) Hôpital Cochin, Paris (L.B-G), Centre Medico-Chirurgical Foch, Suresnes (H.B., M.C., F.R.) Hôpital Saint-Louis, Paris (G.C., A.L.D.), Clinique Chirurgicale Mutualiste, Reims (F.D., M.P., A.P.), Clinique Chantereine, Brou-sur-Chantereine (D.G.), Centre Hospitalier Regional, Creil (R.J.), Hôpital de Juvisy (L.L.), Clinique de l'Archette, Olivet (A.M.), Hôpital R. Ballanger, Aulnay (I.S.), France.

Pharmacokinetic study centres : L. Pendyala, P.J. Creaven, B.H. Meyer.

Roswell Park Memorial Institute, Buffalo, U.S. (LP, PC), Orange Free State University, Bloemfontein, South Africa (BHM).

corticoid therapy, adrenalectomy was performed only at relapse as a second line therapy when effective control of tumor growth by endocrine treatment can no longer be expected, estrogens have recognized cardiovascular effects that can outweigh the overall benefits of therapy, the efficacy of steroid antiandrogens in association with castration has not been evaluated in randomized trials.

It is with the advent of nonsteroid antiandrogens, that do not bind to steroid receptors other than androgen receptors, and of a new method of medical castration by LHRH-analogs that the concept of total androgen blockade gained a new lease of life. The use of nonsteroid antiandrogens alone was not considered optimum since the inhibition not only of androgen action on the prostate but also of the negative control exerted by testosterone on LH and FSH release resulted in an increase in LH and testosterone that counteracted the antiandrogen action on the prostate [21]. The association of a pituitary inhibitor to the antiandrogen was thus deemed necessary [21] and combination treatments with both estrogens and progestins were tested in animal studies [21,26]. However, the final choice fell on the LHRH-analog, buserelin, which was thought to have greater potency and specificity as a pituitary inhibitor [17,31]. Clinical trials have since established that the efficacy of LHRH-analogs (sc, im, nasal or depot) is comparable to that of bilateral orchiectomy [e.g. 4,7,22,29,32,34].

In contrast to the modest benefits afforded by earlier combination endocrine therapies, promising results were noted in open clinical trials with the first combination treatment using a nonsteroid antiandrogen, Anandron, and an LHRH agonist, buserelin, in stage C and D prostate cancer patients [14,15] although the latest results over longer treatment periods appear slightly less spectacular [16]. To establish whether the combination of castration + antiandrogen is truly superior to castration alone we decided to undertake a randomized double-blind trial. However, to avoid evaluating in a first instance the simultaneous effect of two drugs, we decided to use orchiectomy as the most radical means of eliminating testicular androgens. The study was performed in patients with stage D cancer, even though they may be the least responsive to endocrine manipulation, and who had received no previous hormone therapy. Antiandrogen therapy was initiated on the day of castration or shortly after for an optimum response.

Data are also presented on drug monitoring during clinical trials and on recent kinetic studies on Anandron to justify modifications in the existing administration schedule.

PATIENTS AND CLINICAL FOLLOW-UP

In this prospective multicenter double-blind trial, 195 patients with stage D biopsy-proven prostatic carcinoma, who had received no previous surgical, hormonal or radiation treatment for their cancer and with a life expectancy of at least 3 months were randomized into one of three treatment groups: orchiectomy and placebo; orchiectomy and Anandron 150 mg per day; orchiectomy and Anandron 300 mg per day. The test drug was taken orally.

Before study and every 6 months, the work-up included clinical examination, measurement of prostate volume (through transrectal ultrasonography in several centers), chest X-ray, bone scan, bone X-rays, and intravenous pyelogram. Abdominal CT scan and lymphography were performed when necessary to evaluate lymph node involvement. After 1 and 3 months of treatment, a shorter work-up included clinical examination and measurement of prostate volume. At each visit a blood sample was obtained for usual hematology and biochemistry parameters, as well as for radioimmunoassay (RIA) of prostatic acid phosphatases (PAP), of Anandron, and of several hormones using commercially available kits when possible [8,9,24].

The National Prostatic Cancer Project (NPCP) criteria were used to evaluate objective response at each of the 6-monthly visits. The best objective response (at any 6-monthly follow-up), with the time-to-progression and the survival time, were the main efficacy criteria.

Individual subjective and objective criteria (bone pain, performance status, PAP, primary tumor volume, number of areas of increased uptake on bone scan) were analyzed as well. In each centre, successive bone scans were read and compared by independent assessors who did not know to which group the patient belonged.

The patients continued taking the test medication (Anandron or placebo), as long as they tolerated it well and their disease did not progress. When progression occurred, the code was broken and the investigator could then give the patient the treatment he thought most appropriate, including Anandron when the patient had been on placebo.

The statistical methods were the following : For qualitative variables, comparisons between groups were made using a chi-square test. For laboratory data, treatment groups were compared by covariance analysis. For time-to-progression and time-to-death, actuarial rates were computed according to the Kaplan-Meier estimate and compared using the Logrank test. The significance level was $p < 0.05$.

METHODOLOGY OF DRUG KINETICS AND DRUG MONITORING STUDIES

Kinetic Study in Healthy Volunteers

This was an open randomized cross-over study in male volunteers (18 to 40 yrs) receiving a single oral treatment of either 100, 200 or 300 mg of Anandron in tablet form (respectively 2, 4 or 6 50 mg-tablets). The interval between two treatments in the crossover design was 2 weeks. The subjects were fasted for at least 10 h prior to administration of the drug. Blood samples were drawn

before and at 18 time-points during the 168 h following administration. After extraction and separation by high performance
liquid chromatography (HPLC), plasma Anandron was detected and
quantified by UV absorption.

Kinetic Study in Patients

The drug was administered orally to 12 in-patients at the
Roswell Park Memorial Institute. All had a microscopically confirmed diagnosis of Stage D carcinoma of the prostate. Single dose
kinetics of radioactivity and of the unchanged drug were studied
[23,24]. Starting on day 4 in 8 patients and on day 8 in 3 patients, 150 mg of nonradioactive drug (200 mg in one patient) was
given twice daily for 2-7 weeks. The plasma kinetics of the drug
were studied during this period to establish the steady state
levels and time to achieve steady state. With those patients who
were on the multiple dose study for more than 3 weeks, sampling
was carried out every 12 h prior to the drug intake when patients
were still in the hospital and, subsequent to this, on a 1 to 2
week outpatient basis.

Plasma was extracted with chloroform, the chloroform extract
was evaporated and reconstituted in an appropriate volume of
mobile phase. Unchanged Anandron was separated by HPLC and measured by UV absorbance with a detection limit of 50 ng/ml [24].

Drug Monitoring Study

During the clinical trial blood samples were drawn one month
(25 to 40 days), three months (80 to 104 days), six months (160 to
200 days), and/or twelve months (345 to 405 days) after initiation
of treatment.

Anandron was assayed in plasma by RIA. The antibody was raised
in rabbits receiving an antigen prepared by conjugation of the
propanoic derivative (on the N3 of the hydantoin moiety) of
Anandron with BSA. Tritiated Anandron, reference solution or diluted plasma, antiserum and anti-rabbit-γ-globulin antiserum raised
in sheep, were incubated together for 16 h at 4°C. After centrifugation, the radioactivity in the pellet was measured by liquid
scintillation. Each measurement was performed in triplicate. The
sensitivity of the assay is 0.3 ng/ml. The specificity of the
Anandron antibody towards endogenous substances is such that no
extraction procedure is required. The cross-reactions with two
metabolites that have been identified in rat plasma (products of
NO_2 reduction into NH_2 or NHOH) [25] are less than 0.4 %.

The mean plasma concentrations recorded during the clinical
trial were compared : between groups for each time point and
between different times within each group using Student's t test.

RESULTS

Linearity of Plasma Anandron Concentrations as a Function of Dose

Following administration of Anandron to healthy volunteers, it was found that the time to peak (Tmax) and half-life ($t_{1/2}$) are independent of dose whereas the maximum concentration (Cmax) and area-under-the curve (AUC) are proportional to dose (Table 1). The kinetics of Anandron after administration of increasing single doses is therefore linear and, in practice, the plasma concentrations obtained during treatment will be proportional to the dose administered [35].

TABLE 1. Kinetic parameters of Anandron after a single oral dose to 12 healthy volunteers in a randomized cross-over trial

	100 mg	200 mg	300 mg
Tmax (h)	1.8 ± 0.4	1.5 ± 0.3	1.5 ± 0.3
Cmax (mg/l)	0.8 ± 0.1	1.6 ± 0.1	2.3 ± 0.2
AUC (mg/l h)	25 ± 3	56 ± 5	84 ± 7
t 1/2 (h)	43 ± 3	45 ± 4	49 ± 4

mean ± S.E.M.

Anandron Kinetics in Patients

Anandron was about 85 % protein bound in human plasma (unpublished data). Unchanged Anandron accounted for approximately 30 % of total plasma radioactivity. The half-life of elimination of unchanged Anandron in patients ranged from 23 to 87 hours. The negligible excretion of Anandron in the feces and the levels of radioactivity recovered in the urine suggest that Anandron is well absorbed from the gastrointestinal tract [24].

The typical pattern of Anandron accumulation during twice daily dosing for 6 weeks is shown in Figure 1. The steady state levels were attained in approximately 2 weeks from the initiation of the multiple dosing regimen (day 4) and the levels (at a dose of 150 mg every 12 hours) ranged from 4.4 to 8.5 µg/ml [23,24].

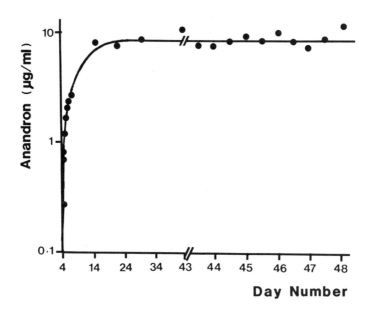

Figure 1. Accumulation of unchanged Anandron in plasma of a
patient receiving twice daily doses of Anandron
(150 mg) for 6 weeks

Clinical Efficacy

One hundred and sixty patients had been entered into the study
between 6 and 33 months before the analysis (median : 20 months)
and were evaluable for tolerance and safety variables. Among them,
33 patients were not evaluable for efficacy, most often because,
in retrospect, it was not absolutely certain that they had metastases at entry or because they had received previous hormonal
treatment. Two patients were lost to follow-up before the 6-month
evaluation, three started treatment more than 3 months after
orchiectomy. Thus 127 patients could be evaluated for efficacy:
  . 43 in the orchiectomy plus placebo group
  . 46 in the orchiectomy plus Anandron 150 mg group
  . 38 in the orchiectomy plus Anandron 300 mg group.
The three groups were similar with regard to their main characteristics: age; number of patients with stage D1 and stage D2
disease; frequency of bone pain and of abnormal PAP levels. The
number of patients with impaired performance status was higher in
the 150 mg group than in the two other groups (Table 2). Median
time between orchiectomy and onset of treatment was 3 days and the
same in the three groups.

TABLE 2. Characteristics of evaluable patients

| | Orchiectomy | | | |
	Placebo	Anandron 150 mg	Anandron 300 mg	p*
Number of patients	43	46	38	
Median age (years)	72.0	72.5	70.0	NS
Stage D1	5	4	1	NS
D2	38	42	37	
Number of patients with bone pain	18	28	17	NS
Number of patients with impaired performance status	12	24	12	< 0.05
Number of patients with abnormal PAP (> 3 ng/ml)	26	30	28	NS

* Chi-Square test - NS = not significant

Among patients who complained of bone pain on entry, a greater percentage was improved in the Anandron 300 mg group at 1, 3 and 6 months of treatment and in the Anandron 150 mg group after 3 and 6 months of treatment than in the placebo group (Table 3).

TABLE 3. Percentage of patients improved among patients with bone pain on entry

| | | Orchiectomy | | | |
		Placebo	Anandron 150 mg	Anandron 300 mg	p*
Number of patients with bone pain on entry		18	28	17	
Percentage improved	Month 1	61 %	67 %	93 %	< 0.10
	Month 3	67 %	81 %	94 %	NS
	Month 6	44 %	71 %	94 %	< 0.01

* Chi-Square test - NS = not significant

Similarly, among patients with impaired performance status on inclusion, all were improved in the Anandron 300 mg group on months 1, 3 and 6 of treatment, compared to 50 to 67 % in the placebo group (Table 4).

TABLE 4. Percentage of patients improved among patients with impaired performance status on entry

| | | O r c h i e c t o m y | | | |
		Placebo	Anandron 150 mg	Anandron 300 mg	p*
Number of patients with impaired performance status on entry		12	24	12	
Percentage improved	Month 1	67 %	57 %	100 %	<0.01
	Month 3	60 %	78 %	100 %	<0.05
	Month 6	50 %	80 %	100 %	<0.01

* Chi-Square test

Although the differences were not statistically significant, there was a tendency for abnormally high PAP values to return to normal levels in a greater percentage of cases in the two Anandron groups than in the placebo group (Table 5).

TABLE 5. Percentage of patients whose PAP became normal among patients with abnormal PAP on entry

| | | O r c h i e c t o m y | | | |
		Placebo	Anandron 150 mg	Anandron 300 mg	p*
Number of patients with abnormal PAP on entry		26	30	28	
Percentage normalized	Month 1	37 %	56 %	58 %	NS
	Month 3	52 %	70 %	78 %	NS
	Month 6	59 %	65 %	72 %	NS

* Chi-Square test — NS = not significant

Using NPCP criteria the best objective response to treatment was regression in 61 % of patients in the two Anandron-treated groups compared to 33 % in the "orchiectomy and placebo" group and the difference was statistically significant. The percentage of patients who did not respond or who had already progressed at the 6-month visit were 20 % and 19 % in the two Anandron groups and 34 % in the placebo group. The remaining patients had stable disease as their best response (Figure 2).

The progression-free actuarial rate was higher at 6 months in the two Anandron groups (83 % and 84 %) than with orchiectomy alone (70 %). However, at 12 and 18 months the rates were similar

in the 3 groups and there was no overall difference (Table 6).
Likewise, the survival rate was similar in the three groups with
medians of the distribution of 24, 22 and 22 months (Table 6).

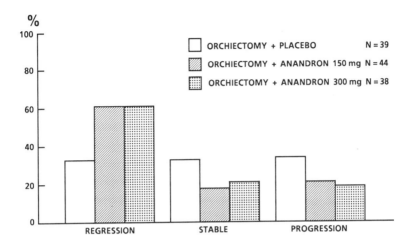

Figure 2. Best objective response according to NPCP criteria
         (6 patients were not evaluable on this basis due to
         a missing parameter, usually bone scan, at month 6).

TABLE 6. Progression and survival data *

| | | Orchiectomy | | |
		Placebo	Anandron 150 mg	Anandron 300 mg
Number of patients		43	46	38
Progression free actuarial rate	Month 6	70 %	83 %	84 %
	Month 12	58 %	57 %	49 %
	Month 18	40 %	42 %	35 %
Median time to progression (months)		13	13	12
Survival actuarial rate	Month 6	98 %	98 %	97 %
	Month 12	83 %	82 %	79 %
	Month 18	70 %	59 %	61 %
Median time to death (months)		24	22	22

* The Logrank test revealed no significant differences among the
  three groups.

Hormone parameters during treatment

Analysis of hormone assay results (Table 7) demonstrated the expected increases in LH and FSH and decreases in testosterone, DHT and estradiol to levels which were similar in the three groups. Prolactin and cortisol did not change in any of the groups while Δ 4-androstenedione, dehydroepiandrosterone and its sulphate decreased in a dose-dependent manner in the groups treated with Anandron compared to the groups treated by orchiectomy alone (not shown). Plasma mean concentrations of Anandron were 7.3 mg/l (s.d. = 3.9, n = 31) in the 300 mg group and 3.5 mg/l (s.d. = 1.2, n = 32) in the 150 mg group. They were stable after 1, 3, 6 and 12 months of treatment.

TABLE 7. Hormone and drug monitoring during treatment (mean ± s.d.)

	Treatmt month	Orchiectomy + Placebo			Orchiectomy +		Anandron 300 mg/day	
					150 mg/day			
Testosterone	0	3.45	±	1.65	4.00 ± 1.49		3.97 ± 1.65	
(ng/ml)	1	0.15	±	0.09	0.16 ± 0.12		0.10 ± 0.04 *	
	3	0.15	±	0.08	0.15 ± 0.07		0.12 ± 0.05	
	6	0.16	±	0.09	0.16 ± 0.09		0.12 ± 0.05	
	12	0.13	±	0.08	0.12 ± 0.04		0.10 ± 0.05	
LH	0	10.9	±	7.8	10.9 ± 8.4		11.7 ± 8.1	
(mUI/ml)	1	29.7	±	15.3	30.8 ± 15.5		28.3 ± 10.0	
	3	31.2	±	16.3	39.5 ± 18.7		31.3 ± 12.9	
	6	38.1	±	18.5	36.6 ± 15.9		34.8 ± 12.5	
	12	26.4	±	6.5	29.3 ± 9.6		26.2 ± 11.5	
Cortisol	0	185	±	81	168 ± 63		172 ± 58	
(ng/ml)	1	153	±	72	186 ± 80		162 ± 56	
	3	152	±	92	187 ± 73		181 ± 61	
	6	202	±	66	190 ± 48		160 ± 60	
	12	210	±	83	204 ± 50		178 ± 44	
Prolactin	0	9.49	±	4.71	8.34 ± 4.88		9.46 ± 4.94	
(ng/ml)	1	7.75	±	3.87	7.08 ± 3.77		8.16 ± 3.79	
	3	6.48	±	2.91	7.03 ± 2.85		8.33 ± 3.76	
	6	6.74	±	3.06	8.07 ± 4.71		10.25 ± 8.37	
	12	8.88	±	3.56	9.07 ± 3.79		7.47 ± 6.21	
Anandron	1	—			3.38 ± 1.12		7.24 ± 3.65	
(μg.ml^{-1})	3	—			3.58 ± 1.23		7.30 ± 3.95	
	6	—			3.73 ± 1.70		7.42 ± 2.91	
	12	—			3.83 ± 0.92		7.04 ± 2.69	

* Covariance analysis ($p < 0.05$): the 300 mg group is significantly different from the placebo and 150 mg groups.

Tolerance

For 8 patients in the higher dose group, 3 in the lower dose group, and none of the placebo group, treatment was stopped because of adverse experiences which were considered drug related in four instances : two cases of interstitial lung disease, one case of visual disturbances and one of nausea, all of which disappeared upon discontinuation of the drug.

There was an overall dose-dependence of the number of inter-current events in the three groups. The most frequently reported adverse events were hot flushes, the frequency of which was about 50 % in each of the three treatment groups. Two symptoms more specific to Anandron were an impairment in visual adaptation to darkness and alcohol intolerance. The former occurred in 19 % of patients in the 150 mg group and 28 % of patients in the 300 mg group and the latter in 17 % of patients of the higher dose group. There were no recorded incidences of gynecomastia.

With regard to hematology and biochemistry parameters, there was no clinically relevant difference among the three groups.

DISCUSSION

The beneficial effects of orchiectomy in curbing the evolution of stage D prostate cancer have been confirmed in this study which shows a 33 % positive response (complete and partial regression) in accord with published data. Smith et al. [33] reported partial or complete regression in 23 % of 32 patients and 32 % of 44 patients included in two separate EORTC studies and treated with DES, 3 mg per day. Murphy et al. [20] found objective regression in 41 % of 83 patients treated with DES or orchiectomy.

The object of the present study was, however, to establish whether this fairly high response rate could be even further improved by the addition of an antiandrogen, in this case Anandron [27]. According to current opinion, adrenal androgens could be converted to active androgens within the prostate and exert a risk-associated trophic effect [10] which orchiectomy alone cannot suppress and which requires the use of an adjuvant therapy such as adrenal biosynthesis inhibitors or antiandrogens.

In view of the difficulty in establishing an unequivocal improvement over an already effective treatment, the study was performed in randomized orchiectomized patients and double-blind versus placebo. Two doses of Anandron (150 and 300 mg) were compared. Kinetic studies showed that time-to-peak and half-life (ca. 2 days in healthy volunteers) were independent of dose whereas, as expected, maximum concentrations and areas-under-the-curve were proportional to dose. Anandron was well absorbed by patients. Steady-state levels were reached in approximately two weeks. Assays of Anandron throughout the clinical trial gave extremely constant results.

The usual changes in pituitary secretion and testicular androgen suppression observed after orchiectomy were not further modified by Anandron administration. Nor did Anandron change plasma cortisol concentrations. However, a reduction in adrenal androgen concentrations was observed as already reported by Bélanger et al [2]. Although the mechanism of this decrease has not yet been elucidated (decreased synthesis, enhanced catabolism or increased elimination), it could also contribute to the antiandrogenic activity of Anandron believed to be primarily due to an interaction with the androgen receptor [19,27].

The results of the trial give good evidence for improvements in both subjective and objective parameters in the Anandron-treated castrated patients compared to those receiving no Anandron. Anandron led to more frequent improvements in bone pain and in performance status, to a greater decrease in tumor masses, and to a more frequent normalisation of prostatic acid phosphatase.

The NPCP criteria were used to evaluate the objective response to treatment, and the categories regression (partial or complete), stable disease and progression were computed separately. Both Anandron-treated groups demonstrated the same percentages of objective regressions (61 %) which were significantly higher than for orchiectomy alone. A difference was also found in the progression-free actuarial rate which at 6 months was 70 % in the orchiectomy alone group and 83 and 84 % in the two Anandron-treated groups. This difference, however, was not maintained after 12 and 18 months of treatment. That the effect of Anandron may be only temporary is not wholly unexpected since, once the cancer has already progressed to stage D, it is unlikely that purely hormonal treatment can curb the evolution of metastatic or autonomous cells. There was no significant difference in survival rate in the "orchiectomy + placebo" and "orchiectomy + Anandron" groups.

Which of the two doses was the more effective ? A greater improvement in pain and performance status was demonstrated after one month of treatment with the higher dose. However, the objective regression rate was the same in both Anandron-treated groups. This, together with the relatively long time needed to attain the steady-state in plasma Anandron concentration, leads us to propose a treatment regimen of 300 mg per day during the first month and 150 mg per day afterwards.

Since both Anandron doses have the same efficacy on tumor regression rate despite the lesser effect of the lower dose on adrenal androgen concentrations, it is probable that the prime mechanism of the antiandrogenic activity of Anandron is through competitive inhibition on the androgen receptor as suggested in experimental animal models.

REFERENCES

1. Allen JM, Kerle DJ, Ware H, Doble A, Williams G, Bloom SR (1983): Br. Med. J., 287:1766.

2. Bélanger A, Dupont A, Labrie F (1984): J. Clin. Endocrinol.
    Metab., 59:422-426.
3. Bhanalaph T, Varkarakis MJ, Murphy GP (1974): Ann. Surg.,
    179:17-23.
4. Borgmann V, Hardt W, Schmidt-Gollwitzer M, Adenauer H,
    Nagel R (1982): The Lancet, 1097-1099.
5. Bracci U, Di Silverio F (1977): In: Androgens and Antiandro-
    gens, edited by L Martini, M Motta, pp. 333-339. Raven
    Press, New York.
6. Bracci U (1979): J. Urol., 5:303-306.
7. Debruyne FMJ, Karthaus HFM, Schröder FH, De Voogt HJ, De
    Jong FH, Klijn JGM (1985): In: EORTC Genitourinary Group
    Monograph 2, Part A : Therapeutic Principles in Metastatic
    Prostatic Cancer, edited by FH Schröder, B Richards,
    pp. 251-270. Alan R. Liss, New York.
8. Fiet J, Gourmel B, Villette JM, Brerault JL, Julien R,
    Cathelineau G, Dreux C (1980): Hormone Res., 13:133-149.
9. Fiet J, Villette JM, Bertagna C, de Géry A, Hucher M, Husson
    JM, Raynaud JP (in press): In: Cancer of the Prostate,
    edited by GP Murphy, S Khoury. Alan R. Liss, New York.
10. Geller J, Albert J, Yen SSC, Geller S, Loza D (1981): J. Clin.
    Endocrinol. Metab., 52:576-580.
11. Geller J, Albert JD (1983): Semin. Oncol., 10:34-41.
12. Geller J (1985): Semin. Oncol. 12, (suppl. 1):28-35.
13. Guliani L, Pescatore D, Giberti C, Martorana G, Natta G
    (1980): Eur. Urol., 6:145-148.
14. Labrie F, Dupont A, Bélanger A, Cusan L, Lacourcière Y,
    Monfette G, Laberge JG, Emond JP, Fazekas ATA, Raynaud JP,
    Husson JM (1982): Clin. Invest. Med., 5:267-275.
15. Labrie F, Dupont A, Bélanger A (1985): In: Important Advances
    in Oncology 1985, edited by VT de Vita, S Hellman, SA
    Rosenberg, pp. 193-217. J.B. Lippincott, Philadelphia.
16. Labrie F, Dupont A, Bélanger A, Poyet P, Giguère M,
    Lacourcière Y, Emond J, Monfette G, Borsanyi JP (1986):
    The Lancet, Jan. 4:49.
17. Lefebvre FA, Seguin C, Bélanger A, Caron S, Sairam MR,
    Raynaud JP, Labrie F (1982): Prostate, 3:569-578.
18. Mellin P (1971): In: International Symposium on the Treatment
    of Carcinoma of the Prostate, edited by G Raspé, W Brosig,
    p. 180. Pergamon Press, Oxford.
19. Moguilewsky M, Fiet J, Tournemine C, Raynaud JP (1986): J.
    steroid Biochem., 24:139-146.
20. Murphy GP, Slack NH and participants in the National Prosta-
    tic Cancer Project (1984): In: Controlled Clinical Trials
    in Urologic Oncology, edited by L Denis, GP Murphy, GR
    Prout, F Schroeder, pp. 119-133. Raven Press, New York.
21. Neumann F, Gräf KJ, Hasan SH, Schenck B, Steinbeck H
    (1977): In: Androgens and Antiandrogens, edited by L
    Martini, M Motta, pp. 163-167. Raven Press, New York.
22. Parmar H, Lightman SL, Allen L, Phillips RH, Edwards L,
    Schally AV (1985): The Lancet, Nov. 30:1201-1205.

23. Pendyala L, Madajewicz S, Creaven PJ (1985): Proc. Am. Assoc. Cancer Res., 26:626.

24. Pendyala L, Creaven PJ, Huben R, Tremblay D, Mouren M, Bertagna C (in press): In: Cancer of the Prostate, edited by G.P. Murphy, S. Khoury. Alan R. Liss, New York.

25. Pottier J, Coussedière D, Raynaud JP (1985): In: Abstracts, 67th Annual Meeting of the Endocrine Society, n° 954, p. 239.

26. Raynaud JP (1979): In: Advances in Pharmacology and Therapeutics, edited by J. Jacob, pp. 259-278. Pergamon Press, Oxford.

27. Raynaud JP, Bonne C, Bouton MM, Lagacé L, Labrie F (1979): J. steroid Biochem., 11:93-99.

28. Sanford EJ, Drago JR, Rohner TJ, Santen R, Lipton A (1976): J. Urol., 115:170-174.

29. Santen RJ, Warner B (1985): Urology, suppl. XXV:53-57.

30. Schröder FH (1985): In: Therapeutic Principles in Metastatic Prostatic Cancer, edited by F.H. Schröder, B. Richards. Prog. Clin. Biol. Res., 185A: 307-317.

31. Seguin C, Cusan L, Bélanger A, Kelly PA, Labrie F, Raynaud JP (1981): Mol. Cell. Endocr., 21:37-41.

32. Smith JA, Glode LM, Wettlaufer JN, Stein BS, Glass AG, Max DT, Anbar D, Jagst CL, Murphy GP (1985): Urology 25:106-114.

33. Smith PH, Pavone-Macaluso M, Viggiano G, de Voogt H, Lardennois B, Robinson MRG, Richards B, Glashan RW, de Pauw M, Sylvester R and the EORTC Urological group (1984): In: Controlled Clinical Trials in Urologic Oncology, edited by L Denis, GP Murphy, GR Prout, F Schroeder, pp. 107-117. Raven Press, New York.

34. Tolis G, Ackman D, Stellos A, Mehta A, Labrie F, Fazekas ATA, Comaru-Schally AM, Schally AV (1982): Proc. Nat. Acad. Sci. (USA), 79:1658-1662.

35. Tremblay D, Dupront A, Meyer BH, Pottier J (in press): In: Cancer of the Prostate, edited by GP Murphy, S Khoury. Alan R. Liss, New York.

36. Worgul TJ, Santen RJ, Samojlik E et al. (1983): J. Urol., 129:51-55.

Hormonal Manipulation of Cancer: Peptides, Growth Factors, and New (Anti) Steroidal Agents, edited by Jan G. M. Klijn et al. Raven Press, New York © 1987.

RU 38486, A PROGESTIN AND GLUCOCORTICOID ANTAGONIST IN THE TREATMENT OF EXPERIMENTAL PITUITARY TUMORS

Steven W.J. Lamberts

Department of Medicine,Erasmus University,Rotterdam,the Netherlands

Progestins like megestrol acetate and medroxyprogesterone have acquired an important place in the treatment of metastatic breast cancer (1). These alkylated and halogenated acetoxyprogesterone derivatives were shown to possess high progestational properties and to have additional anti-estrogenic, anti-gonadotropic, anti-androgenic and especially powerful glucocorticoid-like activities (9).

Recently RU 38486 (Mepifristone, Roussel-UCLAF) was synthesized, a compound which was shown to have a high affinity for the progesterone receptor, but without progestomimetic activity (11). Apart from being a "pure" progesterone-receptor antagonist RU 38486 has also glucocorticoid receptor-blocking activity without agonist effects as proven both by in vitro (9, 12, 7) and in vivo (7, 3) experiments.

In the present study we compared the effects and the mechanisms of action of a "classical" 6-methylated progestin (megestrol acetate : MA) and RU 38486 in three models : I.ACTH release by cultured normal rat pituitary cells; II. The growth of the estrogen/progesterone-receptor positive transplantable Prolactin (PRL)/ACTH secreting rat pituitary tumor 7315a ; III. Hormone release by cultured 7315a tumor cells.

I. A COMPARISON OF THE EFFECTS OF RU 38486 AND MA ON CRF-STIMULATED ACTH SECRETION BY CULTURED NORMAL RAT PITUITARY CELLS.

The cultured cells were prepared from the anterior pituitary glands of normal female rats by methods described before (7). In principle the effect of the addition of 1 nM ovine Corticotropin-Releasing Factor (CRF) on ACTH release was measured for 3 hrs on day 4 of culture. In Fig. 1 the effects on CRF-stimulated ACTH release are shown of pre-incubation of the normal pituitary cells for 72 hrs with increasing concentrations RU 38486 (Fig. 1 left) and MA (Fig. 1 right). Exposure of the cells to RU 38486 resulted in a dose-dependent further stimulation of CRF-stimulated ACTH release, while MA inhibited CRF-stimulated ACTH release in a dose-dependent manner. The glucocorticoid-receptor blocking activity of RU 38486 is further shown in Fig. 2 (left), in which 3 concentrations RU 38486 overcome the inhibitory effect of dexamethasone (10 nM) on CRF-stimulated ACTH release in a dose-dependent manner. The glucocorticoid-agonistic activity of MA is further shown in Fig. 2 (right): both pre-incubation for 72 hrs with 10 nM dexamethasone and with 10 nM MA significantly attenuated CRF-stimulated ACTH release. The combination of both compounds further suppressed CRF-induced ACTH secretion significantly (Fig. 2, right). Finally, we evaluated the interrelationships between MA and RU 38486 on ACTH release (Fig. 3). Pre-incubation of normal rat pituitary cells for 72 hrs with 10 nM MA in combination with three different concentrations of RU 38486 shows a significant inhibition by MA of CRF-stimulated ACTH release, which was overcome completely in a dose-dependent manner by RU 38486.

It is as yet unknown what role the glucocorticoid receptor-blocking or agonistic activities of RU 38486 and MA play in the tumor growth-inhibitory effects of both drugs. This question is of importance, however, because the clinical (side)-effects of both compounds seem to a great extent dependent on the degree of (in)activation of the hypothalamo-pituitary-adrenal axis. Alexieva

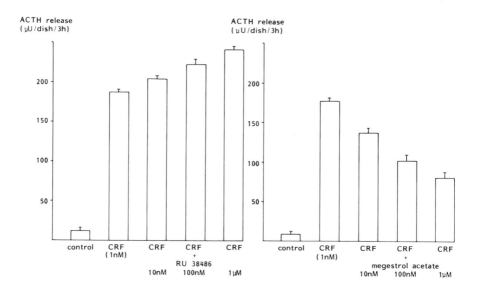

FIG. 1. The effect of preincubation for 72 h. with RU 38496 (left) or MA (right) on CRF-stimulated ACTH release by cultured normal rat pituitary cells.

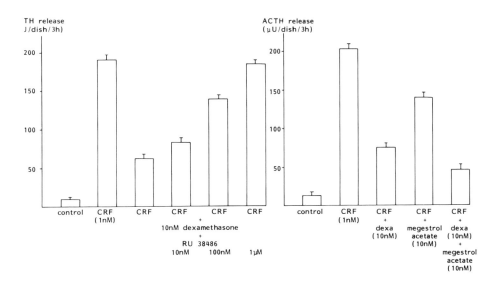

FIG. 2. The effect of preincubation for 72 h with 10 nM dexamethasone with or without RU 38486 (left) or with 10 nM dexamethasone, 10 nM MA and the combination (right) on CRF-stimulated ACTH
       release by cultured normal rat pituitary cells.

et al. (2) showed that treatment of 18 patients with metastatic
breast cancer for 6 weeks with either 90, 180 or 270 mg of MA daily completely suppressed the increment of plasma 11-deoxycortisol
in response to 4.5 g of metyrapone in 15 of 18 patients, while 3
of the 6 patients taking 90 mg of MA daily showed borderline values. Part of the feelings of general well-being, and increase in
appetite and in body weight observed in these patients can be ascribed to the glucocorticoid-like effect of MA. A potential problem is that withdrawal from long-term treatment with MA or medroxyprogesterone should be carried out very slowly in order to
prevent the occurrence of episodes of adrenocortical insufficiency.
    The opposite phenomenon can be expected during treatment with
high doses of RU 38486. Parenteral administration of the drug to
normal rats, monkeys and man acutely stimulated plasma ACTH and
cortisol levels for several hours, which is evidence of the glucocorticoid receptor antagonistic action of RU 38486 after in
vivo administration (5,3). Interestingly these effects in man
are not only dose-dependent, but the time of the day at which RU
38486 is administered also greatly influences the extent of changes in the hypothalamo-pituitary-adrenal axis (4).
    There is evidence that the anti-progestative action of RU 38486
in man can be achieved at a lower dose, than its anti-glucocorticoid activity. Depending on the importance of a combination of

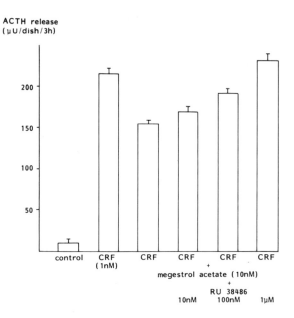

FIG. 3. The effect of preincubation for 72 h with 10 nM MA alone
or in combination with RU 38486 on CRF-stimulated ACTH release by
cultured normal rat pituitary cells.

both blocking activities in order to reach a maximal anti-tumor
effect, the choice of the dose of RU 38486 will determine the occurrence of signs and symptoms of adrenal insufficiency. Substitution therapy with hydrocortisone seems mandatory, however, in
most patients as a safeguard (8).

II. THE EFFECTS OF THE CHRONIC ADMINISTRATION OF RU 38486 AND MA ON THE GROWTH OF THE 7315a TUMOR

The estrogen-induced tranplantable PRL/ACTH-secreting rat pituitary tumor 7315a contains estrogen, progesterone and glucocorticoid receptors. The administration of 2.5 mg/kg RU 38486, 2.5 mg
and 6 mg/kg MA daily for 30 days significantly attenuated tumor
growth (Fig. 4). Part of these results have been published before (7, 6). RU 38486 inhibited tumor growth by 32 ± 3 % (p<0.01
vs. controls), 6 mg/kg MA significantly inhibited tumor size by
29 ± 3 % (p<0.01), while 2.5 mg/kg MA non-significantly affected
tumor size (-16 ± 4 %). The actual tumor weights were suppressed
by 66 % after RU 38486, and by 49 % and 38 % after 6 and 2.5 mg
MA, respectively (p<0.01 vs. control in all instances). In comparison, surgical adrenalectomy inhibited tumor growth by 35 %,and
tumor weight by 69 %.

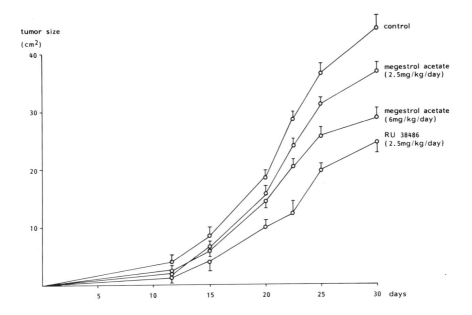

FIG. 4. The effect of the chronic administration of two doses of MA and of RU 38486 on the growth of the PRL/ACTH secreting pituitary tumor 7315a.

III. THE MECHANISM OF ACTION OF THE INHIBITORY EFFECT RU 38486
      AND MA ON PRL RELEASE BY CULTURED 7315a TUMOR CELLS.

We developed a tumor cell clone from the 7315a tumor, which secreted only PRL. Both RU 38486 and MA inhibited PRL release directly in a dose-dependent manner (Table 1). The inhibitory effect of 1 μM RU 38486 could be significant attenuated by 10 nM and 50 nM dexamethasone, but also by 1 nM progesterone. Interestingly , the combination of 50 nM dexamethasone + 1 nM progesterone completely overcame the inhibitory effect of 1 μM RU 38486 (Table 2). The inhibitory effect of MA on PRL release by these cultured 7315a tumor cells could not be counteracted by dexamethasone at low concentrations of 10 nM and 50 nM. In fact 50 nM dexamethasone exerted an additive effect on the inhibitory effect of 50 nM MA. 1 nM progesterone, however, partly attenuated the inhibitory effect of 50 nM MA on PRL release by these tumor cells. In a final experiment it is shown that 100 nM RU 38486 inhibits

TABLE 1. The effect of RU 38486 and megestrol acetate (MA) on PRL release by 7315a tumor cells cultured for 7 days in 10 % charchoal treated fetal calf serum.

Concentration	PRL release as a % of control	
	RU 38486	Megesterolacetate
0.1 nM	98 ± 3	102 ± 3
1 nM	94 ± 4	115 ± 4
10 nM	70 ± 4[a]	92 ± 3
100 nM	56 ± 4[a]	23 ± 3[a]
1 μM	42 ± 3[a]	9 ± 3[a]

[a] p<0.01 vs. control (n=4 dishes per group ; mean ± SEM)

TABLE 2. The effect of dexamethasone and/or progesterone on RU 38486-induced inhibition of PRL release by cultured 7315a tumor cells.

	PRL release (ng/dish/7 days)
Control	410 ± 8
RU 38486 (1 μM)	220 ± 11[b]
RU + dexa (10 nM)	285 ± 6[a,b]
RU + dexa (50 nM)	314 ± 8[a,b]
RU + progesterone (1 nM)	305 ± 6[a,b]
RU + dexa (50 nM) + prog. (1 nM)	386 ± 11[b]

[a] p<0.01 vs. control   [b] p<0.01 vs. RU 38486 (1 μM)
(n=4 dishes per group; mean ± SEM)

PRL release by the 7315a tumor cells in this experiment by 21 ± 3% (Fig. 5). The inhibitory effect of 100 nM MA on PRL release is virtually completely overcome by 100 nM RU 38486.

CONCLUSIONS

Both a classical 6-methylated progestin like megestrol acetate and the newly synthesized steroid RU 38486 inhibit tumor growth by the estrogen/progesterone/glucocorticoid receptor positive transplantable rat pituitary tumor 7315a. Both compounds exhibit profound effects on the progesterone and the glucocorticoid receptors of this tumor, but these effects are strongly contradictory. RU 38486 has both progesterone receptor- and glucocorticoid receptor-blocking activities, which seem both to play an important role in the mechanism of action of the inhibition of tumor growth. Megestrol acetate activity seems mainly to be

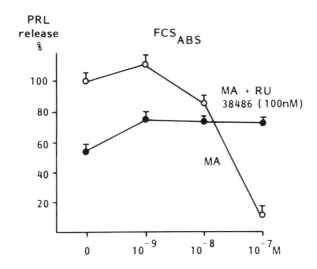

FIG. 5. The effect of different concentrations of MA, and its interrelation with the effect of 100 nM RU 38486 on PRL release by cultured 7315a tumor cells. PRL release as a percentage of control after a 7 day exposure.

mediated via the glucocorticoid agonistic action.

REFERENCES

1. Alexieva-Figusch, J., van Gilse, H.A., Hop, W.C.J., Phoa, C.H., Blonk-van der Wijst, J., and Treurniet, R.E. (1980) : Cancer 46 : 2369-2372.
2. Alexieva-Figusch, J., Blankenstein, M.A., Hop, W.C.J., Klijn, J.G.M., Lamberts, S.W.J., de Jong, F.H., Docter, R., Adlercreutz, H., and van Gilse, H.A. (1984) : Eur. J. Cancer Clin. Oncol. 20 : 33-40.
3. Bertagna, X., Bertagna, C., Luton, J-P., Husson J-M., and Girard , F. (1984): J. Clin. Endocrinol. Metab. 59 : 25-28.
4. Gaillard, R.C., Riondel, A., Muller, A.F., Herrmann, W., and Baulieu, E.E. (1984) : Proc. Natl. Acad. Sci. USA 81 : 3879-3882.
5. Healy, D.L., Chrousos, G.P., Schulte, H.M., Williams, R.F., Gold, P.W., Beaulieu, E.E., and Hodgen, G.D. (1983) : J. Clin. Endocrinol. Metab. 57 : 863-865.
6. Lamberts, S.W.J. Janssens , E.N.W., Bons, E.G., Zuiderwijk, J.M. , Uitterlinden , P., and de Jong, F.H. (1981) : Eur. J. Cancer Clin. Oncol. 17 : 925-931.

7. Lamberts, S.W.J., Uitterlinden, P., Bons, E.G., and Verleun, T. (1985) Cancer Res. 45 : 1015-1019.
8. Lamberts, S.W.J., Bons, E.G., and Uitterlinden, P. (1985) Acta Endocrinol. 109 : 64-69.
9. Moguilewski, M., Deraedt, R., Teutsch, G., and Philibert D. (1982) J. Steroid Biochem. 17 : 68.
10. Neumann, F. (1978) Postgrad. Med. J. 54 : 11-24.
11. Philibert, D., Deraedt, R., Teutsch, G., Tournemine, C., and Sakiz, E. (1982): Endocrinology 110 : A668.
12. Proulx-Terland, L., Coté, J., Philibert, D., and Deraedt, R. (1982): 66.

Hormonal Manipulation of Cancer: Peptides, Growth Factors, and New (Anti) Steroidal Agents, edited by Jan G. M. Klijn et al. Raven Press, New York © 1987.

MIFEPRISTONE IN TREATMENT

OF EXPERIMENTAL BREAST CANCER IN RATS

G.H. Bakker, B. Setyono-Han, F.H. De Jong[+] and J.G.M. Klijn[°]

Departments of Biochemistry and [°]Clinical Endocrinology, Dr. Daniel Den Hoed Cancer Center, P.O. Box 5201, 3008 AE Rotterdam, Department of [+]Biochemistry (Chemical Endocrinology), Medical Faculty, Erasmus University, P.O. Box 1738, 3000 DR Rotterdam, The Netherlands

INTRODUCTION

In the endocrine therapy of breast cancer various hormonal agents have been used, such as oestrogens and antioestrogens, androgens and antiandrogens, progestins, aromatase inhibitors or glucocorticoids. Recently, a steroid molecule with potent antiprogestational and antiglucocorticoid activities was synthesized (6, 7). This steroid, initially indicated by its codename RU38486 and currently named Mifepristone, is the first antiprogestin available for therapy. Inhibitory effects of Mifepristone on the growth of human breast cancer cells in culture have been described (2). Therefore, we have studied the antitumour (1) and endocrine effects of Mifepristone during chronic treatment of rats with dimethylbenzanthracene (DMBA)-induced mammary tumours by measuring the influence of treatment on body weight, reproductive organ weights, plasma hormone concentrations, tumour load and steroid receptor contents of the mammary tumours. The effects of Mifipristone treatment were compared with those of treatment with the LHRH-agonist Buserelin, the progestin megestrol acetate or ovariectomy. The results obtained indicate a strong inhibition of rat mammary tumour growth by Mifepristone, which appears mainly due to its antiprogestational activity.

MATERIALS AND METHODS

Animals, tumours, and related procedures

Female rats of the Sprague-Dawley strain were obtained from the Zentralinstitut für Versuchstiere, Hannover, F.R.G. Rats were kept four or five to a cage on wood shavings and received standard dry pellets (Hope Farms, Woerden, The Netherlands) and tap water ad libitum.

DMBA (Fluka, Basel, Switzerland) was dissolved in olive oil at a concentration of 10 mg/ml by vigorous shaking. The solution obtained was stored in the dark. Induction of mammary tumours was performed with 3 intragastric administrations of 1 ml of DMBA-solution given with weekly intervals to 54-61 days old rats (3).

Micronised Mifepristone was generously provided by Roussel Uclaf, (Dr. R. Deraedt), Romainville, France. Mifepristone was suspended in olive oil at a concentration of 24 mg/ml. Mifepristone was administered s.c. (10 mg/kg/day) for 3 weeks starting from the first day of DMBA injection (prophylactic treatment group) or after tumours had developed (therapeutic treatment group). Therapeutic effects of Mifepristone were compared with those of bilateral ovariectomy or treatment with Buserelin (Hoechst, Frankfurt am Main, F.R.G.; 40 ug/kg/day). In addition, a comparison was made between the effects of 3 weeks of treatment with the antiprogestin (2.5/10/40 mg/kg/day) and of the progestin megestrol acetate (Sigma, St. Louis, U.S.A.; 2.5/10 mg/kg/day). Control rats received a daily injection of physiological saline.

Animals were weighed once a week and palpated twice-weekly to detect the presence of mammary tumours. Treatment started when all rats (apart from the "prophylactic Mifepristone" group) had palpable tumours (105-115 days of age). Rats were anaesthetized with diethyl ether, and the size of individual tumours was calculated as the product of the two largest perpendicular diameters measured with calipers. Total tumour loads for each rat were calculated as the sum of the individual tumour areas.

Rats were divided between control and treatment groups (7-9 rats per group) in such a way, that the same average tumour load was obtained in each group. After therapy for 3 weeks, the tumour load was estimated again with anaesthetized rats after which rats were killed by decapitation. The effects of therapy were determined with respect to changes in tumour load, contents of oestrogen and progesterone receptors in dissected mammary tumour tissue, and organ weights of the pituitary, adrenals, ovaries and uterus. Blood was collected in heparinized tubes and plasma was assayed for its concentration of LH, FSH, ACTH, prolactin, oestradiol, progesterone and corticosterone.

Steroid hormone receptor assays

Oestrogen and progesterone receptors were assayed according to the EORTC procedures (4) by multiple Scatchard analysis, using $(2,3,6,7-^3H)$-oestradiol (85-110 Ci/mmol) and (^3H) ORG 2058 (40-60 Ci/mmol) from Amersham International plc, Bucks., England.

Hormone assays in blood plasma samples

Assay of LH and FSH was performed according to the procedure described by Welschen et al. (8). Oestradiol was assayed with EIR-kits obtained from EIR, Würenlingen, Switzerland. Progesterone was assayed according to de Jong et al. (5). Corticosterone was measured with an antibody kindly provided by Prof. Th.J. Benraad, Catholic University, Nijmegen, The Netherlands).

RESULTS

Prophylactic treatment of rats with Mifepristone for 3 weeks
starting on the first day of DMBA injection significantly delayed
body growth as apparent from the lower body weight of Mifepristone
-treated rats (Fig. 1). Moreover, the tumour latency period was
significantly increased by Mifepristone treatment (control animals: 39±5 days, n=75, range 35-56 days; Mifepristone-treated
animals: 81±16 days, n=17, range 56-114 days; p<0.005).

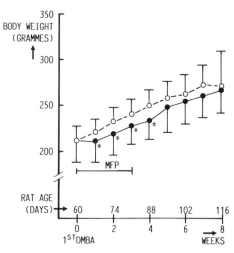

FIG. 1. Effects of 3 weeks treatment with Mifepristone (MFP) from
the time of mammary tumour induction with DMBA (the bar denotes
the prophylactic MFP-period). -o-,
control (n=45-48); -•-, MFP-treat-
ed (n=8). Means±S.D.; *p<0.005.

The effects of treatment with Mifepristone, Buserelin or ovariectomy on tumour load are shown in Table 1. Significant inhibition
of tumour growth was caused by Mifepristone treatment, whereas
ovariectomy and Buserelin treatment resulted in tumour remission.
In a second experiment, a comparison was made between the results
of chronic treatment with Mifepristone and megestrol acetate
(Table 2). Both steroids inhibited tumour growth significantly,
while Mifepristone was more potent than megestrol acetate.

The effects of the various treatments on organ weights and
steroid receptors are shown in Table 3 and 4 respectively.
Mifepristone treatment resulted in increased weights of the
pituitary, ovaries and uterus, whereas no effect on adrenal

TABLE 1. Effects of different treatments on rat mammary
tumour load (mm^2) after three weeks of therapy

Treatment	Initial tumour load	After therapy	% Change
None	783±545 (9)	1748±838 (9)	+123
MFP (10 mg/kg)	791±627 (9)	1044±707 (8)*	+ 32
Ovariectomy	792±646 (9)	252±237 (9)**	- 68
Buserelin (40 ug/kg)	790±611 (9)	508±621 (9)**	- 36

Results are means±s.d. (n); *p<0.05, **p<0.005.

TABLE 2. Relative effects of
treatment with MFP or megestrol
acetate (MA) on rat mammary tumour load after three weeks of
therapy

	After therapy (%)
Control	222±62 (12)
MFP (2.5 mg/kg)	108±46 (17)*[2]
MFP (10 mg/kg)	121±58 (16)*[2]
MFP (40 mg/kg)	118±81 (15)*
MA (2.5 mg/kg)	158±47 (14)*
MA (10 mg/kg)	167±75 (13)*

Initial tumour load=100%. Results
are means±s.d. (n). *p<0.005 vs.
control, [2]p<0.01 vs. resp. MA.

weight was found. In contrast, ovariectomy, treatment with megestrol acetate or Buserelin resulted in reduced weight of the uterus
and ovaries. All treatments resulted in significant reduction of
the amount of assessable progesterone receptor (PR) in the dissected tumours, the effect of megestrol acetate being smaller than
that of the other treatments (Table 4). Megestrol acetate treatment caused no change in the oestrogen receptor (ER) content,
while the other treatments significantly suppressed ER (cf. Table
4). Finally, the effects of Mifepristone, Buserelin and ovariectomy on plasma hormone concentrations are shown in Table 5. Mifepristone treatment caused 2.4 to 8.5-fold increased levels of LH,
oestradiol, progesterone and prolactin (not shown). However,
levels of FSH, corticosterone and ACTH (not shown), were unchanged. On the other hand, ovariectomy and Buserelin treatment gave
rise to significantly increased levels of LH and FSH in combination with castrate levels of oestradiol and progesterone during
Buserelin treatment.

DISCUSSION

The present report describes the results of the first study on
the effects of the new steroid analogue Mifepristone on the growth

TABLE 3. Effects of different treatments on wet weight (mg) of organs isolated from mammary tumour bearing rats at the end of three weeks therapy

	Pituitary	Adrenals	Ovaries	Uterus
Control	16.6±3.5(25)	60±12(26)	161±43(26)	390±108(25)
MFP (2.5 mg/kg)	18.8±4.0(17)[2]	61±13(17)	175±34(17)	381±80 (17)
MFP (10 mg/kg)	19.7±3.3(32)*	62±12(31)	208±50(32)*	518±127(32)*
MFP (40 mg/kg)	19.6±3.8(15)*	64±9 (15)	207±62(15)*	471±144(15)*
Ovex	18.4±1.8(14)	61±8 (14)	-----	297±32 (13)*
Buserelin	15.5±3.3(18)	64±13(18)	110±44(18)*	228±48 (18)*
MA (2.5 mg/kg)	13.2±2.2(15)*	47±17(15)*	120±23(15)*	285±79 (15)*
MA (10 mg/kg)	13.8±2.5(13)[2]	41±9 (13)*	111±19(13)*	361±134(13)

Results are means±s.d. (n); [2]p<0.05, *p<0.005.

TABLE 4. Effects of different therapies on oestrogen (ER) and progesterone receptor (PR) contents (in fmol/mg protein) of rat mammary tumour tissue after three weeks of therapy

	ER	%	PR	%
Control	133±54(24)	100	296±255(23)	100
MFP (2.5 mg/kg)	49±32(17)*	37	80±100(17)*	27
MFP (10 mg/kg)	40±28(29)*	30	2±11 (29)*	1
MFP (40 mg/kg)	60±32(15)*	45	0±0 (15)*	0
Ovex	66±36(12)*	50	9±15 (11)*	3
Buserelin (40 ug/kg)	93±64(15)[2]	70	35±36 (14)*	20
MA (2.5 mg/kg)	159±57(14)	120	145±154(14)[2]	49
MA (10 mg/kg)	157±65(14)	118	169±145(14)[3]	57

Results are means±s.d.(n) and expressed as percentage of the contents in control animals. *p<0.005, [2]p<0.02, [3]p<0.05.

of DMBA-induced rat mammary tumours. The results obtained clearly show that prophylactic treatment of rats with Mifepristone doubled the latency period reflecting a pronounced retardation of mammary tumour growth. Moreover, when Mifepristone was used in therapy of rats bearing mammary tumours the dose of 10 mg/kg/day significantly inhibited tumour growth (75% vs. control; cf. Tables 1 and 2).

TABLE 5. <u>Effects of treatments on blood plasma hormone concentrations</u>

	Control	MFP(10mg/kg)	Ovariectomy	BUS(40ug/kg)
LH (ng/ml)	10±7 (13)	85±71 (16)[2]	602±317(15)*	66±27 (18)*
FSH (ng/ml)	184±76 (13)	190±145(16)	2686±526(15)*	1004±296(18)*
P (nmol/l)	89±61 (13)	212±148(16)*	15±8 (15)*	8±9 (18)*
E2 (pmol/l)	30±33 (13)	102±91 (16)*	20±6 (15)	9±7 (18)*
C (nmol/l)	720±229(12)	775±395(16)	547±236(15)	521±336(18)[3]

Results are means±s.d.(n); BUS=Buserelin, P=progesterone, E2=oestradiol, C=corticosterone. Significance vs. control: *p<0.005, [2]p<0.01, [3]p<0.05.

In the experiments described in this report a higher dose of Mifepristone did not improve inhibition of mammary tumour growth (see: Table 2). Comparison of the effects of progestin and antiprogestin treatment shows that Mifepristone inhibited mammary tumour growth significantly more than megestrol acetate, when used in the same dose. However, no clear dose-response relationship for Mifepristone was found with the dosages used. Organ weights of pituitary, ovaries and uterus were increased after Mifepristone treatment and decreased after megestrol acetate treatment (cf. Table 3). These disparate effects may reflect the progestin and antiprogestin character of both compounds. Mifepristone had a more pronounced effect on the progesterone receptor content of the mammary tumours than megestrol acetate.

The mechanism of action of Mifepristone can be inferred from its effects on blood plasma hormone levels. The considerably increased levels of LH, oestradiol and progesterone, in combination with unchanged levels of FSH and corticosterone, without change in adrenal weight, suggest that the effects of Mifepristone were caused by its antiprogestin activity, rather than its antiglucocorticoid activity. The effects of Mifepristone on plasma hormone levels, organ weights and tumour steroid receptor contents in combination with the reported effects on cultured MCF-7 cells (2), indicate that the main mechanism of action of Mifepristone is a direct antiprogestational effect at the level of the mammary tumour cells via the progesterone receptor.

Mifepristone treatment gave rise to an increased plasma level of oestradiol which may have partly counteracted the inhibitory effect of Mifepristone on mammary tumour growth. On the other hand, as previously reported by Bardon et al. (2), we observed in-vitro a direct action of Mifepristone on MCF-7 cells, i.e. Mifepristone (3.6xExp-8 M) fully inhibited oestradiol-stimulated growth (results not shown). Whether this oestradiol-stimulated growth can be completely blocked in the in-vivo situation remains to be demonstrated. Therefore, further investigations are warranted to find out whether a combination of Mifepristone and other hormonal agents used to inhibit oestrogen activities, can further improve inhibition of mammary tumour growth.

REFERENCES

1. Bakker, G.H., Blankenstein, M.A. and Klijn, J.G.M. (1985):
   Proceedings of the Biennial International Breast Cancer
   Research Conference, London, England (abstract 3-12).
2. Bardon, S., Vignon, F., Chalbos, D. and Rochefort, H. (1985):
   J. Clin. Endocrinol. Metab., 60:692-697.
3. Blankenstein, M.A., Peters-Mechielsen, M.J., Mulder, E. and
   Van der Molen, H.J. (1980): J. Steroid Biochem., 13: 557-
   564.
4. Blankenstein, M.A., Blaauw, G., Lamberts, S.W.J. and Mulder,
   E. (1983): Eur. J. Cancer Clin. Oncol., 19: 365-370.
5. De Jong, F.H., Baird, D.T. and Van der Molen, H.J. (1974):
   Acta Endocrinol., 77: 575-587.
6. Herrmann, W., Wyss, R., Riodel, A., Philibert, D., Teutsch,
   G., Sakiz, E. and Baulieu, E.E. (1982): C.R. Acad. Sci.
   Paris, 294: 933-938.
7. Philibert, D., Deraedt, R., Teutsch, G., Tourneminen, C. and
   Sakiz, E. (1982): Program of the 64th annual meeting of The
   Endocrine Society, San Francisco, U.S.A. (abstract 668).
8. Welschen, R., Osman, P., Dullaart, J., De Greef, W.J., Uilen-
   broek, J.Th.J. and De Jong, F.H. (1975): J. Endocrinol. 64:
   37-47.

Hormonal Manipulation of Cancer: Peptides,
Growth Factors, and New (Anti) Steroidal
Agents, edited by Jan G. M. Klijn et al.
Raven Press, New York © 1987.

ANTIPROLIFERATIVE EFFECT OF PROGESTINS AND ANTIPROGESTINS IN HUMAN BREAST CANCER CELLS

F. Vignon, S. Bardon, D. Chalbos, D. Derocq, P. Gill
and H. Rochefort

INSERM U 148, Unité d'Endocrinologie Cellulaire et Moléculaire,
60 Rue de Navacelles, 34100 Montpellier, France.

The effect of progestins on the growth of mammary adenocarcinoma varies among species. In rodents, it is generally agreed that progestins synergize with estrogens for the growth of mammary tumors (17) and the normal mammary gland (7). In humans, however, progestins have been used successfully in the treatment of breast cancer patients (6). The mechanism by which they prevent breast cancer proliferation is unknown. It had been proposed that progestins were antiestrogenic and prevented the mitogenic activity of estrogens in breast cancer cells on the basis of studies performed on human endometrium (24).

To analyze the mechanism of the effect of progestins on mammary cancer cells, the in vitro experimental systems have been very useful. We have mostly used the MCF7 (22) and T47D (13) cell lines which were both established from pleural effusions of human breast cancers. They both contain estrogen (ER) and progesterone receptors (PgR) (11) and estrogens have been shown to regulate cell growth (14)(3) and the expression of several cellular and secreted proteins and enzymes (12)(9)(28)(16)(2)(21).

Effect of the progestin R5020

In these human cell lines, we have first addressed the 2 following questions :
1. Do progestins directly affect the growth of breast cells or do they mostly act in vivo via the hypothalamo-pituitary axis ?
2. Do progestins act as antiestrogens in human breast cells ?
Using the synthetic progestin, R5020 (18), we have shown that the growth of the human breast cancer cell lines was significantly inhibited when R5020 was added in the presence of estradiol (E2) (25). The effect was more pronounced after 10-12 days of treatment and was dose-dependent. A half-maximal inhibition was obtained with a dose of 1 nM R5020 which suggested that this antiestrogenic action was mediated by the progesterone receptor. In fact, dexamethasone and dihydrotestosterone did not reproduce or inhibit R5020 effect on cell growth. The synthetic progestin was ineffective in a cell line lacking of ER and PgR

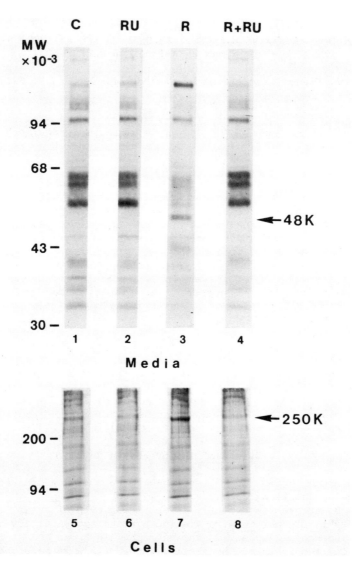

Figure 1
**Effect of RU486 on two progestin-specific proteins : SDS poly-
acrylamide gel.** T47D cells, withdrawn from steroids, were
incubated for 4 days either with vehicle (C,1,5), 10 nM RU486
(RU,2,6), 1 nM R5020 (R,3,7), or 10 nM RU486 plus 1 nM R5020 (R +
RU,4,8). After labeling, the same amount of TCA-precipitable
[35]S-methionine labeled protein from the media (lanes 1 to 4) and
from the cells (lanes 5 to 8) was analyzed on SDS 12%
polyacrylamide gels and fluorographed.
 Reproduced from (1) by permission of the Editor.

but containing androgen and glucocorticoid receptors. The antiproliferative effect of R5020 was associated with a general decrease of secreted proteins in these cell lines (25) and a specific decrease of the production of the estrogen-regulated 52 K glycoprotein (28). Its specific action on the 52 K protein (decrease of production) was comparable with that obtained with the antiestrogen Tamoxifen (28). However, in Tamoxifen-resistant cells, R5020 was still active thus indicating that progestins might be of some benefit after a failure of initial hormonal therapy.

Effect of the antiprogestin RU486

We had therefore shown that a synthetic progestin R5020 has a direct antiestrogenic activity on breast cancer cells in culture, since it both prevented the effect of E2 on the stimulation of cell growth and protein production. We had already provided strong evidence to support that these two effects were mediated by PgR. However, when the synthetic antiprogestin and anti-glucocorticoid RU486 was synthesized and characterized (19)(20)(10) our initial aim was to take advantages of its antiprogestin activity to better understand the progestin inhibitory effect.

Therefore, we have first evaluated the antagonist activity of RU486 in human breast cancer cell lines. D. Chalbos had shown that two proteins were specifically regulated by progestins in breast cancer cells : a 250,000 molecular weight cellular protein (250 K protein) (4) and a 48,000 molecular weight secreted protein (48 K protein) (5). RU486 totally prevented the production of these 2 proteins by R5020 (Fig. 1) and had no agonist activity on these two responses (1) in a wide range of concentrations (Fig. 2). Thus in breast cancer cells, RU486 behaved as a pure antagonist for these 2 responses. Horwitz (12) later showed that RU486 "fails to stimulate insulin receptors and partially blocks their stimulation by R5020" confirming that RU486 had no progestin activity in breast cancer. However, it has not been excluded that RU486 could have an agonist activity on other progestin specific responses such as the 17-ß oxydoreductase (Mauvais-Jarvis and F. Kutten, personal communication).

Nevertheless, contrary to what could be expected from its antagonist activity when we tested the effect of RU486 on the growth of the breast cancer cells, we found out that RU486 did not prevent the progestin inhibitory effect and that it was strongly inhibitory by itself (1) (Fig. 3). The effect was dose-dependent and a half maximal inhibition was obtained with a concentration of 0.1 nM suggesting that the antiproliferative activity of RU486 was probably mediated via the progesterone receptor. In fact, when we tested the antiproliferative activity of RU486 in MCF7 and T47D cells which have different PgR

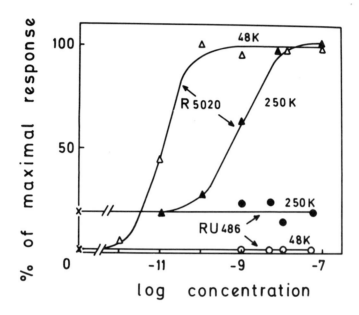

Figure 2
Effect of RU486 on two progestin-specific proteins :   Dose
response curves.   T47D cells were incubated with vehicle (×) or
the indicated concentrations of R5020 (△,▲) or RU486 (o,●).
After [35]S—methionine incorporation, proteins released into the
media and cellular proteins were analyzed on 12% SDS
polyacrylamide gels as described in Fig. 1.   The amounts of
cellular 250 K protein (▲,●) and of released 48 K protein (o, △)
were estimated by densitometer scanning and expressed as
percentages of the maximal response obtained with R5020.
    Reproduced from (1) by permission of the Editor.

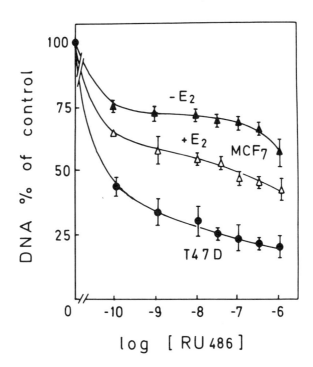

Figure 3
**Effect of RU486 on the growth of T47D and MCF7 cells :   Dose
response curves.** MCF7 cells were grown for 7 days in medium
containing 10% FCS/DCC. They then were trypsinized and cultured
for 5 days in medium containing charcoal-stripped serum (10%
FCS/DCC) with ($\triangle$) or without ($\blacktriangle$) 10 nM E2.   T47D cells ($\bullet$) were
grown for 5 days. Cells then were plated in 24-well dishes at a
density of 20,000 cells per well in medium containing 3% FCS/DCC
without insulin.   Two days later,   cells were treated with
increasing concentrations of RU486 for 10 days, and they were
fixed in situ and processed for DNA assay. Results are expressed
as percentages of control DNA. The absolute values of control DNA
were 17 ± 0.5 (SD) μg, respectively, for untreated MCF7 cells,
11.4 ± 2 μg for E2-pretreated MCF7 cells,   and 12.5 ± 0.4 μg for
T47D cells.
   Reproduced from (1) by permission of the Editor.

concentrations, the efficacy of RU486 was related to PgR concentrations (Fig. 3). Pretreatment of MCF7 cells by E2 resulted in an increase of PgR and a greater inhibition by RU486. Moreover, the inhibitory effect of RU486 was not prevented by the occupation of glucocorticoid or androgen receptors and it was nil in PgR negative cells thus confirming that the antiproliferative effect was mediated by PgR and not by glucocorticoid or androgen receptors (1).

Mechanism of the antiproliferative effect

We therefore found that both the progestin R5020 and the antiprogestin RU486 are antiproliferative in human breast cancer. This shows that the antihormonal and antiproliferative activities are clearly dissociated in this system.

We are addressing the following questions : How can these two compounds modulate the growth of breast cancer cells ? Are they acting through a common mechanism separate from their agonist/antagonist activities or are they intervening through different pathways ?

In favor of a possible common mechanism is the fact that these two compounds similarly decrease the general production of secreted proteins (25)(1). If some of these secreted proteins are necessary mitogens and growth factors for breast cells, as was shown for some estrogen regulated proteins (26)(8)(15), they can both act by decreasing levels of essential growth factors. R5020 was shown to decrease the production of the 52 K glycoprotein which is an autocrine mitogen for MCF7 cells (27).

In parallel with this possible common mechanism mediated by a decrease of positive growth factors the possibility arises of a dissociated or common effect of the two compounds on the stimulation of inhibitory growth factors such as specific progestin or antiprogestin inhibitors (none yet identified) or a common growth inhibitor such as TGFß (23).

Finally though targetted to the responsive cell by the same PgR, R5020 and RU486 can affect differently the cell growth due for example to their structural differences. RU486 shares with the triphenylethylene non-steroidal antiestrogens such as 4-hydroxytamoxifen, a lateral chain in the 11ß position. And in fact, these two antiproliferatives agents appear to display a similar receptor-mediated cytotoxicity in human breast cancer cells (Bardon et al., submitted for publication).

Conclusions

We have found that a progestin R5020 and an antiprogestin RU486 can both inhibit the growth of human breast cancer cells despite their different hormonal/antihormonal activities. The evidence for an antiproliferative effect of R5020 and RU486 in human breast cancer cell lines has provided us with a fundamental tool to evaluate the rationale of progestin treatment and with a new therapeutic agent, an antiprogestin, which is now currently evaluated in Montpellier Cancer Center.

The mechanism by which R5020 and RU486 prevent cell growth : inhibition of breast mitogen, such as the 52 K protein, stimulation of inhibitory factors or other mechanisms (cytotoxicity) remains to be elucidated.

Aknowledgments

We wish to thank D. Philibert and M. Bouton from Roussel Uclaf for providing us with R5020 and RU486.
We aknowledge the skillfull technical assistances of C. Prébois and C. Rougeot and the help of M. Egea and G. Salazar for the preparation of this manuscript.

References

1. Bardon, S., Vignon, F., Chalbos, D., and Rochefort, H. (1978): J. Clin. Endocrin. Met., 60:692–697.
2. Butler, W.B., Kirkland, W.L., and Jorgensen, T.L. (1979): Biochem. Biophys. Res. Commun., 90:1328–1334.
3. Chalbos, D., Vignon, F., Keydar, I. and Rochefort, H. (1982): J. Clin. Endocrin. Met., 55:276–283.
4. Chalbos, D., and Rochefort, H. (1984): Biochem. Biophys. Res. Commun., 121:421–427.
5. Chalbos, D., and Rochefort, H. (1984): J. Biol. Chem., 259:1231–1238.
6. De Lena, M., Brambilla, A., Valagussa, P., and Bonadonna, G. (1979): Cancer Chemother. Pharmacol., 2:175.
7. Delouis, C. (1980): In: Récepteurs hormonaux et pathologie mammaire, edited by P.H. Martin, pp.11, Medsi, Paris.
8. Dickson, R.B., Huff, K.K., Spencer, E.M., and Lippman, M.E. (1986): Endocrinology, 118:138–142.
9. Edwards, D.P., Adams, D.J., Savage, N., and Mc Guire, W.L. (1980): Biochem. Biophys. Res. Commun., 93:804–812.
10. Herrmann, W., Wyss, R., Riodel, A., Philibert, D., Teutsch, G., Sakiz, E., and Baulieu, E.E. (1982): C. R. Acad. Sci., 294:933.
11. Horwitz, K.B., Costlow, M.E., and Mc Guire, W.L. (1975): Steroids, 26:785–795.
12. Horwitz, K.B. and Mc Guire, W.L. (1978): J. Biol. Chem., 253:2223–2228.

13. Keydar, I., Chen, L., Karby, S., Weiss, F.R., Delarea,J., Radu, M., Chaitcik, S., and Brenner, H.J. (1979): Eur. J. Cancer, 15:659–670.
14. Lippman, M., Bolan, G., and Huff, K. (1978): Cancer Res., 36:4595–4601.
15. Manni, A., Wright, C., Feil, P., Baranao, L., Demers, L., Garcia, M., and Rochefort, H. (1986): Cancer Res., 46:1594–1599.
16. Masiakowski, P., Breathnach, R., Bloch, J., Gannon, F., Krust, A., and Chambon, P. (1982): Nucl. Acid Res., 10:7895–7903.
17. Mühlbock, O. (1972): J. Natl. Cancer Inst., 48:1213.
18. Ojasoo, T., and Raynaud, J.P. (1978): Cancer Res., 38:4186–4198.
19. Philibert, D., Deraedt, R., and Teutsch, E. (1981): In: VIII International Congress of Pharmacology, abst. 1463, Tokyo, Japon.
20. Philibert, D., Deraedt, R., Teutsch, E., Tournemine, C., and Sakiz, E. (1982): In: 64th Annual Meeting of the Endocrine Society, abst. 668, San Francisco.
21. Salomon, D.S., Zwiebel, J.A., Bano, M., Lonsonczy, I., Fehnel, P., and Kidwell, W.R. (1984): Cancer Res., 44:4069–4077.
22. Soule, H.D., Vazquez, J., Long, A., Albert, S., and Brennan, M.A. (1973): J. Natl. Cancer Inst., 51:1409–1413.
23. Sporn, M.B., and Todaro, G.J. (1980): New Engl. Med., 303:878–880.
24. Tseng, L., Gusberg, S.B., and Gurpide, E. (1977): In: Biochemical actions of progesterone and progestins, edited by E. Gurpide, vol.286, pp.190, Annals New York Acad. Sci.
25. Vignon, F., Bardon, S., Chalbos, D., and Rochefort, H. (1983): J. Clin. Endocrin. Metab., 56:1124–1130.
26. Vignon, F., Derocq, D., Chambon, M., and Rochefort, H. (1983): C. R. Acad. Sci., 296:151–156.
27. Vignon, F., Capony, F., Chambon, M., Freiss, G., Garcia, M., and Rochefort, H. (1986): Endocrinology, 118:1537–1545.
28. Westley, B., and Rochefort, H. (1980): Cell, 20:353–362.

Hormonal Manipulation of Cancer: Peptides, Growth Factors, and New (Anti) Steroidal Agents, edited by Jan G. M. Klijn et al. Raven Press, New York © 1987.

FIRST CLINICAL TRIAL ON THE USE OF THE ANTI PROGESTIN RU486 IN ADVANCED BREAST CANCER.

T. Maudelonde*, G. Romieu**, A. Ulmann°, H. Pujol**, J. Grenier**, S. Khalaf*, G. Cavalie*, H. Rochefort*

* INSERM U 148, Unité d'Endocrinologie Cellulaire et Moléculaire, 60, rue de Navacelles, 34100 Montpellier, France and Laboratoire de Biochimie Cellulaire et Hormonale, Maternité, Avenue du Professeur Grasset, 34059 Montpellier.

**Centre Paul Lamarque, Hôpital Saint-Eloi, 2 avenue Bertin Sans, 34059 Montpellier, France.

° Laboratoires Roussel Uclaf, 111 Route de Noisy, 93230 Romainville, France.

The antiprogestin and antiglucocorticoid RU486 (mifepristone) has been found to inhibit growth of hormone responsive cell lines in vitro (1,2). This effect appeared to be mediated by the progesterone receptor (PR) but not by the glucocorticoid receptor (GR)(1).

We tested, in this preliminary trial, the long term tolerance and the possible efficacy of RU486 in advanced breast cancer patients who were resistant to tamoxifen.

Patients and methods

Twenty two oophorectomised or post menopausal patients were included in this assay. They all had advanced breast cancer with multiple metastatic sites. Those patients with brain and kidney metastases were excluded. Chemotherapy, radiotherapy, tamoxifen and other hormonal therapy had already been used. RU486 (17ß-hydroxy-11ß, 4 dimethyl aminophenyl 17 propinyl estra 4,9 diene-3-one) was given alone at a dose of 200 mg daily. This dose correspond to 2.5 mg per kilo which was the dose used for experimental studies, particularly for contragestation. One physician (GR) controled all the patients.

Estrogen receptors (ER) were measured by immunoenzymatic assay (3) and progesterone receptor (PR) by dextran coated charcoal assay (4) in the primary tumor or in accessible metastases.

The long term tolerance was assessed by clinical and biogical parameters. We have looked for clinical non specific symptoms (rash, hot flush, dizziness...) and evidence of adrenal dysfunction. Hepatic and kidney function were monitored biochemically. Cortisol and peptide hormones were assayed by RIA before RU486 treatment, during the first four days and at the end of the first and the third month of RU486.

The response to treatment was evaluated by the evolution of metastases and by serial determination of CEA. Partial response was determined as more than 50 % regression of skin, pleural or pulmonary metastases and a decrease of the number of thoracenteses. The sum of products of perpendicular diameters of the greatest dimension has been done in pleuropulmonary metastases. 50% reduction is considered as partial regression. Stabilization was determined as less than 50 % regression or less than 25 % progression.

RESULTS

1. Long term tolerance

The long term tolerance was good, one patient had transient nausea, one had hot flushes and two patients had dizziness at the beginning of the treatment.

We have not seen any symptoms of adrenal dysfunction. Biologically, there was a 10 % decrease of plasma potassium during the first month (Table 1). This modification was well tolerated. In one patient treated concomitantly with furosemide the kalemia decreased to 2.3 mEq/L. However, the blood potassium increased after arrest of the diuretic. Plasma cortisol increased from 235 ± 94 ng/ml to 420 ± 140 ng/ml after four days of RU486($p < 0.001$). This increase was stable during the RU486 treatment. LH, FSH and PRL were not significantly modified for all the treatment period (Table 2).

TABLE 1. Biological long term tolerance

	PLASMA CONCENTRATIONS	
	Before n = 22	After (3 months) n = 5
Potassium (mEq/L)	3.9 ± 0.3	$3.5 \pm 0.5*$
Cortisol (ng/ml)	235 ± 94	$473 \pm 141**$
LH (mUI/ml)	63 ± 33	50 ± 23
FSH (mUI/ml)	49 ± 37	44 ± 29
PRL (µU/ml)	437 ± 541	292 ± 168

− Plasma value of biological and hormonal parameters obtained at day 0 and 90 of RU486 treatment.
− Results are the mean SD. The difference statistically evaluated with t'test was *$p < 0.05$; **$p < 0.001$.

2. Response to therapy

− 12 of the 22 patients had a partial regression or a stabilisation of the lesions following 4 to 6 weeks of treatment.
− In 7 of these patients with high CEA plasma level, a concomitant decreased has been observed.

At 3 months the mean response rate was only 18 % and CEA levels continued to decrease in only two patients. 40% of the 15 patients with cutaneous metastases had partial regression or stabilization for 4   to 6 weeks but the response rate was 7% at 3 months (table 2). Seventeen patients had pleuropulmonary metastases. 18% were stabilized for 3 months or more. The longest period of stabilization was 10 months. A strong analgesic effect was observed in most patients with bone metastases.

TABLE 2. Response rate at different metastatic sites.

	Cutaneous (n=15)	PP (n=17)
a.		
– Total regression	0%	0%
– Partial regression		
6 weeks	20%	0%
3 months	0%	0%
– Stabilization		
6 weeks	20%	18%
3 months	7%	18%
b.		
– Progressive disease	60%	82%

The response rate is determined as the percent of the metastase population responding to RU486.
a) Partial regression or stabilization : Cutaneous metastasis were evaluated from the area of lesions and by photographic comparisons. Pleural and pulmonary (PP) metastases were evaluated by tomograms and frequencies of thoracenteses.
b) Progressive disease : No benefit with RU486.

In 10 of the 22 patients, there was no improvement and the drug was stopped within the first month of the assay for further chemotherapy or a radiotherapy. During the trial 5 patients died. 2 had intercurrent pulmonary infection. Receptor assays were done on eight tumors. Four had ER and PR and were responding to RU486 treatment. Another one had ER only and was resistant to antiprogestin treatment. The three others had neither ER nor PR and were who resistant to RU486.

DISCUSSION

This preliminary trial provides two kinds of information. The most important is that RU486 is well tolerated in long term treatment. 4 patients (18%) had minor side effects and the increased of plasma cortisol was not associated with symptoms of adrenal dysfunction. The 10% decrease of plasma potassium is likely to reflect a hypermineralocorticoid state resulting from

glucocorticoid receptor blokade (5). It requires careful
monitoring in case of diuretic treatment. The second finding is
the favorable response of some patients to RU486. The contrast
between the response rate a 4-6 weeks (50%) and 3 months (18%)
may be due to the selection of patients with very advanced breast
cancer that we had chosen for ethical reasons in this first
trial. Also, the objective effect of RU486 in four patients
(18 %) suggest that it could be useful as second or third line
hormonal therapy. The mechanism of the antitumoral action of
RU486 is unknown. It is likely, as suggested by in vitro
studies(1-2) that the drug acts via the PR of breast cancer cells
similar to the way the antiestrogen tamoxifen acts via the ER
(6-7). If the results are confirmed, RU486 could have a role as
an initial and novel hormonal therapy since current treatment is
based on suppression of estrogen production or action (8). The
observation that 4 patients responded more than 3 months to RU486
after failure of several hormonal therapies is in favor of such a
hypothesis. It also suggests that combined therapy with RU486 and
tamoxifen (which maintains a certain level of PR) could be
beneficial.

In conclusion, RU486 is well tolerated in long term therapy
at 200 mg per day, even in patients with extensive debility. The
response rate in agreement with an antiproliferative effect of
RU486 in breast cancer, first demonstrated in vitro and in a rat
mammary tumor (9).

On the basis of this preliminary study, a controlled clinical
trial has been initiated in order to establish whether this
treatment may be proposed as an additional endocrine therapy of
breast cancer.

REFERENCES

1. Bardon S., Vignon F., Chalbos D., Rochefort H. : RU486, a
   progestin and glucocorticoid antagonist, inhibits the growth
   of breast cancer cells via the progesterone receptor. J.
   Clin. Endocrin. Met., 1985, **60**, 692-697.
2. Horwitz K.B. : The antiprogestin RU38 486 : Receptor-
   mediated progestin versus anti progestin actions screened in
   estrogen-insensitive T47D human breast cancer cells.
   Endocrinology, 1985, **116**, 2236-2245.
3. Nolan C., Przywara L.W., Miller L.S., Suduikis V., Tomita
   J.T.: A sensitive solid-phase enzyme immunoassay for human
   estrogen receptor. In, Current Controversies in Breast
   Cancer, Ames F.C. et al., eds., University of Texas Press,
   Austin, 1984, 433-441.
4. Bressot N., Veith F., Saussol J., Pujol H. et al. :
   Presurgical radiotherapy decreases the concentrations of
   estrogen and progesterone receptors in human breast cancer :
   a 200 patient study. Breast Cancer Res. Treat., 1982, **2**,
   177-183.

5. Chrousos G.P., Vingerhoeds A., Brandon D., Eil C., Pugeat M., De Vroede M., Loriaux D.L., Lipsett M.B. : Primary cortisol resistance in man. A glucocorticoid receptor-mediated disease. J. Clin. Invest., 1982, **69**, 1261-1269.

6. Coezy E., Borgna J.L., Rochefort H. : Tamoxifen and metabolites in MCF 7 cells: Correlation between binding to estrogen receptor and inhibition of cell growth. Cancer Res., 1982, **42**, 317-323.

7. Patterson J., Barry Furr M.B., Wakeling A., Battersby L. : The biology and physiology of Nolvadex (tamoxifen) in the treatment of breast cancer. Breast Cancer Res. Treat., 1982, **2**, 363-74.

8. Hellman S., Harris J.R., Canellos G.P., Fisher B.: Cancer of the Breast. In, Cancer : Principles and Practice of Oncology, De Vita V.T., Hellman S., Rosenberg S.A. eds., J.B. Lippincott Company, Philadelphia, Toronto, 1982, 914-970.

9. Lamberts S.W.J., Uitterlinden P., Bons E.G., Verleun T. : Comparison of the actions of RU 38486 and megestrol acetate in the model of a transplantable adrenocorticotropin-and prolactin-secreting rat pituitary tumor. Cancer Res., 1985, **45**, 1015-1019.

Hormonal Manipulation of Cancer: Peptides, Growth Factors, and New (Anti) Steroidal Agents, edited by Jan G. M. Klijn et al. Raven Press, New York © 1987.

STEROID RECEPTORS IN CEREBRAL TUMOURS

POSSIBLE CONSEQUENCE FOR ENDOCRINE TREATMENT?

M.A. Blankenstein, *†G. Blaauw, †J.W; van 't Verlaat,
C. van der Meulen-Dijk and J.H.H. Thijssen

Departments of Endocrinology and †Neurosurgery,
Academic Hospital Utrecht and *De Wever Hospital Heerlen,
P.O. Box 16250, 3500 CG UTRECHT, The Netherlands.

Cerebral tumours, especially meningiomas, have recently been identified as possible steroid target tissues. Following the first report in 1979 (6), on the presence of oestrogen receptors in human meningiomas, several research groups, including our own (3,4) have tried to confirm these findings. These efforts have resulted in the consensus that investigators using single point assays often find meningiomas to be oestrogen receptor positive, whereas investigators using Scatchard plot analysis report that the majority of meningiomas is oestrogen receptor negative (1,14). From these investigations it became clear that meningiomas contain high amounts of progestin receptors. This was especially remarkable in view of the virtual absence of oestrogen receptors and the causal relationship between the presence of oestrogen and progestin receptors which exists in "classical" oestrogen target tissues like breast and uterus.

Although the criteria for the attribution of the term "receptor" to the progestin binding component present in human meningioma tissue, such as a high binding affinity, a low binding capacity and a high degree of steroid specificity, appeared to be fulfilled (3), there still remained some doubt with respect to the nature of the progestin binding moiety. Schwartz et al (15) for instance reported that, when analysed by sucrose gradient analysis, the progestin binder from meningioma did not behave like the progestin receptor extracted from human breast cancer tissue.

In the present paper we describe our experiments on the further characterization of progestin receptors from human meningioma cytosol, the occurrence of androgen receptors in meningioma tissue and on the occurrence of oestrogen and progestin receptors in non-meningial cerebral tumours. Special emphasis is on the behavior of the progestin receptor on sucrose gradients and gel filtration columns. Our findings are discussed in the light of recent reports on the endocrine treatment of meningiomas with antioestrogens and high dose progestins.

MATERIALS AND METHODS

Meningioma tissues and tissue from other types of cerebral tumours were collected and stored as described before (3,4). Human myometrium tissue was also obtained and stored at -70°C until use. In some experiments a frozen preparation of uterine cytosol was used.

Receptor Assays

Cytosols were prepared according to the recommendations of the EORTC Breast Cancer Cooperative Group (7). Oestrogen and progestin receptors were assayed by Scatchard plot analysis of binding data obtained with a 5-7 point dextran coated charcoal method (3,4). For oestrogen and progestin receptor assays respectively, tritiated oestradiol and ORG.2058 were used as radioactive tracers, whereas diethylstilboestrol (DES) and radioinert ORG.2058 were used as competitors for the assessment of aspecific binding. For the androgen receptor assay, ^{3}H-R1881 was used as a ligand and radioinert R1881 for the assessment of aspecific binding. To prevent binding of R1881 to progestin receptors, 500 nM radioinert ORG.2058 was added to all tubes.

Tissues were considered to be receptor positive, when a statistically significant correlation was observed in the Scatchard plot, when the dissociation constant was below 5 nM and when the receptor content was equal to or higher than 10 fmol/mg protein. For the androgen receptor assay this last criterium was not applied.

Sucrose Gradient Analysis

Cytosol was incubated overnight at 4°C with 5 nM ^{3}H-ORG.2058, either in the presence or in the absence of a 200 fold excess radioinert ligand. After equilibrium was reached, excess radioactivity was removed by a ten minutes treatment with dextran coated charcoal (0.25% Norit and 0.025% Dextran T-70 in cytosol buffer) followed by centrifugation for 10 minutes at 2000xg. Samples were then layered on top of 10-30% sucrose density gradients containing 20 mmole/l sodium molybdate and centrifuged for 2h and 45 min at 65,000 rpm (400,000xg) in a Beckman VTi-65 vertical rotor. After the run, the tubes were pierced, 7-drop fractions (0.15 ml) were collected in scintillation vials and radioactivity was detected following addition of 0.5 ml of distilled water and 4 ml of scintillation fluid (Opti-Fluor, Packard-Becker, Groningen, the Netherlands. Additions to gradients are specified at the individual experiments. Bovine serum albumin (BSA, 4.6S) and Gamma-globulin (7.2S) were run on separate gradients as sedimentation markers.

Gel Filtration

Gel filtration experiments were done at 4°C on Sephadex G-200 (Pharmacia, Uppsala, Sweden) in a 60cm x 9mm column. Elution was done with the same buffer as was used for the preparation of the cytosol. In some experiments, 0.4M KCl and/or 20 mM sodium molybdate were added to the receptor preparation and the elution buffer. Fractions of 1 ml were collected and radioactivity was counted as decribed above. The column was calibrated with thyreoglobulin (670 kD), catalase (232 kD), BSA (67 kD) and chymotrypsin (25 kD).

RESULTS

Occurrence of Steroid Receptors in Cerebral Tumours

At present our series of meningioma tissues consists of 116 samples. All of them have been assayed for progestin receptors, 114 for oestrogen receptors and 21 for androgen receptors. The results of these experiments is depicted in Figure 1. It is clear that most meningiomas contain appreciable amounts of progestin receptors. Oestrogen receptors are only seldomly detectable in meningiomas, whereas androgen receptors take a somewhat intermediate position. Androgen receptors were found in 5 out of 21 tissues, but, as with oestrogen receptors, the receptor levels were relatively low.

In sharp contrast to the meningiomas, other cerebral tumours were found to be virtually devoid of progestin receptors. We studied a series of 9 astrocytomas, 2 ependymomas, 5 gliomas, 6 neurinomas, 3 fibrosarcomas, 2 schwannomas, 1 cerebellar haemangioma, 1 neurofibroma and 7 intracranial metastases of primary tumours located outside the central nervous system. Progestin receptors were found only in 2 neurinomas. The progestin level in these samples was very low, i.e. 12 and 14 fmole/mg protein respectively, when compared to the progestin receptor levels found in meningioma tissue. No oestrogen receptors were found in this series of 36 intracranial non-meningeal tumours.

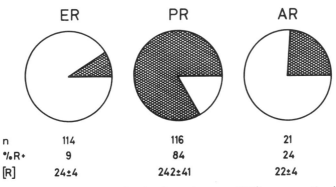

STEROID RECEPTORS IN HUMAN MENINGIOMA

	ER	PR	AR
n	114	116	21
%R+	9	84	24
[R]	24±4	242±41	22±4

FIG.1. Occurrence and content of oestrogen (ER), progestin (PR) and androgen (AR) receptors in meningioma tissue as estimated by Scatchard plot analysis. Cross-hatched areas indicate the proportion of receptor-positive samples. The receptor concentration of the positive cytosols is indicated as means ± S.E.M. and is expressed as fmol/mg cytosol protein.

Sucrose Gradient Analysis

In view of the negative findings of Schwartz et al (15) we studied the sedimentation pattern of the progestin receptor from meningioma in sucrose gradients. Figure 2 shows the sedimentation profile
of progestin receptors from meningioma cytosol in low- and high-
salt sucrose gradients. For comparison, human myometrium cytosol
was also analysed. It is evident that the sedimention constant of the
progestin receptor in both preparations is strongly dependent on the
ionic strength of the gradient. In low-salt gradients a sedimentation
constant of approximately 8S is observed, whereas addition of 0.4M
KCl causes a shift to approximately 4S. The sedimention pattern of
myometrium progestin receptors showed two peaks in low-salt gradients. This was also seen with some meningioma cytosols. Addition
of molybdate had only a marginal effect on the number of receptors, but to a certain extent stabilized the 8S form of the receptor. As a matter of precaution, molybdate was therefore used in
further experiments.

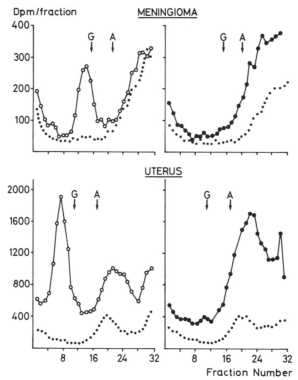

FIG. 2. Sedimentation profiles of progestin receptors from human
meningioma and uterus cytosol in low (o) or high (●) salt sucrose
gradients. The dotted lines represent the sedimentation patterns obtained with a 200 fold molar excess of radioinert ORG.2058. Arrows
indicate the positions of bovine serum albumin (A) and gamma-globulin (G).

Having established the fact that progestin receptors from human meningioma indeed can be successfully analysed on sucrose gradients, we subsequently addressed the ligand specificity of the binding observed on the gradients. For this we used low-salt gradients and the effect of different competitors on the amount of radioactivity sedimenting at 8S was evaluated. Competitors were used in a 200-fold molar excess over 5 nM ^{3}H-ORG.2058. Progesterone and ORG.2058 competed very well for the binding in the 8S region of the gradient. Oestradiol, R2858 (a synthetic oestrogen receptor ligand), cortisol and testosterone showed no competition. The synthetic androgen receptor ligand R1881 caused a 95% displacement of the label, but this competition should probably be attributed to the intrinsic progestational properties of this compound.

Gel Filtration

Initial experiments with Sephadex G-200 gel filtration and elution with cytosol buffer resulted in elution patterns with two peaks: a peak suppressible with a 200-fold molar excess of radioinert ligand in the void volume and a non-suppressible peak representing the remaining free steroid at the end of the elution pattern. This indicated that severe aggregation of receptors must occur under these conditions. Based on the results obtained with sucrose gradient centrifugation (Figure 2), attempts were made to bring the receptor in a smaller form with 0.4M KCl. This had no effect on the sedimentation pattern. Finally, also 20 mM sodium molybdate was also added to the elution buffer. The results obtained in these experiments are exemplified in Figure 3. In the elution pattern of both meningiomal and uterine cytosols, the peak at the void volume was still most prominent, whereas smaller suppressible peaks were observed at larger elution volumes, indicating that at least some of the receptor was in a disaggregated form. It is clear, however, that receptor aggregation has not yet been overcome sufficiently. Nevertheless, it is encouraging to see that also in these experiments no clear differences beteen the progestin receptor in meningioma and that in uterine tissue was found.

DISCUSSION.

Oestrogen Receptors

The present study gives an update and an extension of our series, which was started in 1982. Our initial conclusion that human meningioma tissue is virtually devoid of oestrogen receptors, whereas progestin receptors are abundtantly present (3,4) still remains valid (Figure 1). In attempts to exclude the possibilities that the apparent absence of oestrogen receptors from meningioma is due to metabolic degradation of the ligand or confinement of the receptors to a small subpopulation of cells present in an otherwise receptor-negative tissue, we have employed a recently developed immunocytochemical assay using monoclonal antibodies against the human oestrogen receptor (11). No specific staining was observed (2) which supported our hypothesis that in meningioma tissue the synthesis of the progestin receptor is not mediated through oestrogen receptors.

Progestin Receptors

The main part of the present experiments was devoted to a further characterization of the progestin binding component present in human meningioma tissue. This binder has been termed "receptor" by a large number of investigators (1,3,4,14 and references cited therein), but others (15) doubt whether it is justified to give the progestin binding agent this qualification. Although unequivocal proof

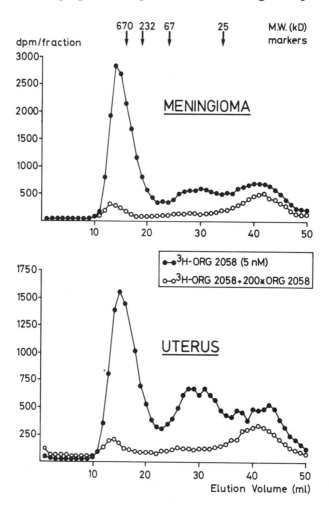

FIG. 3. Elution profiles of human meningioma and uterus cytosol progestin receptors from a Sephadex G-200 column eluted with buffer containing 0.4M KCl and 20 mM sodium molybdate.

that the binding agent is a true receptor will be extremely difficult to obtain, strong indications in further support of this hypothesis have been obtained in this study.

The sedimentation behavior of the progestin binder in meningioma closely resembles that of the human uterine progestin receptor (Figure 2). Progestin binding shows the characteristic 8S to 4S transformation upon an increase of the ionic strength. Moreover, the 8S-form displays a high degree of steroid specificity, comparable to that found earlier with the dextran-coated charcoal technique (3). These findings are consistent with those of Tilzer et al (16), but are in sharp contrast to those of Schwartz et al (15). Some differences exist between the technical approaches used in the present experiments and those used by these authors. They have used, for instance, a different synthetic progestin (R5020) as a tracer, and centrifuge the sucrose gradients at only half the g-value that has been used in our experiments. It is hard to envisage, however, how the use of R5020 would not allow generation of sedimentation patterns like those shown in Figure 2. Although ORG.2058 has a somewhat higher affinity for the progestin receptor than R5020 (4) receptor values obtained with these two tracers did not show differences (data not shown). Theoretically, the use of a ligand with a lower affinity in combination with a longer centrifugation time may result in dissociation of the ligand-receptor complex, but this can not properly be evaluated since Schwartz et al did not include a sample of the gradient patterns obtained in their paper (15).

Further indications that the progestin receptor in meningioma is a "true" receptor comes from the gel filtration experiments. The behavior of uterine and meningiomal receptors was identical, although, admittedly, the elution patterns obtained were not satisfactory. Taken all the indications, present and past, together, we must maintain our earliest conclusion (3) that the progestin binder in meningioma tissue is a true receptor.

For an unequivocal conclusion in this respect, evidence that progestins directly influence the growth of meningioma cells in culture is a prerequisite. Several research groups have tried to obtain such evidence, but the preliminay results do not allow conclusions yet. Grunberg et al (8) repored in an abstract that in a clonogenic assay 3 out of 5 progestin receptor-positive meningiomas were sensitive to progesterone, whereas in 5 progestin receptor-negative meningiomas no response to progesterone was found. In addition, only 1 out of 9 oestrogen receptor-negative meningiomas was found to be sensitive to oestrogens in this type of assay. Unfortunately, the abstract does not state whether the growth rate of the cells increased or decreased in response to these hormones. Weisman et al (18) reported, also in an abstract, that oestrogen increased DNA synthesis in primary cultures of meningioma cells. Remarkably, progesterone and cortisol had no effect, except when added in high concentrations. In a full paper, Jay et al (9) reported that oestradiol in concentrations of 1 and 100 nM stimulated cell growth in 4 meningioma cell cultures. Progesterone and tamoxifen also stimulated cell growth when added alone, but inhibited the oestradiol-induced cell growth. Especially, the putative effects of oestradiol on meningioma cell cultures as reported in these studies is not in agreement with the virtual absence of oestrogen receptors. Moreover the authors did not mention whether progestin receptor levels were measured in the tumours or in the cultured cells. In our very limited experience with primary cultures of meningioma tissue, it appears that progestin receptors may not be expressed in the cultured cells, even if they were present abundantly in the primary tissue specimen. Clearly, much more work is necessary to completely define the effects of steroid hormones on meningioma cells.

Androgen Receptors

Our results, showing the presence of low levels of androgen receptors in only 5 out of 21 meningiomas (Figure 1), are in contrast to those of Poisson et al (13). These authors found that high levels of androgen receptors were present in most meningiomas. We calculated from their data that a statistically significant correlation existed between the level of progestin receptors and the apparent concentration of androgen receptors (r = 0.855, n=25). From this calculation and the observation by Poisson et al (13) that R5020 was a stronger competitor for the binding of ^{3}H-R1881 than testosterone and dihydrotestosterone, we infer that the blocking of progestin receptors with radioinert triamcinolone acetonide may not have been sufficient. This may be due to the high concentration of progestin receptors in the samples. We have used 500 nM radioinert ORG.2058 to block binding of ^{3}H-R1881 to progestin receptors. In competition experiments we found that most of the binding of this label to meningioma cytosol could be displaced by this concentration of ORG.-2058. A small amount of ^{3}H-R1881 could not be displaced by ORG.2058, but was displaced by radioinert R1881, dihydrotestosterone and testosterone, indicating that this represents binding to an androgen receptor. We conclude that low levels of androgen receptors are present in some meningiomas and that the apparent differences between our results and those of Poisson et al (13) must be attributed to methodological differences.

Endocrine Treatment

The possible endocrine treatment of recurrent or inoperable meningiomas would be an attractive consequence of the presence of functioning steroid receptors in these tissues. In spite of the fact that the functional integrity of putative steroid receptors in meningioma cytosols has not been proven yet, several investigators have attempted endocrine therapy for the management of meningioma. Markwalder et al (12) treated six patients with 30 mg tamoxifen daily for a period of 8 to 12 months. No favourable responses were seen. Similar results were quoted in correspondence by Vaquero and Martinez (17) and by Cahill (5). The refractoriness of meningioma to treatment with antioestrogens is in agreement with the absence of oestrogen receptors.

Treatment with high doses medroxyprogesterone acetate had also no effect in 4 slowly growing benign and one rapidly growing anaplastic meningioma (10). The progestin content of the anaplastic tumour was very low (15 fmol/mg protein). It is not clear whether this is related to the unresponsiveness of the tumour. Unfortunately, receptor contents of the other tumours were not available.

Taking the negative results of these pilot studies on the endocrine manipulation of meningiomas together, it appears that research efforts should be directed primarily to the establishment of the functional integrity of the progestin receptor and the hormonal effects on meningioma cells. Based on the outcome of these experiments, more successful clinical trials can hopefully be designed. If, as expected from epidemiologiocal data, progestins indeed can be shown to stimulate the growth of meningioma cells directly, trials with antiprogestins may be more rewarding than trials with antioestrogens or progestins.

ACKNOWLEDGEMENT

The support of this study by the Netherlands Cancer Society (Koningin Wilhelmina Fonds) through Grant UUKC 85-25 is gratefully acknowledged.

REFERENCES

1. Blaauw, G., Blankenstein, M.A., and Lamberts, S.W.J. (1986): Acta Neurochir., 79:42-47.
2. Blankenstein, M.A., Berns, P.M.J.J., Blaauw, G., Mulder, E., and Thijssen, J.H.H. (1986): Cancer Res. (Suppl), 46:In Press.
3. Blankenstein, M.A., Blaauw, G., Lamberts, S.W.J., and Mulder, E. (1983): Eur. J. Cancer Clin. Oncol., 19:365-370.
4. Blankenstein, M.A., Blaauw, G., and Lamberts, S.W.J. (1984): Clin. Neuropharmacol., 7:363-367.
5. Cahill, D.W. (1985): J. Neurosurg., 62:162-163.
6. Donnell, M.S., Glenn, B.A., Meyer, A., and Donegan, W.L. (1979): J. Neurosurg., 50:499-502.
7. EORTC Breast Cancer Cooperative Group (1980): Eur. J. Cancer, 16:1513-1515.
8. Grunberg, S.M., Muensch, H., Daniels, A.M., Daniels, J.R., Kortes, V., Goodkin, R., and Weiss, M.H. (1985): Proc. AACR, 26:204.
9. Jay. J.R., MacLaughlin, D.T., Riley, K.R., and Martuza, R.L. (1985): J. Neurosurg., 62:757-762.
10. Jääskeläinen, J., Laasonen, E., Kärkkäinen, J., Haltia, M., and Troupp, H. (1986): Acta Neurochir. 80:35-41.
11. King, W.L., and Greene, G.L. (1984): Nature 307:745-747.
12. Markwalder, T.-M., Seiler, R.W., and Zava, D.T. (1985): Surg. Neurol., 24:245-249.
13. Poisson, M., Pertuiset, B.F., Hauw, J.-J., Philippon, J., Buge, A., Moguilewsky, M., and Philibert, D. (1983): J. Neuro-Oncol., 1:179-189.
14. Poisson, M., Pertuiset, B.F., Moguilewsky, M., Magdalenat, H., and Martin, P.M. (1984): Rev. Neurol. (Paris), 140:233-248.
15. Schwartz, M.R., Randolph, R.L., Cech, D.A., Rose, J.E., and

Panko, W.B. (1984): Cancer 53:922–927.

16. Tilzer, L.L., Plapp, F.V., Evans, J.P., Stone, D., and Award, K. (1982): Cancer, 49:633–636.

17. Vaquero, J., and Martinez, R. (1985): J. Neurosurg., 62:162.

18. Weisman, A.S., Villemure, J.G., and Kelly, P.A. (1985): 67th Annual Meeting of the Endocrine Society, Abstract 1238.

Hormonal Manipulation of Cancer: Peptides, Growth Factors, and New (Anti) Steroidal Agents, edited by Jan G. M. Klijn et al. Raven Press, New York © 1987.

CURRENT STATUS OF AROMATASE INHIBITORS FOR TREATMENT OF

BREAST CANCER: NEW PERSPECTIVES

Richard J. Santen

Department of Medicine, The Milton S. Hershey Medical Center, The Pennsylvania State University, P.O. Box 850, Hershey, PA   17033

Approximately one-third of human breast cancers are estrogen-dependent (1). New treatment strategies have focused upon the development and use of highly specific antiestrogens and of inhibitors of estrogen production. Knowledge of the various pathways involved in systemic and local estrogen biosynthesis in postmenopausal women is required before studying the specific effects of inhibitors on these pathways.

After the menopause, the ovary produces only minimal amounts of either estrone or estradiol, and the adrenal becomes the major source of estrogen precursors (2-4). While the adrenal does not secrete estrogens directly, it releases the prehormone androstenedione (A), which is then converted into estrone (E_1) in peripheral tissues via the enzyme aromatase. Extraglandular aromatase is present in fat, liver, hair follicles, brain, muscle and in other tissues (5-7). Estrone can be conjugated into estrone sulfate (E_1-S) to form a slowly turning over storage pool with a potential for back conversion to estrone. Alternatively, estrone can be reduced to estradiol (E_2), the major active estrogenic steroid.

A variety of data supports the concept that estrogens can be made in breast cancer tissue in situ from plasma precursors in postmenopausal women (8-10). Local estrogen production can take place via one of two alternative pathways - the aromatase and the sulfatase systems. In our studies, as well as in others (11-17), the aromatase enzyme present in tumor tissue was shown to have a high affinity (i.e. K_m = 0.027µM) and low capacity (i.e. 50-80 pmol/gm protein/hr)(17). Measurable activity was demonstrated in 79 of 128 human breast cancers and was unrelated to the concentration of estrogen receptor or progesterone receptor, size of tumor, presence of local or distant metastases, or the patient's age.

The formation of estrone from its sulfate may be quantitatively more important than production from androstenedione via aromatase (18). We detected one million-fold higher levels of sulfatase (i.e. 0.8-125 µM/g protein/hr) than of aromatase (i.e. 5-80 pM/gm/hr) in breast tumors. The sulfatase enzyme found in human breast tumors (19-20), while of high capacity, is of low affinity (i.e. approximately 10 µM)(18). Studies to compare the amount of estrone synthesized via aromatase with that via sulfatase require use of biologically relevant substrate concentrations which parallel those expected in vivo (18). Human breast tumors, when studied under these in vitro conditions, synthesized 10-fold more estrone via sulfatase than aromatase.

Additional in vitro studies support the biological relevance of the estrone sulfatase pathway. The MCF-7 breast cancer cell line responds to estrone sulfate with an increased rate of synthesis of the 52K estrogen-inducible protein, and with more rapid growth (21). Estrogen-dependent nitrosomethylurea-induced (NMU) rat mammary tumors respond to estrone sulfate when grown in soft agar with an increase in the number of colonies formed (22-23). Preliminary data suggest a dose-response effect of estrone sulfate on the growth of this tumor in ovariectomized rats as well.

In situ production of estradiol by human breast tumors also requires the presence of 17β-hydroxysteroid dehydrogenase, the enzyme which converts estrone to estradiol. We and other investigators detected substantial amounts of this enzyme in all human breast tumors studied. With careful attention to the substrate concentrations used in our in vitro assay, we could detect a high affinity form of the enzyme (i.e., average K_m = 0.47 µM) in approximately 50% of tumors, whereas the other tumors contained only a low affinity form (i.e., average K_m = 22 µM)(23).

Taken together, it appears that human breast tumors contain the enzymes necessary for in situ estradiol synthesis. However, it remains to be established whether the majority of estrogen present in breast tumor tissue is synthesized in situ or is concentrated in the neoplasm after transportation from plasma.

Estrogen formation could potentially be blocked by inhibition of a number of enzymatic steps (24-27). However, blockade of aromatase is theoretically ideal as a means of inhibition of estrogen biosynthesis of estrogens. Its blockade would specifically inhibit estrogen production without exerting effects on glucocorticoid, androgen or mineralocorticoid production.

The most widely studied aromatase inhibitor is aminoglutethimide (28). This compound blocks the three cytochrome P-450-mediated steroid hydroxylation steps required for the aromatization of androgens to estrogens and in so doing, produces a type II binding spectrum. Aminoglutethimide has intermediate potency on the placental microsomal system in vitro when compared to a series of aromatase inhibitors (29). When given to patients at the standard dose level of 1,000 mg daily, aminoglutethimide blocks aromatase by 95-98% (30). As expected, inhibition of this enzymatic step lowers the levels of estrone as well as estradiol and estrone sulfate. The reduction of estrogen levels parallels those produced by surgical removal of the adrenals in postmeno-pausal women (31).

The exact dose-response effects of aminoglutethimide on extra-glandular aromatase activity in women have not been adequately tested as yet. However, a dose of 125 mg of aminoglutethimide given twice daily without hydrocortisone inhibits aromatase to nearly the same extent as larger doses when studied by the direct isotope kinetic technique (32). Consistent with this finding, 125 mg of aminoglutethimide given twice daily also lowers plasma estrogen concentrations to the same extent as does 1,000 mg daily (33).

Aminoglutethimide inhibits the aromatase present in human breast carcinomas as well as blocking this enzyme in other extra-glandular tissues. Concentrations of 10 μM are required to pro-duce a 50% inhibition of this enzyme in tumors (17). Since administration of standard doses of aminoglutethimide produce average plasma drug concentrations of 30 μM, substantial inhibi-tion of local aromatase activity in the tumor tissues would be expected in patients receiving aminoglutethimide (34).

The in situ production of estrogen via the sulfatase pathway is not directly inhibited by aminoglutethimide. However, the reduction of plasma estrone sulfate by aminoglutethimide in-directly lowers the amount of substrate present in tumor tissue for the local sulfatase enzyme (31). Aminoglutethimide is not a specific aromatase inhibitor since it also blocks cholesterol side-chain cleavage.

Inhibitors of aromatase more specific and potent than amino-glutethimide are currently being developed. Most promising are the class of compounds called suicide inhibitors (35). This group of agents undergoes a specific transformation by the enzyme which activates a high affinity site on the inhibitor. This activated site then binds covalently to the enzyme and permanent-ly inactivates it. 4-Hydroxy-androstenedione and 10β-propar-gel-est-4-ene-3,17-dione (PED) and MDL 18,962 are potent suicide inhibitors which are currently under development (36-39).

Aminoglutethimide is the only aromatase inhibitor which has been extensively tested in women with breast cancer. Standard regimens include 1,000 mg of aminoglutethimide daily as well as replacement glucocorticoid (i.e. 40 mg of hydrocortisone daily).

The latter is necessary to prevent a potential state of glucocorticoid deficiency resulting from inhibition of cholesterol side-chain cleavage (28). Approximately 30% of unselected patients and 55% of women with estrogen-receptor positive tumors respond to this regimen. Side effects of AG/HC include lethargy, skin rash, orthostatic dizziness, ataxia and drug fever. Lethargy occurred in approximately 40% of one group of 129 patients reported (40). It is of interest that these side effects diminished during continued drug administration. When side effects are scored as acute (i.e., <6 wk) or chronic (i.e., >6 wk), the frequency of lethargy diminished to 15% of patients and the skin rash disappeared in all but one patient during long-term therapy. Less frequently, hematologic toxicity had been observed. In a group of 1,333 patients, 0.9% developed either thrombocytopenia or granulocytopenia or both (41). These findings occured within the first 6 week of treatment and resolved within one week after discontinuing aminoglutethimide.

The standard aminoglutethimide/hydrocortisone regimen has been compared to surgical ablative methods of reducing estrogen production. AG/HC produced a similar rate of objective tumor regression as did surgical adrenalectomy or hypophysectomy (31,42). Durations of response and of survival after initiation of treatment were also similar when AG/HC was compared to surgical adrenalectomy. Three studies randomly allocated patients to treatment with either AG/HC (aromatase blockade) or antiestrogens in the form of tamoxifen (43-45). A similar percentage of patients experienced objective tumor regression with either regimen in all 3 studies.

The similarity of objective responses observed after blockade of estrogen synthesis or with antiestrogen therapy prompted investigators to choose between aminoglutethimide/hydrocortisone and tamoxifen on the basis of severity of side effects. Clearly, tamoxifen is better tolerated than aminoglutethimide and associated with fewer side effects. The preferred use of tamoxifen as a first-line agent raised the question whether aminoglutethimide might still be effective in patients previously given tamoxifen. Data pooled from several investigators (28) indicated that 31% of 263 women initially given tamoxifen later responded objectively to AG/HC. Of the 94 women who experienced either a complete or partial objective regression in response to initial tamoxifen therapy, 50% underwent a secondary response to AG/HC upon relapse. In contrast, only 25% of the 93 tamoxifen non-responders were found to have a complete or partial objective tumor regression upon cross-over to AG/HC. Based upon these data, the preferred treatment sequence is the use of tamoxifen initially followed by AG/HC later.

At present, the exact sequence of hormonal therapies to be used after initial tamoxifen is not fully established. Choices of different agents depend upon therapeutic efficacy, frequency

of side effects, and major toxicity. These considerations high-
light the fact that clinical trials are now required to compare
AG/HC with high-dose progestins to determine which of these second-line therapies should be used preferentially after tamoxifen.

Development of means to block aromatase more selectively than
with aminoglutethimide is currently an investigative area of
major interest. When used at lower dosage, aminoglutethimide
blocks aromatase selectively without inhibiting glucocorticoid
biosynthesis sufficiently to necessitate glucocorticoid administration. Regimens of 250 mg of aminoglutethimide given alone
have produced objective tumor regression in approximately 20% of
patients with breast cancer in two pilot studies (46,47). Although somewhat lower than observed with 1,000 mg of aminoglutethimide in combination with hydrocortisone, randomized trials
will be necessary to compare the low dose regimen directly with
standard AG/HC therapy.

Selective aromatase inhibition with the suicide inhibitor,
4-hydroxyandrostenedione also appears to be feasible. In a preliminary report, 12 of 40 evaluable patients with breast cancer
responded objectively to 4-hydroxyandrostenedione in a dosage of
500 mg once weekly by intramuscular injection (48). Estradiol
levels fell persistently to 2.8 pg/ml on average during 4 months
of administration. A later study demonstrated the efficacy of
this drug given by the oral route. Other suicide inhibitors such
as PED are now undergoing animal toxicity testing and should soon
be available for clinical trial.

Regimens Using Aromatase Inhibitors for Hormonal Priming for
Chemotherapy:

A logical evolution in the treatment of breast cancer is to
combine chemotherapy with hormonal therapy. However, no study
substantiates a synergistic effect of these combinations which
result in prolonged patient survival (49). One explanation for
this disappointing result is based upon knowledge of the mechanism of action of hormonal therapy. While clearly exerting a
tumoricidal effect on certain cells, hormonal therapy moves
others out of the active cell cycle into a G_0 or resting phase.
Many, if not all, chemotherapeutic drugs are more active against
tumor cells which are actively in cell cycle.

These considerations have led to the use of strategies whereby
tumor cells are primed hormonally prior to each cycle of chemotherapy. With this technique, a phase of hormone depletion is
produced either by administration of antiestrogens or estrogen
biosynthesis inhibitors. Some tumor cells which are completely
estrogen-dependent will be destroyed by this maneuver. Others,
which are sensitive to estrogens but not dependent upon them,
will be moved into the G_0 (resting) phase of the cell cycle.

Upon estrogen repletion, the cells in G_0 will begin to divide in a synchronous fashion. At that time, chemotherapy is administered in order to kill this subfraction of hormone-sensitive cells.

Implementation of this hormone depletion/repletion strategy requires precise control over the biologic effects at the tumor cell level. In other systems, such precise control has been called the "physiological clamp" technique. For breast cancer, we consider the ideal method of producing a physiological clamp on estrogen levels to be the removal of estrogens by the use of hormone synthesis inhibitors or surgical removal of the endocrine gland. This hormonal depletion phase is followed by administration of the physiologic steroid via a physiological route. Use of aromatase inhibitors followed by sublingual (or transdermal) 17β-estradiol provide a practical way of ideally establishing a physiological clamp over tumor tissue estradiol levels.

At the present time, 6 trials (50-55) have tested the concept of hormone depletion/repletion plus chemotherapy. Two of these (50,51) entered heavily pretreated patients (i.e., Bowman et al., Lipton et al.) and demonstrated no beneficial effect of the hormone priming maneuver. Four trials entered previously untreated women to protocols using either tamoxifen/premarin or AG/HC plus estrogen (52-55). The one controlled study indicated a significant survival advantage for patients treated with hormonal priming vs. placebo. The three uncontrolled trials produced a higher than expected rate of complete objective tumor regression in treated patients (i.e., 40%, 37% and 36%).

These studies are examining cell kinetic parameters such as percent S phase in tumor biopsies to document the effects of hormonal priming. It should be recognized that tumor heterogeneity, difficulties in monitoring cell kinetic parameters accurately, possible alterations of the metabolism of chemotherapeutic agents induced by hormones, and other problems will complicate the ideal design and interpretation of such studies. However, this strategy may ultimately provide a new approach to combined modality therapy.

This work was partially supported by NCI Grant CA 40011.

REFERENCES

1. McGuire, W.L. (1975): In: Selected Topics in the Clinical Sciences/Annual Review of Medicine, 26:353-363.

2. Rizkallah, T., Tovell, H.M., Kelly, J. (1975): J Clin Endocrinol Metab, 40:1045-1056.

3. Judd, H.L., Lucas, W.E., Yen, S.S.C. (1976): J Clin Endocrinol Metab, 43:272-278.

4. MacDonald, P.C., Edman, C.D., Hemsell, D.L., Porter, J.C., Siiteri, P.K. (1978): Am J Obstet Gynecol, 130:448-455.

5. Longcope, C., Pratt, J.H., Schneider, S.H., Fineberg, S.E. (1978): J Clin Endocrinol Metab, 46:146-152.

6. Smuk, M., Schivers, J. (1977): J Clin Endocrinol Metab, 45: 1009-1012.

7. Berkowitz, G.D., Fujimoto, M., Brown, T., Brodie, A.M.H., Migeon, C.J. (1984): J Clin Endocrinol Metab, 59:665-700.

8. Edery, M., Goussard, J., Dehennin, L., Scholler, R., Reiffsteck, J., Drosdowsky, M.A. (1981): Eur J Cancer, 17: 115-120.

9. Fishman, J., Nisselbaum, J.S., Menendez-Botet, C.J., Schwartz, M.K. (1977): J Steroid Biochem, 8.893-896.

10. Millington, D.S. (1975): J Steroid Biochem, 6:239-245.

11. Miller, W.R., Forrest, A.P.M. (1974). Lancet, ii. 866-868, 1974.

12. Abdul-Hajj, Y.J., Overson, R., Kiang, D.T. (1979): Steroids, 33: 205-222.

13. de Thibault de Boesinghe, L., LaCroix, E., Eechante, W., Leusen, I. (1974): Lancet, ii:1268.

14. Li, K., Chandra, D.P., Foo, T., Adams, J.B., McDonald, D. (1976): Steroids, 28:561-574.

15. Valera, R.M., Dao, T.L. (1978): Cancer Res, 38: 2429-2433.

16. Perel, E., Wilkins, D., Killinger, D.W. (1980): J Steroid Biochem, 13: 89-94.

17. Tilson-Mallett, N., Santner, S., Feil, P.D., Santen, R.J. (1983): J Clin Endocrinol Metab, 57:1125-1128.

18. Santner, S.J., Feil, P.D., Santen, R.J. (1984): J Clin Endocrinol Metab, 59:29-33.

19. Wilking, N., Carlstrom, K., Gustafsson, S.A., Skoldefors, H., Tollbom, O. (1980): Eur J Cancer, 16:1339-1344.

20. Tseng, L., Mazella, J., Lee, L.Y., Stone. M.L. (1983): J Steroid Biochem, 19:1413-1417.

21. Vignon, F., Terqui, M., Westley, B., Derocq, D., Rochefort, H. (1980). Endocrinology, 106:1079-1086.

22. Manni, A., Wright, C. (1984): J Natl Cancer Inst, 73: 511-514.

23. Santner, S.J., Leszczynski, D., Wright, C., Manni, A., Feil, P.D., Santen, R.J. (1986): Breast Cancer Res Treat, 7:35-44.

24. Santen, R.J., Misbin, R.I. (1981): Pharmacotherapy, 1: 95-120.

25. Potts, G.O., Creange, J.E., Harding, H.R., Schane, H.P. (1978): Steroids, 32:257-267.

26. Santen, R.J., Van den Bossche, H., Symoens, J., Brugmans, J., DeCoster, R. (1983): J Clin Endocrinol Metab, 57: 732-736.

27. Thomas, J.L., LaRochelle, M.C., Covey, D.F., Strickler, R.C. (1983): J Biol Chem, 258.11500-11504.

28. Santen, R.J., Henderson, I.C. (Eds) (1982): Pharmanual: A Comprehensive Guide to the Therapeutic Use of Aminoglutethimide. S. Karger, A.G. Basel/New York.

29. Santner, S.J., Rosen, H., Osawa, Y., Santen, R.J. (1984): J Steroid Biochem, 20:1239-1242.

30. Santen, R.J., Santner, S., Davis, B., Veldhuis, J., Samojlik E., Ruby, E. (1978): J Clin Endocrinol Metab, 55:1257-1265.

31. Santen, R.J., Worgul, T.J., Samojlik, E., Interrante, A., Boucher, A.E., Lipton, A., Harvey, H.A., White, D.S., Smart, E., Cox, C., Wells, S.A. (1981): N Engl J Med 305:545-551.

32. Dowsett, M., Jeffcoate, S.L., Santner, S., Santen, R.J., Stuart-Harris, R., Smith. D.E. (1985): Lancet, i:175-176.

33. Harris, A.L., Dowsett, M., Smith, I., Jeffcoate, S. (1983): Br J Cancer, 47:621-627.

34. Murray, F.T., Santner, S., Samojlik, E.A., Santen, R.J. (1979): J. Clin Pharmacol, 19:704-711.

35. Sjoerdsma, A. (1981): Pharmacol Ther, 30:3-22.

36. Brodie, A.M.H, Garrett, W.M., Hendrickson, J.R., Marcotte, P.A., Tsai-Morris, C.H., Robinson, C.H. (1981): Steroids, 38:693-702.

37. Covey, D.F., Hood, W.F., Parikh, V.D. (1981): J Biol Chem, 256:1076-1079.

38. Marcotte, P.A., Robinson, C.H. (1982): Biochemistry, 21: 2773-2778.

39. Johnston, J.O., Wright, C.L., Metcalf, B.W. (1984): Endocrinology, 115:776-785.

40. Santen, R.J., Worgul, T.J., Lipton, A., Harvey, H., Boucher, A., Samojlik, E., Wells, S.A. (1982): Ann Int Med, 96: 94-101.

41. Messeih, A.A., Lipton, A., Santen, R.J., Harvey, H.A., Boucher, A.E., Murray, R., Rayaz, J., Buzdur, A.U., Nagel, G.A., Henderson, I.C. (1985): Cancer Treat Rep, 69:1003-1004.

42. Harvey, H.A., Santen, R.J., Osterman, J., Samojlik, E., White, D.S., Lipton, A. (1979): Cancer, 43:2207-2214.

43. Lipton, A., Harvey, H.A., Santen, R.J., Boucher, A., White, D., Bernath, A., Dixon, G., Richards, G., Shafik, A. (1982): Cancer Res (Suppl) 42: 3434s-3436s.

44. Smith, I.E., Harris, A.L., Morgan, M., Gazet, J.-C., McKinna J.A. (1982): Cancer Res, (Suppl) 42:3430s-3433s.

45. Gale, K., Gelman, R., Tormey, D., Cummings, F. (1983): In: Proceedings of the 19th Annual Meeting of the American Society of Clinical Oncology, Abst C-409.

46. Murray, R., Pitt. P. (1985): Eur J Cancer Clin Oncol 21: 19-22.

47. Stuart-Harris, R., Dowsett, M., Bozek, T., McKinna, J.A., Gazet, J.C., Jeffcoate, S.L., Kurkure, A., Carr, L., Smith, I.E. (1984): Lancet, 2:604-607.

48. Coombes, R.C., Gross, P., Dowsett, M., Powles, T., Brodie, A.M.H. (1985): In: Proceedings of the 67th Annual Meeting of The Endocrine Society, Baltimore, MD, Abstr 762.

49. Lippman, M.E. (1983): Breast Cancer Res Treat, 3:117-127.

50. Bowman, D. (1983): In: Proceedings of the American Society of Clinial Oncology, Abstr C-413.

51. Lipton, A., Santen, R.J., Harvey, H.A., Manni, A., Simmonds, M.A., White, D.S., Boucher, A., Walker, B.K., Dixon, R.H., Valdevia, D.E., Gordon, R.A. (1986): Am J Clin Oncol, in press.

52. Lippman, M.E., Cassidy, J., Wesley, M., Young, R.C. (1984): J Clin Oncol, 2:28-36.

53.   Allegra, J.C. (1983):   Sem Oncol, 10 (Suppl 2):23-28.

54.   Sorace, R., Lippman, M., Bagley, C., Lichter, A., Danforth,
      D. (1984): In: Proceedings of the American Society of
      Clinical Oncology, Abstr C-462.

55.   Paridaens, R., Blonk van der Wijst, J., Julien, J.P.,
      Ferrazzi, E., Clarysse, A., Heuson, J.C., Rotmensz, M.
      (1983): J Steroid Biochem, 19 (Suppl):207S, Abstr 579.

56.   Dowsett, M., Santner, S.J., Santen, R.J., Jeffcoate, S.L.,
      Smith, I.E. (1986): Brit J Cancer, in press.

57.   Corkery, J., Leonard, R.C.F., Henderson, I.C., Gelman, R.S.,
      Hourihan, J., Ascoli, D.M., Salhanick, H.A. (1982): Cancer
      Res, 42 (Suppl):3409s-3414s.

58.   Ingle, J.N., Green, S.J., Ahmann, D.L., Edmonson, J.H.,
      Nichols, W.C., Frytak, S., Rubin, J. (1982): Cancer Res, 42
      (Suppl):3461s-3467s.

59.   Murray, R.M.L., Pitt, P. (1982): Cancer Res, 42 (Suppl):
      3437s-3441s.

60.   Buzdar, A.U., Powell, K.C., Blumenschein, G.R. (1982):
      Cancer Res, 42 (Suppl):3448s-3450s.

61.   Harvey, H.A., Lipton, A., White, D.S., Santen, R.J.,
      Boucher, A.E., Shafik, A.S., Dixon, R.J., and members of the
      Central Pennsylvania Oncology Group (1982): Cancer Res, 42
      (Suppl):3451s-3453s.

Hormonal Manipulation of Cancer: Peptides, Growth Factors, and New (Anti) Steroidal Agents, edited by Jan G. M. Klijn et al. Raven Press, New York © 1987.

CLINICAL STUDIES WITH 4-HYDROXYANDROSTENEDIONE
IN BREAST CANCER PATIENTS

R.C. Coombes, T.J. Powles, P.E. Goss, D. Cunningham, G. Hutchison, M. Dowsett, and A.M.H. Brodie

Ludwig Institute for Cancer Research (London Branch), St. George's Hospital Medical School, London, SW17 ORE (RCC); St. George's Hospital, London, SW17 OQT (DC,GH); Royal Marsden Hospital, Sutton, Surrey SM2 5PT (RCC,TJP,PEG); Chelsea Hospital for Women, London SW3 6LT, UK (MD); University of Maryland, Baltimore, MD 21201, USA (AMHB).

INTRODUCTION

It is widely accepted that estrogen deprivation is the major mechanism by which both medical and surgical endocrine treatment of breast cancer is effective (19). One means by which this can be achieved is by reduction of estrogen production and during the last few years we have developed a number of selective inhibitors of aromatase (estrogen synthetase) (17). Several of these appear to act both by competition with the substrate and inactivation of the enzyme. 4-Hydroxyandrostenedione (4-OHA) is the most potent inhibitor of this type that we have evaluated (1,3). Another drug, aminoglutethimide (AG), inhibits the peripheral aromatase enzyme system and reduces plasma estradiol levels in postmenopausal women (15) and the clinical effectiveness of AG in postmenopausal breast cancer patients supports the concept that aromatase inhibition is a viable approach to the treatment of breast cancer (11,20,21). The inhibition of aromatase by AG is dependent on its interaction with cytochrome P_{450} (9) which results in inhibition of other steroidogenic enzymes (7,9,23). The combination of AG with glucocorticoid is necessary for maximal plasma estrogen suppression (8) and possibly for therapeutic safety (14).

4-OHA is a more potent inhibitor of aromatase <u>in vitro</u> than AG (25) and has been shown to inhibit ovarian estrogen synthesis in rats (4,25) and peripheral aromatisation in rhesus monkeys (2). The additional observation that 4-OHA inhibits the growth of estrogen-dependent mammary tumor growth in rats (4,25) has led to the clinical trial of 4-OHA in postmenopausal breast cancer patients.

PATIENTS AND METHODS

Patients

All patients were either postmenopausal (at least 2 years' amenorrhoea) or surgically ovariectomized women who had histologically or cytologically proven progressive metastatic breast cancer. No patient had received endocrine or cytotoxic chemotherapy within 4 weeks of starting treatment. Informed consent was obtained for all patients and the study was approved by the Royal Marsden Hospital's Ethics Committee and the Office for Protection from Research Committe, University of Maryland, USA. Patients were free to withdraw from the study at any time.

4-OHA was provided by Ciba Geigy Pharmaceuticals as a sterile micro-crystalline formulation (CGP 32349) in ampoules and was stored at 4°C. The powder was suspended in physiological saline (125 mg/ml) immediately prior to i.m. injection and in water or saline (50 mg/ml) for oral administration. In patients receiving chronic parenteral therapy the injection sites were varied to minimise local side effects.

58 patients received parenteral 4-OHA at a dose of 500 mg once weekly. 31 further patients received oral 4-OHA at a dose of 250 mg daily for the first month and thereafter at a dose of 500 mg daily. Assessment was carried out at 3 months according to UICC criteria.

RESULTS

Response to Therapy

Parenteral Administration (Goss et al, submitted)

Six of the 58 patients entered into the trial were not assessable because 4-OHA was administered for less than 3 weeks. Table 1 gives the pretreatment characteristics of all the patients entered. Most patients were heavily pretreated, 29 (50%) having received at least 2 previous endocrine therapies. Only 8 patients had not received any previous endocrine therapy.

Overall evaluation of 52 assessable patients (Table 2) revealed that 14 (27%) had objective complete (2) or partial (10) responses to treatment. In 10 (19%) patients the disease stabilized for at least 8 weeks on therapy and in 28 (54%) patients the disease progressed. Of the 22 estrogen receptor (ER) positive patients, 6 responded to 4-OHA, 3 had static disease and in 13 the disease progressed. Of the 3 patients with ER negative tumors 1 responded and 2 had progressive disease. Twenty four patients had previously responded to endocrine therapy, and 7 of these responded to 4-OHA, whilst in 3 the disease stabilized. There was no difference (p = 0.4) in disease free interval (ie the time from primary diagnosis to first relapse) between responders and non-responders. The responses seemed to occur most often in soft tissue and lymph nodes affected by breast cancer, with only one response in a visceral site. There were no responses in liver metastases (n = 11). Only 4 of 35 (11%) patients' skeletal metastases responded although bone pain was alleviated in 5 out of 8 patients with this symptom. Of the 14 patients who responded to 4-OHA, 4 have since relapsed at 3, 4, 4 and 13 months. Ten patients remain in remission for periods between 2 and 18 months. Mean duration of response and response to subsequent therapy cannot yet be adequately evaluated.

TABLE 1. Pretreatment Characteristics of Patients Treated with 4-hydroxyandrostenedione (from Goss et al, submitted)

No. of patients entered	58
Age (yr)$^+$ Median	64
Range	37 – 84
ER status – positive	24
– negative	3
– unknown	31
Pretreatment sites of disease (No.)	
Local disease	31
Skin, other than chest wall	20
Lymph nodes	26
Bone	35
Bone pain	8
Lung parenchyma	8
Pleural effusion	3
Liver	11
Central nervous system	2
No. of patients who received 2 or more previous endocrine therapies	29 (50%)
Objective response to prior endocrine therapy	27 (47%)

TABLE 2. Response to 4-hydroxyandrostenedione According to ER Status and Previous Response to Endocrine Therapy

	Response to 4-OHA				
	CR	PR	NC	PD	NA
Overall response	4	10	10	28	6
			14		
ER status – Positive	1	5	3	13	2
Negative	0	1	0	2	0
Unknown	3	4	7	13	4
Previous response to endocrine therapy					
Responders	2	5	3	14	3
Non-responders	2	2	3	9	0
No previous therapy or response not assessable	0	3	4	5	3

CR = complete response   PR = partial response   NC = no change
PD = progressive disease   NA = not assessable

Oral administration (Cunningham et al, submitted)
All 31 patients receiving oral 4-OHA had assessable disease. Sites of disease were bone (18 patients), visceral (14 patients) and soft tissue (20 patients). 25 (81%) of patients had received previous hormone therapy and in all, 33 courses had been given. Twenty one courses had been followed by definite evidence of response to therapy (Table 3).

TABLE 3. Oral 4-hydroxyandrostenedione - Details of Previous Hormone Therapy

	No. of Patients	No. Responding
Tamoxifen	22	15
MPA	3	1
Aminoglutethimide	3	1
Decadurabalon	2	2
Danazol	2	1
Norethisterone Acetate	1	1

Concerning response to 4-OHA (Table 4) 8/31 (26%) showed evidence of partial response and 4 (13%) showed stabilisation of disease.

TABLE 4. Oral 4-hydroxyandrostenedione - Response to Treatment

	No.	%
Partial Response	8	26
Stable Disease	4	13
Progression	11	36
Non-evaluable	8	25

Side effects

Parenteral administration
Sterile abcesses were seen in 6 patients and this caused treatment to be discontinued in 2 patients. Four patients experienced mild lethargy which appeared treatment related. One patient developed an anaphylactoid reaction immediately after injection.

Oral administration
25/31 patients experienced no toxicity. One developed a skin rash, one developed facial swelling and one complained of lethargy. In no patient was this severe enough to warrant discontinuation of therapy. A single patient developed mild leucopenia (WBC = $2.5 \times 10^9/1$), necessitating discontinuation of treatment. No deterioration of liver function was seen in any patient unless documented liver metastases were present.

DISCUSSION

Approximately 30-40% of postmenopausal patients with advanced breast cancer respond to hormonal manipulation if selected randomly without regard to the ER status of their tumors (12). AG is an example of an agent in current clinical use (18,24). It is thought to exert its anti-tumor effect by suppressing circulating estrogens through its inhibitory action on the enzyme complex aromatase (6). However, it also inhibits earlier steps in the steroid biosynthetic pathway (5) depleting corticosteroids, and requiring their replacement (16). In addition, AG causes substantial drowsiness in approximately 40% of patients and a morbilliform, maculopapular skin rash in approximately one third of patients (24). Our study addressed the question of whether a more powerful and selective aromatase inhibitor than AG could produce improved response rates without adverse side effects.

The observed overall response rate of 27% is similar to other major forms of endocrine treatment although there was a bias in favour of ER positive tumors in our study which might have favoured higher response rates (13). However most patients had advanced metastatic disease and most had already received several endocrine therapies prior to receiving 4-OHA. A number of these patients had been resistant to their previous therapy which would reduce the likelihood of their response to subsequent endocrine treatment (12). In addition the optimum dose, route of administration and dose scheduling have not yet been determined. A comparison of 4-OHA to other forms of endocrine therapy is now needed to define its exact role in breast cancer management.

As regards toxicity, the most frequent side effect was development of local sterile abscesses and moderately painful lumps at the injection sites. The incidence of painful lump decreased as the technique of administration was modified. A slow rate of injection through a narrow bore needle together with careful selection of the injection site, tended to alleviate this problem.

Concerning the tolerability of oral therapy, 25/31 patients had no side-effects. The most serious problem encountered was transient leucopenia in a single patient.

In conclusion, 4-OHA, a potent new aromatase inhibitor, is capable of markedly reducing plasma estradiol levels and producing tumor regression in postmenopausal patients with advanced breast cancer. This is the first direct evidence that selective inhibition of estradiol synthesis is important in the endocrine therapy of breast cancer. Optimum dose, route of administration and dose scheduling are now being investigated.

REFERENCES

1. Brodie, A.M.H., Garrett W.M., Hendrickson, J.R., Tsai-Morris, C.H. and Williams, J.G. (1983): J. Steroid Biochem., 19:53-58.
2. Brodie, A.M.H., and Longcope C. (1980): Endocrinology, 106:19-21.
3. Brodie, A.M.H., Schwarzel, W.C. and Brodie, H.J. (1976): J. Steroid Biochem., 7,787-793.
4. Brodie, A.M.H., Schwarzel, W.C., Shaikh, A.A. and Brodie, H.J. (1977): Endocrinology, 100:1684-1695.
5. Camacho, A.M., Cash, R., Brough, A.J. and Wilroy, R.S. (1967): J. Am. Med. Assoc., 202:20-26.
6. Chakraborty, J., Hopkins, R. and Parke, D.V. (1972): Biochem. J., 130:19-20.
7. Cohen, M.P. (1969): Proc. Soc. Exp. Biol. Med., 127:1086-1090.
8. Dowsett, M., Harris A.L., Stuart-Harris, R., Hill, M., Cantwell, B.M.J., Smith, I.E. and Jeffcoate, S.L. (1985): Br. J. Cancer, 52:525-529.
9. Faglia, G., Gattinoni, L., Travaglini P., Neri V., Acerbi, L., and Ambrosi, B. (1971): Metabolism, 20:266-272.
10. Harris, A.L., Dowsett, M., Jeffcoate, S.L. and Smith, I.E. (1983): Eur. J. Cancer Clin. Oncol., 19:493-498.
11. Harris A.L., Dowsett M., Smith I.E. and Jeffcoate S.L. (1983): Br. J. Cancer, 47:621-627.
12. Kennedy, B.J., (1965): Cancer, 18:1551-1557.
13. McGuire, W.L., Carbone, P.P., Sears, M.E. and Escher, G.C. (1975): In: Estrogen Receptors in Human Breast Cancer, edited by W.L. McGuire, pp17-30. Raven Press, New York.
14. Murray, R.M.L., and Pitt, P. (1984): In: Aminogluthimide as an Aromatase Inhibitor in the Treatment of Cancer, edited by G.A. Nagel and R.J. Santen, pp.109-122. Hans Huber, Berne.
15. Santen, R.J., Santner S., Davis B., Veldhuis J., Samojlik E. and Ruby E. (1978): J Clin Endocrin Metab, 47:1257-1265.
16. Santen R.J., Wells, S.A., Runic, S. (1977): J. Clin. Endocrinol. Metab., 45:469-479.
17. Schwarzel, W.C., Kruggel, W. and Brodie, H.J. (1973): Endocrinology, 92:866-880.
18. Smith, I.E., Fitzharris, B.M., McKinna, J.A. et al (1978): Lancet, 2:646-649.
19. Stoll, B.A. (1981): In: Hormone Management of Endocrine-Related Cancer, edited by B.A. Stoll, pp 77-91. Lloyd Luke, London.
20. Stuart-Harris, R., Dowsett M., Bozek T., McKinna J.A., Gazet, J-C., Jeffcoate, S.L., Kukure, A., Carr, L. and Smith, I.E. (1984): Lancet, 2:604-607.

21. Stuart-Harris, R., Dowsett, M., D'Souza, A., Donaldson, A., Harris, A.L., Jeffcoate, S.L. and Smith, I.E. (1985): Clin. Endocrinol., 22:219-226.
22. Thompson, E.A. Jr., Siiteri, P.K., (1974): J. Biol. Chem., 249:5353-5358.
23. Touitou, Y., Bogdan, A., Legrand, J.C. and Desgrez, P. (1975): Acta Endocr. Copenh., 80:517-526.
24. Wells, S.A., Santen, R.J., Lipton, A. et al (1978): Ann. Surg., 187:475-484.
25. Wing L-Y, Garrett W.M., Brodie A.M.H. (1985): Cancer Res., 45:2425-2428.

Hormonal Manipulation of Cancer: Peptides,
Growth Factors, and New (Anti) Steroidal
Agents, edited by Jan G. M. Klijn et al.
Raven Press, New York © 1987.

SECOND LINE ENDOCRINE THERAPY IN ADVANCED BREAST CANCER. A RANDOMIZED PHASE II STUDY, COMPARING AMINOGLUTETHIMIDE PLUS HYDROCORTISONE vs. MEDROXY-PROGESTERONE ACETATE vs. TRILOSTANE PLUS HYDROCORTISONE VS. HYDROCORTISONE: AN E.O.R.T.C.STUDY.

C.Rose(1), H.T.Mouridsen(1), J.Wildiers(2), R.Paridaens(3), R.Sylvester(4) and N.Rotmensz(4).

1: The Finseninstitute, DK 2100 Copenhagen, Denmark.
2: St. Rafael, Leuven, The Netherlands.
3: Institute Jules Bordet, Bruxelles, Belgium.
4: The E.O.R.T.C. Data Center, Bruxelles,Belgium.

INTRODUCTION

It has been demonstrated in randomized trials in advanced breast cancer that there is a partial cross-sensitivity and a lack of complete cross-resistance between the different endocrine treatment modalities (3). It appears from these trials that a response to first line endocrine therapy seems to predict a response rate in the order of 50 % with second line endocrine therapy. In contrast only 10-20 % of the patients who failed to respond to first line endocrine therapy will obtain a subsequent response to other competitive, additive or inhibitive endocrine therapies. This experience of cross-sensitivity and non-cross resistance between different endocrine treatment modalities emphasizes the clinical significance of defining the best and the less toxic second line endocrine therapy.
The E.O.R.T.C. Breast Cancer Cooperative Group has therefore conducted a randomized phase II study in postmenopausal patients with advanced breast cancer in order to evaluate the relative efficacy and toxicity of 4 different endocrine therapies: Aminoglutethimide plus Hydrocortisone (AG+H), Medroxy-progesterone acetate (MPA), Trilostane plus Hydrocorisone (T+H) and Hydrocortisone alone (H).

MATERIALS AND METHODS

192 patients admitted consequtively to the participating centres from October 1983 to November 1985 entered this trial.

Criteria of eligibility: (1) histological evidence of breast cancer; (2) postmenopausal patients less than 76 yr.Postmenopausal status is defined as at least 1 yr. after spontaneous or artificial menopause; (3) progressive disease with measurable and/or evaluable lesions according to UICC criteria (2); (4) a performance status of < 3 (6); (5) ER positive or ER unknown status of the primary tumour or a metastasis. ER positive is defined as > 15 fmol/mg cytosol protein; (6) one course of prior endocrine therapy ; (7) informed consent.
  Criteria of ineligibility; (1) previous treatment with the agents used in the study either as an adjuvant or for advanced disease ; (2) treatment for the present disease by endocrine ablative procedureswithin 12 weeks ; (3) previous or concomitant malignancies with the exception of exicional biopsy of in situ carcinoma of the cervix uteri or adequately treated basal- or squamouscell carcinoma of the skin ; (4) patients in whom pleural effusion, ascites, metastases in the central nervous system or osteoblastic bone lesion were the sole manifestations of the disease.

Trial design.
Patients were stratified according to institution, ER-status and dominant site of disease and were randomly allocated by the E.O.R.T.C. Data Center to one of the following 4 treatment groups: AG+H, MPA, T+H, and H alone.

Therapeutic regimens.
The patients were treated with AG 250 mg q.i.d.and H 40 mg daily, MPA 100 mg t.i.d., T 240 mg q.i.d., and H 40 mg daily, or H 40 mg daily. The dose of AG and T respectively was escalated to full dose over a period of 10 days.

Treatment duration.
The treatment was continued until progression of the disease. However, it was aimed to give a minimum of 12 weeks of treatment.

Pretreatment and follow-up investigations.
Pretreatment examinations included physical examination, chest x-ray, bone x-rays or bone scintigraphies, and clinical chemical tests.These were repeated during therapy with intervals of 1-3 months.

Definition of response.
Patients were assessed 4 weeks after start of therapy and at 2 - 3 months interval thereafter.
Assessement of response, time to treatment failure, and duration of survival were defined according to the UICC-criteria (2).
As of May 1986, 156 out of 192 patients have been extramurally reviewed for patient eligibility. So far, none of the patients have been reviewed for response to treatment.

Definition of toxicity.
Toxicities were graded according to WHO criteria (6).

Statistical techniques.
Time to progression and survival curves were calculated according to the Kaplan-Meier product-limit method and were compared using the log-rank test. All p-values correspond to a two-tailed test. The 95 % confidence limits (95 % C.L.,%) are given for the response rates.

RESULTS
From October 1983 to November 1985 a total of 14 institutions entered 192 patients of whom 48 patients were randomized to each group. This analysis is based on all data available as of May 1986.
As shown in table 1, 138 patients were eligible and 125 patients were evaluable for analysis of both response, time to progression, survival and toxicity.

The characteristics for the 125 fully evaluable patients are given in table 2. The 4 treatment groups are well balanced with respect to median age, dominant site of disease, ER-status, performance status and prior therapy.

Table 1
EORTC 10834: PATIENTS EVALUABILITY

TOTAL NUMBER OF PATIENTS ENTERED:	192
REVIEWED:	156
NUMBER OF ELIGIBLE PATIENTS :	138
NUMBER OF NON ELIGIBLE PATIENTS :	18
NUMBER OF FULLY EVALUABLE :	125
NUMBER OF PARTLY EVALUABLE :	7
NUMBER OF NON EVALUABLE	6
TOO EARLY :	36

Table 2.
EORTC 10834 : PATIENTS CHARACTERISTICS (pts.)

	MPA	AG+H	T+H	H	TOTAL
AGE (yrs.)					
median	62	63	63	62	-
DOMINANT SITE					
SOFT TISSUE	9	13	8	9	39
BONE	11	10	7	11	39
VISCERAL	13	11	10	13	47
ESTROGEN RECEPTORS					
POSITIVE	11	13	9	10	43
UNKNOWN	33	34	25	33	82
PERFORMANCE STATUS					
0 OR 1	26	28	20	26	100
2 OR 3	7	6	5	7	25
PRIOR THERAPY					
SURGERY	30	32	23	28	113
RADIOTHERAPY	27	27	23	30	107
CHEMOTHERAPY	22	23	22	20	87

Figure 1 gives the time to progression for all fully evaluable patients in each treatment group. It appears that the time to progression is comparable in each of the four groups with an overall p-value of 0.42.

Figure 2 presents the duration of survival in the 125 evaluable patients. The median duration of survival is about 11 months in all four groups, and approximately 40 % of the patients are alive after 1 year.

The overall response data in the fully evaluable patients are shown in table 3. Only 9 patients obtained a remission upon treatment with AG+H, T+H or H alone. It appears from the 95 % C.L. that none of the response rates differs significantly from each other.

The toxicities observed during treatment are summarized in table 4. Nearly all the side-effects recorded were mild or moderate and only a few percent were recorded as grade 3 effects. Toxicity was more frequent and severe in the T+H treated group of patients, and expecially the episodes of diarrhoea seems to be of importance.

Table 3.
EORTC 10834: RESPONSE RATE (125 PTS.)

	MPA	AG+H	T+H	H	TOTAL	(%)
COMPLETE RESPONSE	-	1	-	-	1	(1)
PARTIAL RESPONSE	-	5	1	2	8	(6)
NO CHANGE	13	9	6	8	36	(29)
PROGRESSIVE DISEASE	20	17	15	20	72	(58)
EARLY DEATH		2	3	3	8	(6)
TOTAL	33	34	25	33	125	(100)
95 % C.L., %	0-11	7-35	0-20	1-20	3-13	

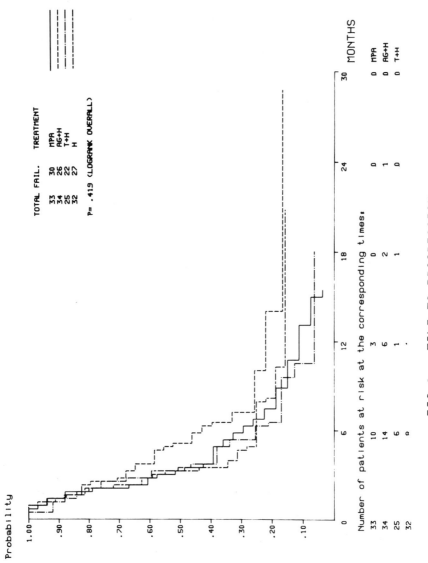

FIG 1., TIME TO PROGRESSION

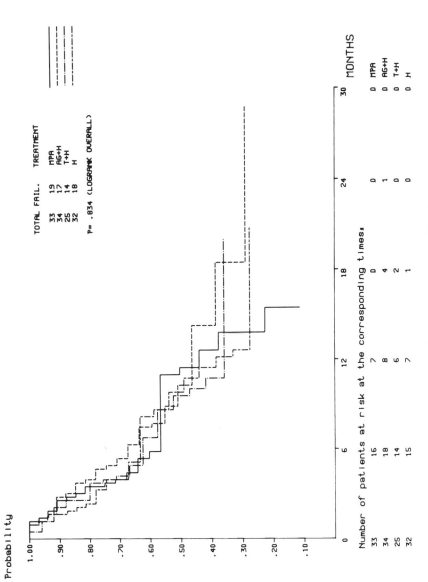

Probability

1.00

.90

.80

.70

.60

.50

.40

.30

.20

.10

0   6   12   18   24   30 MONTHS

TOTAL FAIL.   TREATMENT

33   19   MPA
34   17   AG+H
25   14   T+H
32   18   H

P= .834 (LOGRANK OVERALL)

Number of patients at risk at the corresponding times,

33	16	7	0	0	0 MPA
34	18	8	4	1	0 AG+H
25	14	6	2	0	0 T+H
32	15	7	1	0	0 H

FIG. 2., DURATION OF SURVIVAL

Table 4.
EORTC 10834: SIDE EFFECTS IN PERCENT.

	MPA (N=40)	AG+H (N=42)	T+H (N=40)	H (N=36)
NAUSEA/ VOMITING	14(3)	22	18	14
CUTANEOUS	3	26(2)	10(5)	3
WEIGHT GAIN	13	10	24(3)	25
ORAL	3	2	11(5)	-
CARDIAC	5	2	-	6
DIARRHEA	-	-	14(8)	3(3)
LEG CRAMPS	-	-	10	-

( ) PERCENTAGE WITH GRADE 3 SIDE EFFECTS.

DISCUSSION

The preliminary results from this randomized phase II trial in postmenopausal patients with progressive breast cancer demonstrate a low overall response rate to second line endocrine therapy. No responses were seen in the MPA treated group and this is in contrast to the results obtained in a previous E.O.R.T.C. trial where 300 mg of MPA daily were compared to 900 mg. The patients eligibility criteria were comparable to those used in the present study and a response rate of 15 % was obtained in 136 patients treated with 300 mg daily (4).
Beardwell et al. found a response rate of 26 % to Trilostane in combination with Hydrocortisone or Dexometasone in postmenopausal patients not selected on the basis of ER-status. (1). They used a different schedule for excalation to full dose, and this fact might explain while the frequency of gastrointestinal disturbances were lower than in the present study.

A response rate of 17 % in the AG+H treated patients is in aggrement with other reports concerning second line endocrine therapy with this combination (5). To our knowledge, no randomized studies have so far compared AG+H treatment with H therapy alone.
Since the present study demonstrates that time to progression and survival is comparable in these two treatment groups, the E.O.R.T.C.Breast Cancer Cooperative Group has decided further to evaluate the effect of different doses of AG with and without Hydrocortisone replacement.

REFERENCES

1.
Beardwell,C.G., Hindley, A.C., Wilkinson,P.M., Todd, I.D.H., Ribeiro, G.G. and Bu'Lock, D.(1983):Canc.Chemother.Pharmacol.10:158-160.
2.
Hayward, J.L., Carbone, P.P., Heuson, J.C., Kumaoka, S., Segaloff, A., Rubens, R.D. (1977): Cancer 39: 1289-1294.
3.
Rose,C., Mouridsen, H.T.(1984): Recent Results in Cancer Research, 91: 230-242.
4.
Rose,C., Mouridsen, H.T., Engelsman, E., Nooi, M, Sylvester, R., Rotmensz, N. for the E.O.R.T.C. Breast Cancer Cooperative Group. (1985): Proceedings ASCO, 4:abstr. C 217.

5.
Stuart-Harris, R.C., Smith I.E. (1984): Cancer Treatment Reviews, II: 189-204.
6.
WHO Handbook for Reporting Results of Cancer Treatment. (1979): WHO Offset Publication, Geneva, 48.

Hormonal Manipulation of Cancer: Peptides,
Growth Factors, and New (Anti) Steroidal
Agents, edited by Jan G. M. Klijn et al.
Raven Press, New York © 1987.

SEX-STEROID RECEPTORS AND ANTISTEROIDAL AGENTS IN THE

TREATMENT OF PANCREATIC ADENOCARCINOMA

P.J. Johnson and T.P. Corbishley

The Liver Unit, King's College Hospital School of Medicine
and Dentistry, Denmark Hill, London SE5 9RS, U.K.

Several lines of evidence suggest that pancreatic adenocarcinoma, a major cause of cancer-related death, may be a
sex-steroid responsive tumour. The aim of this chapter is to
review this evidence as it relates to man and human derived
material (cell-lines) and to consider early reports that it
may be possible to influence the growth rates of these tumours
by various hormonal manipulations and, as such, may have
important implications for therapy.

Sex-Steroid Binding Proteins in Normal Human Pancreatic Tissue

Sex-steroid hormones effect both exocrine and endocrine
pancreatic function. Small amounts of oestrogen receptor
(ER), progesterone receptor (PR), and androgen receptor (AR),
have been demonstrated in homogenates of normal adult pancreas
(6) but no investigation of their distribution in isolated
purified cell populations has been reported. These receptors
may be important modulators of hormone action in normal pancreatic tissue but they are of high affinity (K_a, 10^9 l/mol)
and low capacity and thus can only retain very small amounts
of steroid hormone within the pancreas. A much larger capacity
oestrogen binding protein (EBP) of moderate affinity (K_a,
10^6 l/mol) which makes up 4% of the total soluble protein of
the pancreas has been described in the rat and in man (13, 14,
16). This protein, which in the rat is localised in the exocrine cells (4), may account for the high retention of
systemically injected radiolabelled oestrogens in the pancreas
reported over 20 years ago (17, 20). An accessory protein,
probably a small water soluble peptide, is required to
express its full oestrogen binding capacity and it has been
suggested that this factor may be somatostatin and that the

accessory factor-EBP complex may be involved in the regulation of pancreatic secretion (1, 3, 14).

Sex-steroid binding in pancreatic adenocarcinoma tissue

Substantial levels of ER have been described in human pancreatic adenocarcinoma tissue and pancreatic cell-lines (Colo-357, Mia Pa Ca 2, RWP-1, RWP-2 and Ger) (2, 6). In our initial report we detected ER in 5 of 6 specimens of human pancreatic adenocarcinoma tissue obtained at autopsy (8) and these numbers have now been extended to 15 of 16. The characteristics of ER from this source were identical to those of ER derived from premenopausal uterus and could be clearly distinguished from sex-hormone binding globulin (SHBG). The observation that both cytosolic and nuclear receptors could be detected was taken as evidence that this pathway might be physiologically active and the suggestion was further supported by the detection of progesterone receptors in the same tissues. Using the synthetic progesterone analogue promegestone saturable high affinity binding was detected in all 5 ER positive tissues tested and it is of interest that the one ER negative tumour was also PR negative (5).

Androgen receptor

Using a Sephadex LH20 based assay technique we were originally unable to detect any AR in normal or malignant pancreatic tissue (8). The development of a new sensitive micro-assay technique which enables more dilute cytosols to be utilized in which endogenous hormone is diluted and there is greater exchange of ligand from occupied receptors (12) has allowed the detection of AR in both tumour and normal tissue (6). There were no significant differences between the AR of prostatic and pancreatic origin, in terms of binding affinity, sedimentation behaviour, and in competitive binding studies. Similar amounts of binding were detected in the two cell-lines studied (Mia Pa Ca 2 and Ger) but binding in normal pancreas was only just detectable (6).

Sex-steroid metabolising enzymes in normal and malignant human pancreatic tissue

The presence of the sex-steroid conversion enzymes aromatase and 5αreductase was demonstrated in homogenates of pancreatic tumour tissue by the conversion of testosterone to 17β oestradiol and 5αdihydrotestosterone (DHT) respectively (11). Substantially lower activity of both of these enzymes could also be detected in normal adult tissue. Using whole cell monolayers of the Mia Pa Ca 2 and Ger pancreatic cancer cell-lines we have recently demonstrated substantial activity of 5α reductase and 3$\alpha\beta$ hydroxysteroid oxidoreductase producing 5αDHT and 3$\alpha\beta$androst-17-diols from testosterone. No aromatase or 17β hydroxysteroid oxioreductase activity could be detected in any of these experiments.

Serum levels of sex-steroid hormones in patients with
pancreatic adenocarcinoma

Patients with pancreatic adenocarcinoma, like most other
cancer patients, have low levels of circulating total androgens (T and DHT) and moderately raised levels of SHBG resulting in very low physiologically active fractions of the
androgens (7, 10). In contrast to observations in patients
with primary malignancies at other sites, pancreatic adenocarcinoma patients of both sexes have elevated serum oestradiol
concentrations and therefore have the balance of their serum
sex-steroids tilted strongly in favour of the oestrogens (7).

The detection of oestrogen, androgen, and progesterone
receptors together with activities of aromatase and 5α
reductase all at a significantly higher level than found in
the normal gland formed a rational basis for studies in
animal models aimed at determining whether manipulation of
the sex-steroid environment might influence the growth rate
of these tumours.

HORMONE MANIPULATION IN PANCREATIC ADENOCARCINOMA CELL-LINES AND ANIMAL MODELS

The growth of 4 human pancreatic cancer cell-lines was
inhibited by progestagens, oestradiol and tamoxifen at high
pharmacological doses but at concentrations 2 to 5-fold less
than that required by 5-fluorouracil (5-FU) to produce an
equitoxic effect. A synergistic cytotoxic effect was noted,
with a combination of progesterone and 5-FU showing the greatest
synergistic action (2). The growth of one cell-line was
also reported to be sensitive to a 5 reductase inhibitor (2).

Growth of both the DNCP-322 azaserine induced rat acinar
cell pancreatic tumour in Wistar/Lewis rats and duct type
pancreatic adenocarcinoma in Syrian hamsters has been shown
to be reduced by somatostatin and LH-RH analogues (15). The
LH-RH agonists significantly reduce tumour volume and weight,
probably by reducing circulating testosterone levels. The
same authors also showed that castration of male hamsters
4 days after transplantation of the tumour reduced both weight
and volume of the tumours. The somatostatin analogues have
a similar effect on tumour growth but are speculated to act
either by reducing gastrointestinal hormone secretion or by
acting as an accessory factor in the binding of oestrogens
by the pancreatic oestrogen binding protein.

In another series of experiments, 2 human pancreatic
adenocarcinoma xenografts (Ca Pan 4 and Ca Pan 5) and one
cell-line (GTCC) which had been serially passaged in nude
mice were used (9). Homogenised tumour was implanted subcutaneously in the right flank of each mouse and tumour
volume measured weekly. Following a pilot study which showed

a trend for tumours treated with cyproterone acetate to grow more slowly than those in control animals a definitive study using several combinations of cyproterone acetate, aminoglutethamide and hydrocortisone was embarked upon. (Because the preliminary studies with tamoxifen looked unpromising, this agent was not used alone in the definitive study, though a subsequent reanalysis of the data showed it to be at least as effective as cyproterone acetate). In both Ca Pan 4 and GTCC cyproterone acetate inhibited tumour growth to a significant degree compared to the control animals (tumour/control (T/C) values were 0.33 and 0.23 on day 23 for cyproterone acetate 50 and 75 mg/kg respectively, $p < 0.01$). There was also a trend for testosterone (40 mg/kg) to stimulate tumour growth in GTCC which reached a maximum T/C value of 1.6. The growth rate in Ca Pan 4 was near maximum (doubling time 4 days) and probably not capable of further stimulation.

TRIALS OF HORMONE MANIPULATION IN HUMANS

Theve et al (18) treated 14 patients (aged 40 to 82 years, 8 female) with unresectable, histologically confirmed pancreatic adenocarcinoma, with tamoxifen 20mg twice daily. They compared survival times of this group with those of the 629 patients diagnosed with the same tumour over the previous 13 years. Median survival time for the historical control group was 2.5 months and none survived longer than 21 months. The median survival figure for those receiving tamoxifen was 8.5 months and 3 patients survived more than 22 months.

Similar findingswere reported by Tønneson and Kamp-Jensen (19) who found a median survival of 7 months in 10 patients receiving tamoxifen 10mg three times a day compared to 3 months in an untreated group of 14 patients who were operated upon in the period immediately prior to the treated group. The two groups appeared well-matched and whilst all patients in the untreated group were dead within 9 months of diagnosis, survival was almost 50% in the treated group at 9 months.

These encouraging studies have led several groups to undertake prospective clinical trials with contemporary, untreated control patients.

On the Liver Unit at King's College Hospital, London we are coordinating a prospective randomised controlled clinical trial comparing tamoxifen (20mg twice a day) to cyproterone acetate (100 mg three times a day), to a control group receiving supportive therapy only. To show a statistically significant improval in median survival time of the same order as that described in the above trials (i.e. a doubling), 35 patients in each group were required. This number has now been achieved, and analysis is being undertaken, but an unexpectedly high death rate in the first few weeks

following primary procedures to relieve the obstructive
jaundice means that the numbers may need to be increased.

REFERENCES

1. Andren-Sandberg, A. (1986): Scand. J. Gastroenterol.,
   21:129-133.

2. Benz, C. (1986): Organ Syst. Newsletter, 2:18.

3. Boctor, A.M., Band, P., and Grossman, A. (1981): Proc.
   Natl. Acad. Sci. USA, 78:5648-5651.

4. Boctor, A.M., Band, P., and Grossman, A. (1983):
   Endocrinology, 113:453-462.

5. Corbishley, T.P., Iqbal,M.J., Johnson, P.J., and Williams,
   R. (1984): IRCS Med. Sci., 12:575-576.

6. Corbishley, T.P., Iqbal, M.J., Wilkinson M.L., and
   Williams, R. (1986): Cancer, 57:1992-1995.

7. Corbishley, T.P., Iqbal, M.J., Wilkinson, M.L., and
   Williams, R. (1986): Anticancer Research (In Press).

8. Greenway, B., Iqbal, M.J., Johnson, P.J., and Williams,
   R. (1981):Brit. Med. J., 283:751-753.

9. Greenway, B., Duke, D., Pym, B., Iqbal, M.J., Johnson,
   P.J., and Williams, R. (1982):Br. J. Surg., 69:
   595-597.

10. Greenway, B.A., Iqbal, M.J., Johnson, P.J., and Williams,
    R. (1983): Br.Med.J., 286:93-94.

11. Iqbal, M.J., Greenway, B., Wilkinson, M.L., Johnson, P.J.,
    and Williams, R. (1983):Clin.Sci.,65:71-75.

12. Iqbal, M.J., Corbishley, T.P., Wilkinson, M.L., and
    Williams, R.S. (1985): Analyt.Biochem., 144: 79-85.

13. Pousette, A., Carlström, K., Sköldefors, H., Wilking, N.,
    and Theve, N.O. (1982): Cancer Res., 42: 633-637.

14. Pousette, A., Fernstad, R., Theve, N-O., Sköldefors, H.,
    and Carlström, K. (1985): J. Steroid Biochem. 23:
    115-119.

15. Redding, T.W., and Schally, A.V. (1984): Proc. Natl. Acad. Sci. USA, 81:248-252.

16. Rosenthal, H.E., and Sandberg, A.A. (1978): J. Steroid Biochem., 9:1133-1139.

17. Sandberg, A.A., and Rosenthal, H.E. (1974): J. Steroid Biochem., 5:969-975.

18. Theve, N-O, Pousette, A., Carlström, K. (1983): Clin. Oncol., 9: 193-197.

19. Tønnesen, K., and Kamp-Jensen, M. (1986): Eur. J. Surg. Oncol., 12:69-70.

20. Ullberg, S., and Bengtsson, G. (1963): Acta Endocr. Copenh., 43: 75-86.

Hormonal Manipulation of Cancer: Peptides, Growth Factors, and New (Anti) Steroidal Agents, edited by Jan G. M. Klijn et al. Raven Press, New York © 1987.

AMINOGLUTETHIMIDE IN THE MANAGEMENT OF PROSTATIC CANCER: A REVIEW

M.R.G. Robinson, Pontefract General Infirmary, Friarwood Lane, Pontefract, West Yorks, U.K.

It is more than 40 years since Huggins and Scott (1945) introduced adrenalectomy to treat carcinoma of the prostate which has escaped the control of primary endocrine therapy by orchidectomy or oestrogens. This was based on the rationale that to remove the extratesticular androgens, which may keep the prostatic cancer cells stimulated, could be of benefit (Blandy 1983). Murphy (1978) reviewing the literature reported a subjective response, maintained for more than 3 months in 58 (46%) of 128 patients. This palliation is considered worthwhile in patients with uncontrolled pain for metastases even though in very few patients it is accompanied by objective responses. Unfortunately bilateral adrenalectomy is a major surgical procedure with considerable morbidity and mortality in old men with advanced malignant disease and therefore the concept of producing a medical adrenalectomy by using drugs to suppress the androgen production of the adrenal cortex has attracted the interest of clinicians in recent years. Many drugs are known to inhibit adrenal androgens synthesis. These include Spirolalactone, Cyproterone Acetate, Cyanoketone, Estradiol 17B, Hydroxymethylene, Medrogesterone and Aminoglutethimide (Robinson 1981).

Aminoglutethimide was introduced in the USA in 1959 to treat children with convulsions. It was soon withdrawn because of its endocrine side-effects, including hypothyroidism and adrenal insufficiency. Following its administration, the adrenal glands of both rats and humans exhibit cellular hypertrophy, cytoplasmic vacuolation and accumulation of lipids (Block et al 1984, Morales et al 1971).

In 1967 Cash reported that Aminoglutethimide blocked the conversion of cholestrol to delta-5-pregnenolone, the first step in the production of adrenal cortical steroid hormones, thus inhibiting the production of aldosterone, cortisol, androgens and oestrogens. It does not inhibit the production of testosterone by the testes (Gaunt 1968).

In 1974 we reported the results of treating 26 patients who had
carcinoma of the prostate which had progressed on Stilboestrol
therapy with Aminoglutethimide in divided daily doses of
500-1000 mg (Robinson et al 1974). They continued to
receive 1 mg Stilboestrol three times a day. Four patients
initially did not receive steroid replacement therapy. Three
of these after 1-2 week's treatment developed hypotension
and clinical evidence of acute adrenal failure. Subsequently
these and all ther other patients were given daily Cortisone
Acetate 20-25 mg and Fludrocortisone 0.1 mg. Eight of these
patients had complete relief of metastatic pain and 9 had
partial relief. Objectively, as was observed in a later
review of this study, the patients were not assessed by
response criteria which are currently acceptable (Robinson 1980).
Nevertheless, 13 patients had an elevated acid phosphatase and
in 4 of these, the levels fell to normal during therapy. One
patient with a normal acid phosphatase demonstrated a clear
reduction of the activity of bone metastases on repeated
scintigrams and another had a marked reduction of prostatic
size on rectal examination. Relief of upper urinary tract
obstruction on an intravenous urogram was also demonstrated
in one patient.

Table 1 compares our clinical results with those of
different studies reported during the last 5 years. The
therapeutic regimes used were very similar. Aminoglutethimide
was given in doses which were increased over a period of a
few weeks from 500 to 1000 mg daily, together with Corticosteroid
treplacement using Cortisone Acetate or Hydrocortisone alone or
in combination with Fludrocortisone. Exact comparison cannot
be made between the response rates because different response
criteria have been used. Only Drago et al (1984) and Murray
and Pitt (1985) have used the accepted National Prostatic
Cancer Project Criteria of Response and Ponder et al (1984)
have evaluated their patients only for subjective response.
Amongst the total of 199 patients studied, only one complete
objective response has been reported (Drago et al 1984) and
the main clinical value of Aminoglutethimide appears to be a
subjective improvement in symptoms, particularly in terms of
pain relief. Drago et al (1984) and Murray and Pitt (1985)
have reported a significant increase in the length of survival
of responders compared with non-responders. Block et al (1984)
however, have been unable to report any response at all in
their series of 20 patients.

TABLE I

	No of Patients	Stable Disease	'Objective' Response	'Subjective' Response
Robinson et al 1974	26	-	7	17
Rostrom et al 1982	12	-	0	9
**Drago et al 1984	43	10	7*	-
Ponder et al 1984	40	-	-	19
Block et al 1984	20	-	0	0
**Murray & Pitt 1985	58	8	11	17

TOTAL NUMBER OF PATIENTS   199

* Including 1 complete response
** National Prostatic Cancer Project Criteria of Response used.

CLINICAL RESPONSE OF CARCINOMA OF THE PROSTATE TO
AMINOGLUTETHIMIDE AND CORTICOSTEROIDS IN DIFFERENT
PUBLISHED STUDIES.

In our study (Robinson et al 1974) in some patients we were
able to demonstrate, using the laboratory method of Robinson
and Thomas (1971) a fall in plasma testosterone levels in
patients on Stilboestrol who were given Aminoglutethimide.
This was not confirmed in other patients in the same study using
the method of testosterone measurement described by Shearer
et al (1973).

Rostom et al (1982) reported a fall of testosterone and
androstenedione levels in 6 of 8 patients with a good subjective
response and a fall of dehydroepiandrosterone in 4 of the same
8 patients. Ponder et al (1984) found significant decreases
in testosterone, Δ^4 androstenedione and dehydroepiandrosterone
with no difference between subjective responders and non-
responders. They also report a statistically non-significant
decrease in 5α Dihydrotestosterone. They speculate that the
beneficial effect of Aminoglutethimide may not be mediated
by adrenal androgen suppression. It may be due to the
inhibition of oestrogen production by inhibition of the aromatase
enzyme (Santen et al 1978; Harris et al 1983). Animal
experiments suggest that oestrogen may be important to maintain
prostatic androgen receptors. Alternatively, the effect may
be due to the inhibition by Aminoglutethimide of the cytochrome
P-450 dependant cyclo-oxygenase which is involved in the
arachidonic acid metabolism and prostaglandin synthesis
(Harris et al 1983). Analgesics which are inhbitors of
prostaglandins do give pain relief in bone metastatic disease,
and an argument against this theory of the effect of
Aminoglutethimide is that many of the patients given the drug

have previously been taking these analgesics without benefit. It is also possible that it is the Corticosteroid replacement therapy, not Aminogluthemide, which is beneficial to patients. Several older studies have reported a favourable response to corticosteroid therapy alone in the management of relapsed prostatic cancer (Sprague et al 1940; Muller and Hinman 1954; Greyhack 1959).

The toxicity of Aminoglutethimide combined with steroid replacement therapy that has been reported for patients with advanced carcinoma of the prostate in the studies reviewed in Table 1 is listed in Table 2. Treatment was withdrawn because of toxicity in only 12 of the 199 patients. The most frequent side effects were lethargy, skin rashes which were usually transient, depression and nausea and vomiting. Some of the toxicity such as osteoporosis, hirsuitis and Cushingoid Habitus is probably related to steroid replacement therapy. Hypothyroidism, one of the expected side effects, has only been reported in one patient.

Thrombocytopenia has been observed in three patients. Messeih et al (1985) reported in a review of 1333 patients receiving Aminoglutethimide that 12 had marked leucopenia and/thrombocytopenia. By February 1985, the Committee for the Safety of Medicines in Great Britain had documented 4 cases of bone marrow depression and aplasia, 7 of agranulocytosis and graanulocytopenia and 1 of thrombocytopenia associated with Aminoglutethimide. There were 6 deaths (Vincent et al 1985).

TABLE II

AMINOGLUTETHIMIDE AND CORTICOSTEROID REPLACEMENT TOXICITY

199 PATIENTS

Lethargy	65	Stiffness	2
Skin Rashes	25	Skin Irritation/No Rash	1
Depression	14	*Warfarin Resistance	1
Nausea and Vomiting	8	Hypothyroidesm	1
Hypotension	7	Hirsutism	1
Hepatic Enzyme Elevatin (SGOT)	7	Cushingoid Habitus	1
Vertigo and Ataxia	6		
Electrolyte Disorders	3		
Oedema	3		
Thrombocytopenia	3		
Osteoporosis	2		

*Patient on Anticoagulants

This review of the use of Aminoglutethimide with steroid replacement therapy in the management of carcinoma of the prostate which has relapsed on standard hormonal therapy would indicate that it is of benefit to some patients especially in terms of the subjective relief of symptoms. Although based upon the concept that the reduction of adrenal androgens should be beneficial in this situation, the mode of action of this treatment is not clear. Phase III trials of Corticosteroids alone versus Aminoglutethimide plus Corticosteroids are needed to help to clarify the situation. There is also a need to evaluate the clinical benefit and toxicity of Aminoglutehimide and Corticosteroids against Pituitary Ablation and cytotoxic chemotherapeutic agents in the management of advanced uncontrolled cases of prostatic cancer.

References

1. Blandy JP (1983). NATO ASI Series 355-357 Plenum Press New York.

2. Block M, Trump D, Rose D P, Cummings KB, Hogan T F. (1984). Cancer Treatment Reports Vol 68 No 5: 719-722.

3. Cash R, Brough A J, Cohen MNP, Satah PS (1967). Journal of Clinical Endocrinology & Metabolism 27:1239.

4. Drago J R, Santen R J, Lipton A, Worgal T J, Harvey H A, Boucher A, Mann A, Rohner T J (1984). Cancer 53: 1447-1450

5. Gaunt R, Steinitz BG, Chart J J (1968). Clinical Pharmacology and Therapeutics 9: 657

6. Greyhack J T (1959). Surgical Clinics of North America 39:13.

7. Harris A L, Mitchell M P, Smith K, Powles T J (1983) British Journal of Cancer 48: 595

8. Harris A L, Dowsett M, Smith I E, Jeffcoat S L (1983) British Journal of Cancer 47: 621(1983)

9. Huggins and Scott W W (1945). Annals of Surgery 122:1031

10. Messeih A A, Lipton A, Santen R J, Harvey H A, Boucher A E, Murray R, Ragaz J, Buzdar A U, Nagel G A & Henderson I C. Cancer Treatment Reports 69: 1003-1004 (1985)

11. Morales A, Connolly J G, Mobbs B G (1971)
    Canadian Journal of Surgery 14: 154-160

12. Murray R and Pitt P (1985). European Journal of Cancer
    21: 453-458

13. Muller S M and Harrison F (1954)
    Journal of Urology 72: 485

14. Murphy G P (1978). Management of Advanced Cancer of the
    Prostate in "Genito-Urinary Cancer". Ed. D G Skinner and
    J B de Kernion. W B Sanders Co Philadelphia p 397.

15. Ponder B A J, Shearer R J Pocock R D, Miller J, Easton D,
    Chilvers C E P, Dowsett M, Jeffcoat S L (1984)
    British Journal of Cancer 50: 757-763

16. Robinson M R G, Thomas B S (1971). British Medical
    Journal 45:556

17. Robinson M R G, Shearer R J, Ferguson J P (1974)
    British Journal of Urology 46: 555

18. Robinson M R G (1983)
    Carcinoma of the Prostate: Adrenal Inhibitors
    In "Cancer of the Prostate and Kidney", Ed M Pavone-Macaluso
    and P H Smith, NATO ASI Series 349-353. Plenum Press
    New York.

19. Rostom A Y, Folkes, A, Lord C, Notley R G, Schweitzer F A W,
    White W F (1982). British Journal of Urology 54: 552-555

20. Santen R J, Santer S, Davis B, Veldhuis J, Samojlik E,
    Ruby E (1978). Journal of Clinical Endocrinology and
    Metabolism 47: 1257

21. Shearer R J, Hendry W F, Fergusson J D and Sommerville I F
    (1973). British Journal of Urology 115: 170-174

22. Sprague R G, Power M H, Mann H L, Albert D, Mattison D R,
    Herch P S, Kendall E C, Slocomb C H, Pulley H F.
    Archives of Internal Medicine 85: 199 (1950).

23. Vincent M D, Clink H M, Coombes R C, Smith I E, Kandler R.
    Powles T J (1985). Letter to British Medical Journal 291:
    105-106

Hormonal Manipulation of Cancer: Peptides, Growth Factors, and New (Anti) Steroidal Agents, edited by Jan G. M. Klijn et al. Raven Press, New York © 1987.

KETOCONAZOLE IN THE TREATMENT OF PROSTATIC CANCER.

L. Denis, C. Mahler and *R. De Coster.

Depts of Urology and Endocrinology.
A.Z. Middelheim, 2020 Antwerp / Belgium.
*Endocrine Research Laboratories.
Janssen Pharmaceutica, 2340 Beerse / Belgium.

INTRODUCTION

Ketoconazole (K) is an orally active antifungal agent, belonging to the imidazole group. In antimycotic therapy it is usually effective at a single dose of 200 mgr daily, but in some systemic diseases such as coccidiodomycosis it is administered in doses up to 1200 mgr a day (13, 17, 35). In 1981 De Felice et al (11) reported gynecomastia and loss of libido in some of their patients. Pont and co-workers (21-23) noticed the same side-effects and demonstrated a reversible, dose related drop of Testosterone (T) levels after intake of 200-400 or 600 mgr K. The same investigators concluded after in vitro studies that K interfered with testicular and adrenal androgen synthesis.
Their reports triggered renewed research in the endocrine effects of Ketoconazole High Dosis (KHD) and the mecanism of its action. It was shown that KHD through interaction on the cytochrome P-450 dependent enzymes, inhibits the 17-20 lyase that converts progesterone in to androgens in testes and adrenals. Further studies demonstrated that at still higher doses other cytochrome P-450 dependent enzymes such as the 20-22 desmolase, the 17 α hydroxylase and also the 11 β hydroxylase are affected (5-9, 18, 24, 25, 28, 31, 32).

KETOCONAZOLE AND PROSTATIC CANCER

Androgen suppression is the established hormonal treatment in disseminated prostatic cancer for four decades (4-15), and some reports on total androgen withdrawal (16) even claim superior results.
Therefore KHD-suppressing T production both in testes and adrenals, seemed a promising drug in the therapy of advanced prostatic cancer. In 1983 Trachtenberg (27) published the first encouraging results in three patients treated with KHD 400 mgr tid. Since then KHD has been used as firstline in previously untreated, and as secondline therapy in relapsed patients.
Based on the EORTC and the NPCP criteria (20) the effects of KHD as firstline medication were evaluated in 68 patients (3, 14,

29, 30, 33). In 38 patients treated for at least one year four
of them were in complete remission, fourteen in partial remission,
thirteen considered in stable disease and seven in progression.
T values dropped to castrate levels when plasmatic K levels were
maintained above 5 ng/ml. Acid phosphatases, when enhanced before
start of therapy dropped to normal levels in most patients.
Pain and Karnofsky index also improved in most patients (2).
Allen et al (1) published also promising results in relapsed
prostatic cancer patients. This report was confirmed by a compiled
series of 75 evaluable cases according to the same EORTC and NPCP
criteria.
This report claimed one complete remission, 15 patients with
partial remission, 26 patients with stable disease while 33
patients progressed.
However the improvement in pain and performance status was the
striking subjective response, stressed in most reports (2).

PERSONAL EXPERIENCE

Our own experience with KHD started in 1983. We treated a
first group of 12 patients with advanced prostatic cancer with
KHD 400 mgr tid. Seven of them were previously untreated, five
in relapse. After a complete diagnostic work-up the virgin group
was treated for four weeks. Biochemical, hormonal and subjective
parameters were documented once weekly. Serum T levels dropped
to castrate range within three-four days in five of the seven.
Concomitant monitoring of K plasmatic levels showed a lack of
compliance in the two non-responders, as well as variations in T
levels when the strict treatment regimen of 8 hours was not
respected.
Luteinizing hormone, progesterone and 17 α hydroxyprogesterone
values increased according to expectations. Prolactine secretion
was not affected and there was no significant change in oestradiol
values. Cortisol levels decreased in three patients. One of them
died on the fourth day of treatment with a dramatic drop of cortisol value in the serum.
Prostatic acid phosphatases, elevated in three patients, decreased.
In three patients with pain, improvement was spectacular within
two days. At the end of this study all surviving patients were
orchidectomized.
In the five patients in progression after previous hormonal
therapy no significant hormonal change was seen. Pain relief was
striking. Treatment had to be discontinued in two patients because
of gastro-intestinal side-effects. One patient died after four
weeks and two patients remained in subjective remission for six
and eight months.
As far as side-effects were concerned gastro-intestinal upset
was commonly experienced. In two patients there was a transitory
rise of hepatic transaminases. No other reported side-effects
(skin reactions, gynecomastia) were seen (7, 12).

EFFECTS OF KHD ON ACTH STIMULATED ADRENAL STEROIDOGENESIS

The changes in cortisol levels we had seen in some of our patients prompted us to investigate the effects of KHD on adrenal
ACTH stimulated steroidogenesis.
Fifteen previously orchidectomized patients with metastatic prostatic carcinoma relapsing after a mean period of 22 months (16-
18) were treated at least 28 days by KHD (300 mgr tid).
Dexamethasone 0,25 mgr bid was added during the last 14 days.
ACTH challenges (0,25 mgr IV) were performed on days 0, 14 and
28. Plasma was taken 20 minutes, just before and 30, 60, 90, 120,
180 and 240 minutes after onset of ACTH infusion.
Non-routine hormonal assays as well as controls of our routine
hormonal assays were performed in the research laboratories of
Janssen Pharmaceutica. All investigations were completed in eight
out of these fifteen patients. KHD lowered basal levels of the
adrenal androgens by about 70%, their stimulation by ACTH was
completely inhibited. Progesterones increased twicefold. Cortisol
values were slightly decreased after KHD alone but its response
to ACTH was blunted. There was no significant change in aldosterone levels.
11-Deoxycortisol, 11-deoxycorticosterone and corticosterone
values, both basal and after stimulation increased significantly
under KHD.
    With the combined KHD dexamethasone regimen there was a further
decrease of adrenal androgens and steroids. 17-Hydroxyprogesterone
and to a lesser extent progesterone rose more markedly after
ACTH challenge in the combination treatment then after KHD alone.
11-Deoxycortisol, 11-deoxycorticosterone and corticosterone were
lowered by the KHD dexamethasone association.
    We conclude from this study that KHD in vivo inhibits nearly
completely the biosynthesis of adrenal androgens but that it also
interferes, allthough to a lesser extent with the mineralo- and
glucocorticoids synthesis.
ACTH stimulation is unable to overcome the androgen synthesis inhibition and its effect on cortisol synthesis is blunted. Our
study confirms the manifest hypocorticism reported in a few cases
(19, 26, 29, 34).
This hypocorticism results from a partial inhibition of the 11 β
hydroxylase and is responsible for the rise of pituitary ACTH
in longterm treated patients with KHD.
    In order to prevent Addisonian crisis in seriously ill
patients, treated with KHD, we feel that combination therapy with
corticosteroid substitution is advisable.
Despite some supplementary advantages (enhanced inhibition of
adrenal androgens synthesis, reduction of the excess of some
mineralocorticoids) combination therapy however has also some inherent disadvantages (side-effects of corticoids).
    None of the fifteen patients showed objective responses. Seven
patients died with a mean survival of five months. Five patients
are alive with a mean survival of three months.

Remarquable pain relief was obtained in eight out of the fifteen patients.

CONCLUSION

Allthough KHD is without any doubt an active drug, able to induce remissions in metastatic prostatic cancer we do not feel that it has particular advantages in regard to other available medications but we look forward to the development of more specific and potent derivatives of this molecule.

REFERENCES

1. Allen, J.M., Kerle, D.J., Ware, H., Doble, A., Williams, G., and Bloom, S.R. (1983): Combined treatment with ketoconazole and luteinizing hormone releasing hormone analogue: a novel approach to resistant progressive prostatic cancer. Br.Med.J. 287: 1766.

2. Amery, W.K., De Coster, R., and Caers, I. (1986): Ketoconazole from an antimycotic to a prostate cancer drug. (in press).

3. Ang, K.K., Drochmans, A., Vantongelen, K., and Van der Schueren, E. (1986): Feasibility of high-dose ketoconazole for the management of advanced prostatic cancer. Int.J. Urology (in press).

4. Byar, D.P. (1973): The Veterans Administration Cooperative Urological Research Group's Studies of Cancer of the Prostate. Cancer 32, 1126-1130.

5. De Coster, R. (1984): Effect of ketoconazole in testosterone biosynthesis in short term cultures of dispersed rat testicular cells. Proc. 7th Int. Congress. Endocrinology, July 1-7, Quebec p. 559 (abstract). Elsevier, Excerpta Medica, Amsterdam, Oxford, Princeton.

6. De Coster, R., Beerens, D., Dom, J., and Willemsens, G. (1984): Endocrinological effects of single daily ketoconazole administration in male beagle dogs. Acta Endocrinologica 107, 275-281.

7. De Coster, R., and Denis, L. (1985): High dose ketoconazole therapy blocks testosterone biosynthesis in patients with advanced prostatic carcinoma: site of action. Presented at XX Congress of the International Society of Urology, Vienna, June 23-28, 1985.

8. De Coster, R., and Van den Bossche, H. (1985): Ketoconazole: mechanism of action. Presented at the symposium on treatment of advanced prostatic cancer and the role of LHRH-superagonists. Baden near Vienna, June 20-21, 1985.

9. De Coster, R., Denis, L. and Mahler, C. (1985b): Ketoconazole blocks both basal and stimulated androgen secretion in castrated patients with prostatic cancer. Presented at the 3rd International Forum of Andrology, Paris, June 17-18,1985.

10. De Coster, R., Denis, L., Mahler, C., Coene, M.C., Haelterman, C., and Beerens, D. (1985b): Effects of ketoconazole on ACTH-stimulated adrenal steroidogenesis in orchiectomized prostatic cancer patients. J. Steroid Biochem. 23 suppl.: 36.

11. De Felice, R., Johnson, D.G., and Galgiani, J.N. (1981): Gynecomastia with ketoconazole. Antimicrob. Agents Chemother. 19: 1073-1074.

12. Denis, L., Chaban, M., and Mahler, C. (1985): Clinical applications of ketoconazole in prostatic cancer. In: "Therapeutic Principles in Metastatic Prostate Cancer", Schröder, F.H., and Richards, B. (Eds), New York: Alan R. Liss Inc., pp. 319-326.

13. Graybill (1983): Summary: potential and problems with ketoconazole. American Journal of Medicine 74: 86-90.

14. Heyns, W., Drochmans, A., Van der Schueren, E., and Verhoeven, g. (1985): Endocrine effects of high-dose ketoconazole therapy in advanced prostatic cancer. Acta Endocrinol. 110: 276-283.

15. Huggins, C., and Hodges, C.V. (1941): Studies on prostatic cancer. I. The effect of castration, of estrogen and of androgen injection on serum phosphatases in metastatic carcinoma of the prostate. Cancer Res. 1: 293-297.

16. Labrie, F., Dupont, A., Belanger, A., Lacoursiere, Y., and Members of the Laval University Prostate Cancer Program (1984): Complete androgen blockade at start of treatment causes a dramatic improvement of survival in advanced prostate cancer. In: LHRH and its analogues. Labrie, F., Belanger, A., and Dupont, A. (Eds), Elsevier Science Publishers B.V., 368-379.

17. Levine, H.B. (1982): Ketoconazole in the management of fungal disease. New York, Adis Press, 1-162.

18. Loose, D.S., Kan, P.B., Hirst, M.A., Marcus, R.A., and Feldman, D. (1983): Ketoconazole blocks adrenal steroidogenesis by inhibiting cytochrome P-450-dependent enzymes. J. Clin. Invest. 71: 1495-1499.

19. Mahler, C., Denis, L., and Chaban, M. (1985): Ketoconazole in der Behandlung des Prostatakarzinoms. Abstract Book of the XXXVII Kongress der Deutscher Gesellschaft für Urologie, Mainz 2-5 Oktober 1985, p. 299.

20. Newling, D. (1985): Criteria for response to treatment of metastatic prostatic cancer. In: EORTC GU Monograph 2, Part A: Therapeutic Principles in Metastatic Prostatic Cancer, Alan R. Liss Inc., p. 205-220.

21. Pont, A., Williams, P.L., Azhar, A., Reitz, R.E., Bochra, C., Smith, E.R., and Stevens, D.A. (1982a): Ketoconazole blocks testosterone synthesis. Archives of International Medicine 142, 2137-2140.

22. Pont, A., Williams, P.L., Loose, D.S., Feldman, D., Reitz, R.E., Bochra, C., and Stevens, D.A. (1982b): Ketoconazole blocks adrenal steroid synthesis. Annals of Internal Medicine 97: 370-372.

23. Pont, A., Graybill, J.R., Craven, P.C., Galgiani, J.M., Dis-

mukes, W.E., Reitz, R.E., and Stevens, D.A. (1984): High-dose ketoconazole therapy and adrenal and testicular function in humans. Archives of Internal Medicine 144, 2150-2153.

24. Santen, R.J., Vanden Bossche, H., Symoens, J., Brugmans, J., and De Coster, R. (1983): Site of action of low-dose keto-conazole on androgen biosynthesis in men. Journal of Clinical Endocrinology and Metabolism 57 (4), 732-736.

25. Schürmeyer, Th., and Nieschlag, E. (1984): Effect of keto-conazole and other imidazole fungicides on testosterone bio-synthesis. Acta Endocrinol. 105: 275-280.

26. Tapazoglou, E., Subramanian, M.G., Al-Sarraf, M., Kresge, C., and Decker, D. (1986): High dose ketoconazole therapy in patients with metastatic prostate cancer. Cancer Treatm. Rep. (in press).

27. Trachtenberg, J. (1983): Ketoconazole: a novel and rapid treatment for advanced prostatic cancer. The Journal of Urology 130, 152-153.

28. Trachtenberg, J. (1984): The effects of ketconazole on testosterone production and normal and malignant androgen dependent tissues on the adult rat. The Journal of Urology 132, 599-601.

29. Trachtenberg, J., and Pont, A. (1984): Ketoconazole therapy for advanced prostate cancer. Lancet ii: 433-435.

30. Trachtenberg, J. (1985): High dose ketoconazole in the treatment of stage D2 prostatic cancer. Presented at: American Urological Association Meeting, Boston, October, 1985.

31. Vanden Bossche, H., Lauwers, W., Willemsens, G., and Cools, W. (1985b): The cytochrome P-450 dependent C_{17-20}-lyase in subcellular fractions of the rat testis: Differences in sensitivity to ketoconazole and itraconazole. In: Microsomes and Drug Oxidations, Boobis, A.R., Caldwell, J., de Matteis, F., and Elcombe, C.R. (Eds), pp. 63-73, Tayler and Francis, London.

32. Vanden Bossche, H., Lauwers, W., Willemsens, G., and Cools, W. (1985c): Ketoconazole, an inhibitor of the cytochrome P-450-dependent testosterone synthesis. In: EORTC Genito-urinary Group, Monograph 2, Part A: Therapeutic Principles in Metastatic Prostatic Cancer, Schröder, F.H., and Richards, B. (Eds), pp. 187-196, Alan R. Liss, New York.

33. Van der Schueren E., Drochmans, A., Heyns, W., Verhoeven, G., Ang, K.K., and Van Tongelen, K. (1985): High dose ketocona-zole in the treatment of metastatic carcinoma of the prostate: clinical and biochemical effects. Presented at: 3rd European Conference on Clinical Oncology and Cancer Nursing, Stockholm, June 16-20.

34. White, M.C., and Kendall-Taylor, P. (1985): Adrenal hypo-function in patients taking ketoconazole. The Lancet i, 44-45.

35. Willemsens, G., Cools, W., and Vanden Bossche, H. (1980): Effects of miconazole and ketoconazole on sterol synthesis in a subcellular fraction of yeast and mammalian cells. In: The

host invader interplay, Vanden Bossche, H. (Ed), pp. 691–704, Elsevier Biomedical Press, Amsterdam.

Hormonal Manipulation of Cancer: Peptides, Growth Factors, and New (Anti) Steroidal Agents, edited by Jan G. M. Klijn et al. Raven Press, New York © 1987.

A STUDY OF THE ROLE OF ADDITIONAL ANDROGEN DEPLETION FOR PRIMARY THERAPY OF PATIENTS WITH ADVANCED LOCAL OR METASTATIC CARCINOMA OF THE PROSTATE

Gordon Williams, M.B., F.R.C.S., Eamonn A. Kiely, M.B., F.R.C.S.(I), Raj Kapadia, M.B., F.R.C.S., Andrew Doble, M.B. F.R.C.S., Howard Ware, M.B., F.R.C.S., and Anthony Timoney, M.B., F.R.C.S.(I)

Department of Urology, Hammersmith Hospital, London W12 OHS, England

PATIENTS AND METHODS

Fifty new patients with advanced local or metastatic prostatic cancer were randomised to receive either orchidectomy alone or orchidectomy plus Ketoconazole, orchidectomy plus Dexamethazone or orchidectomy plus Cyproterone acetate. Ketoconazole was given in a high dose of 400 mg three times a day, Dexamethazone 0.5 mg in the morning and 0.3 mg in the evening and Cyproterone acetate 100 mg three times a day. The mean follow-up is 12.4 months with a range of 1 - 18 months. Pre-operative staging and follow-up examinations have included clinical examination, digital rectal examination, acid phosphotase and bone scans. These have all been repeated regularly throughout the period of follow-up. In addition, the following serum endocrine studies have also been performed at each visit; testosterone; dihydrotestosterone; androstenedione; progesterone; cortisol and lutienising hormone. Following the manufacturers' advice that high dose Ketoconazole had been associated with an unacceptable incidence of septicaemia in other studies this arm of the trial was withdrawn in February 1986 and results presented are up to that date.

119

INTRODUCTION.

Between 60 - 80% of men with advanced prostatic cancer will respond to conventional endocrine therapy using orchidectomy or oestrogens.   There is still no convincing evidence, however, that such treatment prolongs life and approximately half of those who originally respond will relapse within two years, and from relapse, have a median survival of only six months (1, 7) Why patients fail to respond or relapse is poorly understood.   If it is due to the emergence of androgen resistant cells, different primary therapies which produce differing levels of androgen ablation should not differ in their response.   However, it has been reported by Labrie et al, (8) that total androgen ablation using a specific anti-androgen (Flutamide) in combination with an LHRH analogue or orchidectomy does produce an increase in primary response rates, prologation of survival and decreased mortality.

There is also data to suggest that some tumours are relatively and not absolutely androgen independent(4) In some patients whose disease has progressed after androgen deprivation there is frequently disease activation if they are treated with exogenous androgens(5) These observations provide theoretical support for treatment with an LHRH analogue or orchidectomy to reduce levels of testosterone and a pure anti-androgen to neutralise the effects of adrenal androgens and those produced by peripheral conversion of precursor steroids.   As we were unable to obtain the specific anti-androgen Flutamide, we have studied alternative ways of reducing androgen availability to the prostate by combining in a prospective randomised study, orchidectomy with the addition of Dexamethazone or Ketoconazole or Cyproterone acetate to patients with locally advanced or metastatic prostatic cancer.   Dexamethazone inhibits ACTH production and decreases adrenal androgen and progesterone production.   Ketoconazole inhibits both testicular and adrenal androgen production and leads to elevated levels of serum progesterone. Cryproterone acetate inhibits testosterone production and also acts by inhibiting the uptake of 5 alpha dihydrotestosterone by the cytoplasmic receptor in the prostatic cell.   In theory a combination of orchidectomy and one of these agents should produce an effect over and above that of orchidectomy alone.

RESULTS

Endocrinology

The mean pre-treatment values for the four groups and those at six months are shown in Table 1. At six months there was a significant reduction of testosterone in the orchidectomy plus ketoconazole group compared to orchidectomy alone ($P < 0.05$). There was a significant reduction of dihydrotestosterone in the orchidectomy plus ketoconazole group compared to orchidectomy alone ($P < 0/001$). There was a significant elevation of progesterone in the orchidectomy plus ketoconazole group compared to orchidectomy ($P < 0.001$) and a significant decrease in the dexamethasone and orchidectomy compared to orchidectomy ($P < 0/01$). Cortisol was significantly suppressed in the orchidectomy plus dexamethasone group compared to orchidectomy ($P < 0.001$). Androstenedione was significantly reduced in the orchidectomy plus ketoconazole group compared to orchidectomy alone ($P < 0.05$) and highly significantly reduced in the orchidectomy plus dexamethasone group compared to orchidectomy ($P < 0.001$). LH was significantly elevated in the orchidectomy plus Cryproterone group compared to orchidectomy alone ($P < 0.01$). This trend in endocrine data has been continued at 12 months though the numbers are too small for adequate statistical evaluation.

Clinical Response

This was assessed according to the criteria of the British Prostate Group (3) and are summarised in Table II.

Withdrawals and Adverse Effects

From the 19 February 1986 the Ketoconazole limb of the study has been withdrawn due to the reported incidence of septicaemia occuring in patients receiving high dose Ketoconazole therapy for carcinoma of the prostate. Five patients were withdrawn from the Ketoconazole arm, two due to nausea and vomiting, two due to the development of peptic ulceration and one who died two weeks after commencement of the drug from advanced prostatic cancer. No patient was withdrawn from the orchidectomy arm. Two patients in the Dexamethazone arm died from advanced cancer

at 10 weeks, one of whom was non-compliant. Two patients
randomised to Cyproterone died of prostatic cancer at two and
three months and one died from a non cancer death at two months.

DISCUSSION

There is considerable evidence to show that carcinoma of the
prostate responds not only to androgen withdrawal, but also to
progestogens (6), cortisone (2) and anti-androgens (9). To
determine whether or not added benefit could be obtained over
conventional therapy, 50 patients have been randomised to receive
either an orchidectomy alone or orchidectomy plus Ketocanazole,
a drug which in high dose reduces both androstenedione and
testosterone production and leads to an elevation of serum
progesterone. Dexamethazone decreases androstenedrone by a
central action and also reduces progesterone and cortisone.
Cyproterone acetate, a progestational anti-androgen blocks uptake
of dihydrotestosterone by the intra-cellular receptor.

This study has clearly shown significant alterations in the
endocrine status of these patients with advanced progressive
prostatic cancer when treated with these combinations of
therapy. However, the numbers of patients studied are too small
to draw any conclusions with regard to possible therapeutic
benefit resulting from these changes. High dose Ketoconazole
cannot be considered as a drug for the treatment of prostatic
cancer because of the reported adverse events. However, other
possible less toxic Imidazde derivatives are being developed
and may be worthy of further study. Low dose Dexamethazone
sufficient to produce cortisol inhibition was well tolerated
and associated with a high partial response rate. A large multi-
centre trial comparing orchidectomy with orchidectomy plus
Dexamethazone may be justified. Previous workers have shown no
significant advantage to the addition of Cyproterone to
orchidectomy and this appears to be confirmed in the small
numbers in this study.

In conclusion, for any meaningful data to be produced on the
value of new therapies for the management of carcinoma of the
prostate, large, long term, multi-centre studies are required.

This study has shown a possible benefit from the addition of
Dexamethazone to orchidectomy and further studies may be
indicated.

Key   *n   **mean   ***sem

TABLE 1

		PRE-TREATMENT				6 MONTHS			
		O	O + K	O + D	O + C	O	O + K	O + D	O + C
Testosterone (nmol/1)	*	9	8	10	11	9	5	9	8
	**	19.34	14.84	16.93	17.42	0.79	0.50	0.54	0.82
	***	2.98	2.10	2.32	2.29	0.08	0.06	0.11	0.19
Dihydrotestosterone (nmol/1)		10	8	10	11	9	5	9	8
		3.21	3.85	2.51	2.88	0.51	0.48	0.51	0.49
		0.49	0.35	0.24	0.41	0.06	0.10	0.05	0.07
Androstenedione (nmol/1)		10	8	10	12	9	5	7	10
		6.24	5.13	6.02	5.28	4.67	2.55	0.95	3.60
		0.86	0.46	0.74	0.59	0.62	0.49	0.19	0.51
Progesterone (nmol/1)		10	6	9	12	8	5	8	7
		2.07	1.91	3.56	2.68	2.23	5.58	0.88	2.06
		0.27	0.23	0.50	0.34	0.23	0.40	0.16	0.30
Cortisol (nmol/1)		10	8	10	11	9	5	7	9
		494.7	405.1	594.2	498.0	449.8	487.4	60.0	454.4
		46.6	71.5	55.6	34.8	38.6	68.7	5.0	28.7
Luteinising hormone (iu/1)		9	8	10	12	9	5	7	9
		6.80	8.65	9.47	10.47	36.28	29.76	33.26	13.71
		1.01	2.83	2.10	1.85	3.55	5.90	4.61	4.66

TABLE 2

RESPONSE TO THERAPY

	6 MONTHS			No.	12 MONTHS		
	Partial	Stable	Progressive		Partial	Stable	Progressive
O (10)	3	4	3	(6)	3	1	2
O + K (14)	4	3	1	(4)	1	2	1
O + D (14)	7	3	0	(4)	4	0	0
O + C (12)	2	4	1	1			

O = Orchidectomy
K = Ketoconazole
D = Dexamethasone
C = Cyproterone

REFERENCES

1. BRENDLER, H. 1969. Cancer of the urogential tract.
   Prostatic cancer therapy with orchidectomy or
   oestrogen or both.   JAMAM 210: 1074

2. BRENDLER, H. 1973. Adrenalectomy and hypophysectomy for
   prostatic cancer. Urology. 2: 99-101

3. CHISHOLM, G.D., BEYNON, L.L. 1983. The response of the
   malignant prostate to endocrine treatment. In
   The Endocrinology of Prostate Tumours. 241-262.
   Ed. R Ghanadian. Published MTP Press Ltd, Lancaster.

4. FOWLER, J. E. Jr, WHITMORE, W. F. 1981.
   The response of metastatic adenocarcinoa of the
   prostate to exogenous testosterone.
   J. Urol. 126: 372-375

5. FOWLER, J., WHITMORE, W.F. 1982.
   Considerations for the use of testosterone with
   systemic chemotherapy in prostatic cancer.
   Cancer. 49: 1373-1377

6. GELLER, J., ALBERT, J., YEN, S.S.C. 1978.
   Treatment of advanced cancer of prostate with megestrol
   acetate. Urology. 12: 537-41

7. JORDAN, W.P. JR, BLACKARD, C.E., BYAR, D.P. 1977.
   Reconsideration of orchidectomy in the treatment of
   advanced prostatic cancer. South Med. J. 70: 1411-1413

8. LABRIE, F., DUPONT, A., BELANGER, A. 1985.
   Complete androgen blockage for the treatment of
   prostatic cancer in Vincent T De Vita.
   S. Hellman and S A Rosenburg (Eds) (193-217).
   Important Advances in Oncology. J. B. Lippincott Co.
   Philadelphia.

9. WEIN, A.J., MURPHY, J.J. 1973.
   Experience in the treatment of prostatic carcinoma
   with cyproterone acetate. J. Urol. 109: 68-70

Hormonal Manipulation of Cancer: Peptides, Growth Factors, and New (Anti) Steroidal Agents, edited by Jan G. M. Klijn et al. Raven Press, New York © 1987.

THE USE OF SYNERGISTIC HORMONAL COMBINATIONS IN THE TREATMENT OF ADVANCED PROSTATIC CANCER: CYPROTERONE ACETATE PLUS MINI-DOSE DIETHYLSTILBESTROL

S.L. Goldenberg, N. Bruchovsky, P. S. Rennie, C. M. Coppin, E. M. Brown

Divisions of Urology,(S.L.G), Medical Oncology (C.M.C.), Radiation Oncology (E.M.B.), and Department of Cancer Endocrinology (S.L.G., N.B., P.S.R.), University of British Columbia and Cancer Control Agency of British Columbia, 600 West 10th Avenue, Vancouver, B.C., Canada, V5Z 4E6

SUMMARY

Using a short-term screening procedure which measures changes in cellular concentrations of dihydrotestosterone and androgen receptors, we treatments to mimic the effects of surgical castration on the rat prostate. The agents tested included cyproterone acetate, mini-dose diethylstilbestrol, cyproterone acetate plus mini-dose diethylstilbestrol, megestrol acetate plus mini-dose diethylstilbestrol and LHRH-agonist plus RU23908. Castration-like changes were most pronounced with the synergistic combination of cyproterone acetate plus mini-dose diethylstilbestrol. This observation served as a starting point for a clinical trial employing the two agents in the treatment of advanced prostatic cancer. Forty-seven previously untreated symptomatic men with stage D2 disease received cyproterone acetate 100 mg twice daily and diethylstilbestrol 0.1 mg once daily. On the basis of NPCP criteria the objective response rate was 98% (13% CR, 74% PR and 11% stable). Survival at 12 and 18 months was 80% and 67% (Kaplan-Meier). These results are virtually identical to those obtained with alternative medical castration therapies such as LHRH agonists alone or in combination with antiandrogens. Thus, cyproterone acetate plus mini-dose diethylstilbestrol affords another means of attaining rapid and potent androgen-withdrawal effects in cases where surgery or the use of estrogens in conventional doses is not acceptable. Moreover, since this therapy is easily administered and well tolerated by patients, it may be utilized to facilitate the application of chemo-hormonal treatment.

INTRODUCTION

Withdrawal of testicular androgens is the accepted standard treatment of Stage D prostatic cancer. Disadvantages related to surgical orchiectomy and medical castration with estrogen therapy have prompted the development of alternate drugs with fewer side effects and better patient tolerance. We have studied the ability of a variety of these agents to mimic the intracellular effects which are seen following orchiectomy in the rat model. We were particularly interested in studying a combination of the progestational antiandrogen, cyproterone acetate (CPA), plus a mini-dose of diethylstilbestrol (DES), anticipating a synergistic action on androgen suppression. A combined effect of progesterone and estrogen on the suppression of monkey plasma gonadotrophin was first described in 1952 by Salhanick et al. (5). More recently Geller et al.(2) combined megestrol acetate (MA) with a mini-dose of DES, maintaining castrate levels of plasma testosterone in men for up to 12 months.

Studies on the normal rat ventral prostate have yielded many observations on the outcome of hormonal manipulations. Following castration the concentration of androgen receptors in the nucleus undergoes a rapid decrease, matched by an increase of similar velocity and magnitude in the concentration of cytosolic receptor. However, both prostatic weight and the number of cells in the prostate do not drop significantly below the normal level until the 4th day after orchiectomy. These then decline rapidly to 30% and 15% of normal by day 7 (4). This period of rapid involution represents the activation of a specific killing mechanism triggered by the withdrawal of androgen, termed "autophagia". The cells which survive (androgen independent) possess the capacity of self-renewal under androgen replacement (ie. they are androgen stimulated) and in this way may be considered to be stem cells.

We have studied the ability of CPA, DES, CPA plus DES, MA plus DES and LHRH-agonist plus the non-steroidal antiandrogen RU23908, to mimic the early effects of surgical orchiectomy on the rat prostate. The results of this study served as the basis of a clinical trial of the combination of CPA plus DES in the treatment of men with stage D2 prostatic cancer. Descriptions of both the experimental and clinical studies are given below.

EXPERIMENTAL STUDY

Materials and Methods

Groups of 5 to 7 male Wistar rats weighing 250 to 350 g were either castrated on day 1 or received daily injections of drugs or vehicle on days 1-3. Table 1 shows the drug doses used. On day 4 ventral prostate tissue was collected,

TABLE 1. Drug Dosages

Drug	Dose per 100 g body weight
Cyproterone acetate	300 ug
Megestrol acetate	300 ug
Diethylstilbestrol	300 ng
LHRH-agonist (Buserelin or Leuprolide)	80 ng
RU23908	300 ug

weighed, and analysed for DNA content and concentrations of dihydrotestosterone (DHT) and androgen receptors. DHT levels were determined by extraction with ethyl acetate/ hexane, purification using Water's Sep Pak^R prepacked silica columns and quantitation by RIA. Nuclei were prepared by discontinuous sucrose gradient centrifugation. Purified nuclei were assayed for androgen receptor content by labelling receptor with tritiated DHT and separating free from bound with PD10-G25 gel-chromatography. Non-specific binding was determined using unlabelled DHT as a competitor. Cytosol preparations were assayed for androgen receptor by labelling with tritiated R1881 (plus a 500-fold excess of triamcinolone acetonide) and separating bound from free R1881 with PD10-G25 gel-chromatography. Non-specific binding was determined by competition with unlabelled DHT.

Results

Changes in Prostatic Weight

Four days after castration prostatic tissue wet weight was reduced to 80% of the normal value. After the CPA plus DES and MA plus DES regimens, the weight of the prostate was reduced to 81% and 72% of normal, respectively. Injection with LHRH-agonist plus RU23908 failed to decrease prostatic weight.

Changes in Whole Tissue DHT

Castration, CPA plus DES, and MA plus DES reduced whole tissue DHT levels to near 0. The synergistic effect of CPA plus DES was clear, since at these concentrations, neither drug alone effectively reduced whole tissue DHT levels to background. No reduction in whole tissue DHT levels was apparent after treatment with LHRH-agonist plus RU23908.

Changes in Nuclear DHT

Treatment with CPA plus DES reduced nuclear DHT levels to background and the two drugs again appeared to work synergistically. MA plus DES did not completely reduce nuclear DHT levels to castrate levels, and treatment with LHRH-agonist plus RU23908 appeared to be even less effective.

Changes in Nuclear Receptor Levels

As with nuclear DHT levels, nuclear receptor levels were reduced to background by castration, or CPA plus DES. Again, the synergistic effect of combination treatment was seen. A reduced response to LHRH-agonist plus RU23908 was consistent with previous data.

Changes in Cytosolic Receptor Levels

After castration the levels of cytosolic receptor rose most prominently after CPA plus DES treatment.

CLINICAL STUDY

On the basis of the synergism demonstrated in the foregoing experiments, we initiated a phase-2 clinical study using CPA (200 mg daily) and mini-dose DES (0.1 mg daily) in 47 previously untreated, symptomatic stage D2 prostate cancer patients. The combined therapy reduced the concentration of serum testosterone to castrate levels in 65% of patients by 7 days and in 92% by 28 days. The mean time to castration levels was 17 days. Serum acid phosphatase as measured by RIA was elevated in 43 out of 45 patients, with a mean level of 45 ng/dl (normal < 3.2). By day 1 the mean had dropped to 13.2 and by 2 months the mean was 4.3 ng/dl. As expected, serum luteinizing hormone and follicle stimulating hormone levels decreased and eventually remained at

50% of initial values. Serum prolactin levels increased with treatment to 250% of the initial value. Of the 47 patients, however, only 12 developed hyperprolactinemia. In this subgroup of patients, 7 (58%) went on to disease progression while 5 (42%) remained responders (3 partial and 2 complete). On the basis of NPCP criteria the overall initial objective response rate was 98% (13% CR, 74% PR and 11% stable). One patient failed to respond to treatment and, eventually, 19 (40%) "escaped" with a mean time to progression of 10 months (range 4 - 17 months).

In Table 2 the bone scan, serum acid phosphatase and prostatic soft tissue responses to treatment are summarized.

TABLE 2. Response to Treatment*

n=47	Bone scan	PAP	Soft tissue	Response
No.abnormal	45	43	44	47
CR/PR	22	40	38	41(87%)
Stable	22	2	6	5 (11%)
Progression < 3 months	1	1	0	1 (2%)
Progression > 3 months	19	19	4	19(40%)

* NPCP criteria

We observed a pronounced resolution of soft tissue disease (prostate and lymph nodes) and a rapid relief from pain. Skeletal metastases seemed to be less responsive. Amongst the 19 progressors, all developed new bone lesions while only 4 relapsed with advancing soft tissue disease. Kaplan-Meier predictions at 12 and 18 months showed survivals of 80% and 67% and free from progression rates of 68% and 43%, respectively.

The drugs were well tolerated by all patients. Side effects attributable to androgen withdrawal were loss of libido, impotence and reduced energy. Symptoms related to the use of DES were nipple tenderness, with or without breast engorgement, and dyspnea on exertion. These rarely appeared during the first 3 months of therapy and for the most part were reversed when estrogen was discontinued or reduced in dosage.

The clinical combination of CPA plus mini-dose DES demonstrated the same synergistic action on hormone suppression as was seen in the rat prostate. Whenever the DES was discontinued serum testosterone levels increased and could only be totally suppressed again when the DES was reinstituted. This type of response was observed in 7 patients.

Thus, the combination of CPA plus mini-dose DES yielded a prompt, synergistic suppression of plasma testosterone with a high initial objective response rate, particularly in the PR category. We observed excellent resolution of soft tissue disease, decrease of acid phosphatase levels and relief of pain symptoms. Survival rates at 12 and 18 months were similar if not identical to those reported elsewhere in these Proceedings for alternative forms of medical castration therapy utilizing LHRH agonists alone or in combination with antiandrogens.

DISCUSSION

Androgen withdrawal therapy is incapable of curing prostatic carcinoma. As emphasized earlier, when the normal prostate is deprived of androgen, a cellular autophagic mechanism is activated and the hormone-dependent tissue involutes, leaving a surviving population of stem cells capable of regenerating the gland upon androgen replacement. We have no reason to exclude the possibility that prostatic cancer similarly is composed of stem cells and differentiated progeny. The latter are selectively killed when androgens are withdrawn leaving a stem cell population which is immune to death by this process. Any differentiation of stem cells that might occur after androgen withdrawal would not be associated with the expression of autophagic control and for practical purposes the property of androgen dependence is permanently lost from the tumour. This is consistent with the observation that secondary hormonal therapy after manifestations of a response to primary ablative treatment is seldom effective in producing an objective regression of a recurrent tumour (1).

If the object of treatment is cure rather than palliation, then it is necessary to adopt strategies whose success would depend upon the eradication of the stem cell compartment of the tumour. Experience with combination drug-hormone therapy, both in clinical (6) and experimental situations (3), strongly suggests that androgen withdrawal and effective chemotherapy should be instituted concurrently and as early as possible in the treatment history of the tumour. Synergistic hormonal combinations, are an excellent means of obtaining rapid androgen withdrawal and may be used to facilitate the implementation of chemo-hormonal therapy.

Acknowledgments
    Part of this work was supported by grants from the National Cancer Institute of Canada and the Medical Research Council of Canada. We thank Cynthia Wells for typing the manuscript.

REFERENCES

1. Catalona, W.J. (1984): "Prostatic Cancer." Orlando: Grune and Stratton, pp. 145-171.

2. Geller, J., Albert, J., Yen, S.S.C., Geller, S., and Loza, D. (1981). Medical Castration with megestrol acetate and minidose of diethylstilbestrol. Urol. Supp., 17:27-33.

3. Isaacs, J.T. (1984). The timing of androgen ablation therapy and/or chemotherapy in the treatment of prostatic cancer. The Prostate 5:1-17.

4. Lesser, B., and Bruchovsky, N. (1973). The effects of testosterone, 5 alpha-dihydrotestosterone and adenosine 3',5'-monophosphate in cell proliferation and differentiation in rat prostate. Biochem. Biophys. Acta. 308:426-437.

5. Salhanick, H.A., Hisaw, F.L., and Zarrow, M.X. (1952). The action of estrogen and progesterone on the gonadotropin content of the pituitary of the monkey. J. Clin. Endocrinol. Metab., 12:310.

6. Servadio, C., Mukamel, E., Lurie, H., and Nissenkorn, I. (1983). Early combined hormonal and chemotherapy for metastatic prostatic carcinoma. Urol. 21:493-495.

Hormonal Manipulation of Cancer: Peptides, Growth Factors, and New (Anti) Steroidal Agents, edited by Jan G. M. Klijn et al. Raven Press, New York © 1987.

HORMONAL ASPECTS AND TREATMENT OF ENDOMETRIAL CARCINOMA

J.A. Wijnen, M.D.

Department of Gynecological Oncology, University Hospital Rotterdam-Dijkzigt, and The Dr Daniel den Hoed Cancer Center / Rotterdam Radio-Therapeutic Institute, Groene Hilledijk 301, 3075 EA Rotterdam, The Netherlands

INTRODUCTION

Presently in the Western world about 3% of all newborn women will develop endometrial cancer. At the moment this is 3.5 times less than breast cancer (43). Considering the estimated cancer death rates, it is suggested that endometrial carcinoma is a relatively benign malignancy with an excellent prognosis. However, the overall 5-year survival rates as presented in the 1985 Annual Report of the FIGO over 13.581 patients was not better than 67.7% (Table I) (15). This figure has changed very little over the past 20 years (15). For a long time no sense of urgency has appeared to critically evaluate the treatment of this disease because 3/4 of all cases are diagnosed at an early stage and the degree of curability is relatively satisfactory.

PROGNOSTIC FACTORS

The increasing incidence of endometrial cancer (7,11,33) and a better understanding of prognostically important factors (1,3,12,21) initiated a collaborative clinical-pathological study of the Gynecologic Oncology Group in the United States, in patients with early stage endometrial adenocarcinoma. The results of this study (6) clearly demonstrate that the biologic behavior of this tumor and the prognosis of the patient is determined by the histopathologic differentiation grade and depth of myometrial invasion, expressed by incidence of pelvic and para-aortic lymph node metastases and recurrences (Table II). As a consequence of preoperative clinical staging, according to the FIGO-classification, surgical- pathological data should not be incorporated. However, in 14-19% of clinically stage I disease, which encompasses 76% of all patients with endometrial cancer, the tumor appeared to have spread outside the uterus (6,9,15) (Table III). Extrauterine and especially extra-pelvic tumor localizations in patients with clinically early stage disease will have their impact on prognosis and treatment. Collected data as reported by Morrow

Table I   Endometrial Carcinoma
                      Incidence per FIGO stage and survival

FIGO stage	% of patients per stage	% 5-yr survival	
		Ann.Rep.FIGO 1985 N = 13.581	Aalders 1982 N = 909
I	76	75.1	90
II	14	57.8	85
III	7	30.3	16
IV	3	10.6	10
Total	100	67.7	75

Table II   Endometrial Carcinoma FIGO stage I (N = 222)

Histologic grade	Deep myometrial infiltration		Lymph node metastases	Recurrences	
	N =	%	%	N =	%
1	93	4	2	4	4
2	88	15	11	13	15
3	41	39	27	17	42
Total	222			34	15

Adapted from Boronow 1984, and Di Saia et al. 1985.

Table III   Endometrial Carcinoma
              Extra-uterine tumor spread: FIGO stage I (N = 222)

	% total	% micros- copic only
Adnexal spread	7.2	5.9
Pelvic nodes	10.4	4.9
Aortic nodes*	7.2	3.6
Tumor cells in peritoneal washings	13.5	
Peritoneal implants	2.7	

* para-aortic nodes sampled in 157 patients

Adapted from Boronow et al. 1984.

(31) and Rutledge (40) indicated 25-30% 5-year survival rates in patients with stage I disease and histopathologically proven pelvic lymph node metastases. However, these figures also demonstrate that treatment of pelvic nodes can be beneficial.

SURGICAL TREATMENT

Fortunately, more than 2/3 of all patients with endometrial cancer will have well differentiated (grade I), only superficially invading adenocarcinomas without extra-corporal spread (14) contributing favorably to the overall 5-year survival rates of 75-90% in this stage (2,15). Those patients are most likely cured by surgery only and it will be very difficult to demonstrate any benefit of adjuvant treatment whether it is radiotherapy, hormonal or cytotoxic chemotherapy in this prognostically favorable group.

In order to identify endometrial cancer patients with prognostically unfavorable factors who will need adjunctive treatment and saving others from unnecessary overtreatment, a stepwise Evaluation and Surgical Treatment Protocol based on the results of the GOG 33 study was developed in conjunction with the Dutch Gynecologic Oncology Group (WOG) (47,48). Following this protocol it is estimated that only 1/3 of all clinically early stage endometrial cancer patients will have to be more extensively surgically staged, to identify patients at high risk for residual or recurrent disease.

ADDITIONAL TREATMENT

Until now, the additional treatment of choice is radiotherapy. Although the incidence of local recurrences will be reduced by additional radiotherapy, there are remarkably few prospective randomized studies that have tested the value of this adjunctive treatment. To date there are no firm data that adjunctive pelvic and/or aortic radiation or systemic therapy would increase significantly the 5-year survival rates in these patients. Especially by including a para-aortic field in this patient population with a mean age from 60.6 years in stage I to 66.5 years in stage IV (15) that tend to have other concurrent medical problems, the morbidity is considerable. Moreover, by evaluating the recurrence pattern in stage I endometrial carcinoma, collected data from 3 reports indicate recurrences in 63-79% outside the pelvis (2,14).

The 5-year survival rates in these advanced or recurrent cases is 10% or less (15,37). Adequate control of local disease can be achieved by individualized treatment, however, the prevention of recurrence at distant sides remains a major problem. Systemic treatment might have the potential to prevent these distant recurrences and this mode of treatment should be considered for the high risk patient.

HORMONAL ASPECTS OF ENDOMETRIAL ADENOCARCINOMA

It is now more than 50 years since the first animal experiments showed that estrogenic substances were possible carcinogens (10). In 1941, Greene (18) described endometrial hyperplasia and adenocarcinoma in a group of estrogen treated rabbits. Since then numerous studies have confirmed the link between uninterrupted, unopposed (exogenous) estrogen exposure and the increased risk of endometrial adenocarcinoma and its precursors.

One of the now well documented effects of estrogens on endometrium is the enhanced synthesis of estrogen receptors (20,30). By binding free steroids, the receptors form hormone-receptor complexes. These complexes function via translocation and subsequent nuclear regulation of protein synthesis. The result of this process is cellular proliferation.

Together with the estrogen receptors, progesterone receptors are synthesized (16,41).

Endometrial cancer appears to be a great exception in women with a normal menstrual cycle and before climacteric age. Apparently the cyclical production of estrogens and progesterone prevents the development of this disease. The effectiveness of progestogens in reversing adenocarcinoma and its precursors has been reported since 1959 (23,25,26).

Progesterone interrupts estrogen-receptor synthesis directly, but also indirectly by inducing the enzyme estradiol-dehydrogenase which, by metabolizing intracellular estradiol to estron, effectively lowers the estrogenic potency within the cell (19,24). These changes form the basis for the anti-estrogenic effects of progesterone, which culminates in diminished DNA synthesis and cell multiplication in post- as well as premenopausal epithelium.

In the postmenopausal situation, with low serum estradiol levels, the concentration of endometrial estrogen and progesterone receptors and consequently the sensitivity of these cells to estrogen, decreases. However, in postmenopausal women the incidence of endometrial cancer rises. This controversy can be explained by the observation that in some women large quantities of estrogen are produced by so-called extraglandular conversion of weak adrenal and ovarian androgens (22,42). These estrogens lead to chronic proliferation of the endometrium unopposed by progestogens. This situation counts as a causative effect for endometrial changes like cystic and adenomatous hyperplasia and adenocarcinoma. High levels of estrogen and progesterone receptors demonstrated in hyperplastic endometrium, are consistent with this observation (29,44,45,49).

Conflicting results have been published about estrogen and progesterone receptor levels in endometrial cancer (29,39,44). The autonomy of the cancer cells, especially in the differentiated tumors might be the result of destruction of the receptor system. Progressive loss of progesterone binding activity from the well differentiated to the more anaplastic forms of endometrial cancer have been reported (13,38,39,45,49). Heterogeneity of cells in a tumor is probably a major factor responsible for conflicting results, reported concerning this subject (32).

HORMONAL TREATMENT

Progestogens have a privileged position as a systemic therapy for endometrial cancer. Its popularity is due to the relative ease of administration, good tolerance and objective response rates generally reported as 30-50% in patients with metastatic or recurrent endometrial cancer (37). Clinical experiences of gynecological oncologists are usually less favorable than the up to 53% reported responses in the literature (5).

In 1980 Piver et al (36) reported in 114 patients only 15.8% objective responses, with 7.0% being complete. The only significant factor was that patients whose disease recurred 3 or more years after initial therapy had a significant increase in response (33.3%) compared to those with recurrence less than 3 years after their original treatment (8.3%).

In 1985 Podratz (37), in reviewing the results of progestational agents in 155 patients with advanced primary or recurrent endometrial carcinoma between 1968 and 1980 in the Mayo Clinic, reported an objective response in only 11.2% of patients. Response rates decreased with decreasing tumor differentiation from 40% in well differentiated tumors to 0% in undifferentiated lesions. There was no significant advantage for anyone of 3 progestational agents used in this period and survival after initiation of hormone therapy was 40% at one year, 19% at two years and 8% at five years. Survival was highly dependent on the degree of tissue differentiation and was influenced significantly by the estimated tumor volume at the start of the therapy and by the time interval from primary treatment to the beginning of hormone therapy.

These results are consistent with the recent observations that well differentiated endometrial carcinomas are more likely to contain progesterone receptors and show better responses to progestogen therapy (13,38).

Unfortunately progesterone binding results in decreased estrogen en progestogen receptor synthesis. As this may eventually result in the elimination of progestogen receptors, it could be responsible for the limited duration of clinical response.

The anti-estrogen tamoxifen binds to estrogen receptors, but exhibits a different estrogenic response in that it continues to stimulate progestogen receptor production, but decreases estrogen receptor production; it does not stimulate protein synthesis or cellular proliferation (8). Theoretically this would be an attractive drug in endometrial carcinoma; unfortunately a combination of tamoxifen and progestogen achieved only a tumor response rate of 33% in a few selective patients (8).

Adjuvant hormonal treatment

The benefit of adjuvant progesterone treatment in early stage endometrial cancer has not been established yet. Only few well designed studies have been published and no improvement of recurrence or survival rates could be reported. Recently De Palo et al. (35) presented results of a prospective, randomized study on adjuvant medroxyprogesterone acetate in a group of carefully surgically staged and according to risk factors stratified patients with early stage endometrial carcinoma. After 2 years no significant differences in recurrence and survival rates could be demonstrated in any of the three risk categories. If progestogen receptors are more prevalent, and clinical responses more common in well differentiated tumors, then it seems unlikely that adjuvant progestogens would have a great impact on survival figures which, for the most part, reflect poor control of the higher grade, more aggressive carcinomas.

CONCLUSIONS

It seems that the occasional dramatic clinical regression or prolonged stabilization occurring during progesterone therapy and the good tolerance of this treatment justifies a continued, but more limited and selective role for these agents. Optimal doses, sequencing and combinations with other hormone substances and/or cytotoxic agents have to be established. Standardization of definitions of response and rigid adherence to objectivity seem to be of utmost importance in reporting results of medical treatment of endometrial carcinomas.

For the future more efforts should be directed towards:

1. The prevention of endometrial cancer. Use of the progestogen challenge test in both estrogen users and untreated post-menopausal women has identified many women at increased risk to develop endometrial adenocarcinoma (17). Eliminating the prescription of unopposed estrogen substitution and controlling body weight, could be other contributions to the prevention of this disease.

2. The development of more sensitive biochemical techniques to identify hormone responsive tumors.

3. Methods for conditioning neoplasms not, or no longer responsive to hormones, to rendering them responsive.

4. Well-designed studies to aid in identifying more effective cytotoxic agents and effective multi-modality therapy in advanced or recurrent endometrial adenocarcinoma and in early stage patients at high risk for recurrent or persistent

disease. Experiences with chemotherapy in endometrial cancer thus far is limited and restricted to advanced or recurrent disease, but results are promising (4,27,34,46).

REFERENCES

1. Aalders, J., Abeler, V., Kolstad, P., Onsrud, M. (1980): Obstet.Gynecol. 56:419.
2. Aalders, J.G. (1982): Doctoral thesis. Dijkstra Niemeyer B.V., Groningen.
3. Aalders, J.G., Sijde, R. van der, Poppema, S., Szabo, B.G., Janssens, J. (1984): Int.J.Radiat.Oncol.Biol.Phys. 10: 2083.
4. Audet-Lapointe, P., Ayoub, J., Méthot, Y., Déry, J.P., Michon, B., Chemaly, R., Guay, J.P., Stanimir, G., Simard, A., Hanley, J., Labrie, F. (1985): In: New surgical trends and integrated therapies in gynecological malignancies, edited by A. Onnis, pp 15-21. Eur.J.Gynaecol.Oncol. series.
5. Bonte, J., Decoster, J.M., Ide, P., and Billiet, G. (1978): Gynecol.Oncol. 6:60-75.
6. Boronow, R.C., Morrow, C.P., Creasman, W.T., Di Saia, P.J., Silverberg, S.G., Miller, A., Blessing, J.A. (1984): Obstet.Gynecol. 63:825-832.
7. Cancer registration in Norway (1973): The incidence of cancer in Norway 1969-1971. The Norwegian Cancer Soc., Oslo.
8. Carlson, J.A., Allegra, J.C., Day, T.G., and Wittliff, J.L. (1984): Am.J.Obstet.Gynecol. 149:149-153.
9. Chen, S.S. (1985): Gynecol.Oncol. 21:23-31.
10. Cook, J.W., and Dodds, E.C. (1931): Nature 131:205.
11. Cramer, D.W., Cutler, S.J., and Christine, B. (1974): Gynecol.Oncol. 2:130.
12. Creasman, W.T., Boronow, R.C., Morrow, C.P., Di Saia, Ph.J., Blessing, J. (1976): Gynecol.Oncol. 4:239.
13. Creasman, W.T., Soper, J.T., McCarty Jr., K.S., McCarthy Sr., K.S., Hinshaw, W., and Clarke-Pearson, D.L. (1985): Am.J.Obstet.Gynecol. 151:922-932.
14. DiSaia, P.J., Creasman, W.T., Boronow, R.C., and Blessing, J.A. (1985): Am.J.Obstet.Gynecol. 115:1009-1015.
15. FIGO (1985): In: Annual Report, edited by F. Patterson, P. Kolstad, H. Ludwig, H. Ulfelder, vol.19, pp 123-136.
16. Freifeld, M.L., Feil, P.D., Bardin, C.W. (1974): Steroids 28:93.
17. Gambrell, R.D., Massey, F.M., Castaneda, T.A., Ugenas, A.J., Ricci, C.A., Wright, J.M. (1980): Obstet.Gynecol.147:872.
18. Greene, H.S.N. (1941): J.Exp.Med. 73:273.
19. Gurpide, E., Holinka, C.F., Deligdisch, L. (1983): In: Steroids and Endometrial Cancer, edited by V.M. Iasonni, I. Nenci, C. Flamigni, pp 127-136. Raven Press, New York.
20. Hsueh, A.J.W., Peck Jr., E.J., Clark, J.H. (1975): Nature 254:337.

21. Jones, H.W. (1975): Obstet.Gynecol.Survey 30:147.
22. Judd, H.L., Shamouki, I.M., Frumar, A.M., Lagasse, L.D. (1982): Obstet.Gynecol. 59:680.
23. Kelley, R.M., and Baker, W.H. (1961): N.Engl.J.Med. 264:216.
24. King, R.J.B., and Whitehead, M.I. (1983): In: Steroids and Endometrial Cancer, edited by V.M. Iasouni, I. Nenci, C. Flamigni, pp 105-116. Raven Press, New York.
25. Kistner, R.W. (1959): Cancer 12:1106.
26. Kjorstad, K.E., Welander, C., Halvorsen, T., Onsrud, T.G. (1978): In: Endometrial Cancer, edited by M.G. Brush, R.J.B. King, R.W. Taylor, p 188. Baillière Tindall, London.
27. Koretz, M., Ballon, S., Friedman, M., Donaldson, S. (1980): NCOG. Proceedings Am.Soc.Clin.Oncol., no. 874.
28. Kottmeier, H.L. (1966): Annual report on the results of treatment in carcinoma of the uterus and vagina (FIGO), vol.14.
29. McLaughlin, D.T., and Richardson, G.S. (1976): J.Clin.Endocrinol.Metab. 42:667-668.
30. O'Malley, B.W. (1971): N.Engl.J.Med. 284:370.
31. Morrow, C.P., Di Saia, P.J., Townsend, D.E. (1973): Obstet. Gynecol. 42:399.
32. Mortel, R., Zaino, R., and Satyaswaroop, G. (1984): Cancer 53:113-116.
33. National Cancer Institute Monograph 41 (1975): Third National Cancer Survey: Incidence Data DHEW Publication No. (NIH) 75-787.
34. de Oliveira, C.F., Burg, M.E.L. van der, and Vermorken, J.B. (1986): EORTC 55833, personal communication.
35. de Palo, G., Merson, M., del Vecchio, M., Mangioni, C., and Periti, P. (1985): Proceedings of ASCO, vol.4, March.
36. Piver, M.S., Barlow, J.J., Lurain, J.R., and Blumenson, L.E. (1980): Cancer 45:268.
37. Podratz, K.C., O'Brien, P.C., Malkasian, G.D., Decker, D.D., Jefferies, J.A., and Edmonson, J.H. (1985): Obstet. Gynecol. 66:106-110.
38. Quinn, M.A., Pearce, P., Fortune, D.W., Koh, S.A., Hsieh, C., Cauchi, M. (1985): Br.J.Obstet.Gynaecol. 92:399-406.
39. Rubin, B.L., Gusberg, S.B., Butterfly, J., Han, T.C., Maralit, M. (1972). Am.J.Obstet.Gynecol. 114:660.
40. Rutledge, F. (1974): Gynecol.Oncol. 2:331.
41. Schmidt-Gollwitzer, M., Genz, T., Schmidt-Gollwitzer, K., et al. (1978): In: Endometrial Cancer, edited by M.G. Brush, R.J.B. King, T.W. Taylor, pp 227-241. Ballière Tindall, London.
42. Siiteri, P.K., MacDonald, P.C. (1973): In: Handbook of Physiology, Secretion 7, Endocrinology, edited by S.R. Geiger, E.B. Astwood, R.O. Greep, American Physiology Society, Washington DC.
43. Silverberg, E. (1986): CA-A Cancer J. for Clin. 36:9-23.
44. Spona, J., Ulm, R., Bieglmayer, C., Husslein, P. (1979).

Gynecol.Obstet.Invest. 10:71-80.

45. Syrjälä, P., Kontula, K., Jänn, O., Kauppilla A and Vihko (1978): In: Endometrial Cancer, edited by M.G. Brush, R.J.B. King, T.W. Taylor, pp 227-241. Ballière Tindall, London.

46. Turbow, M.M., Thornton, J., Ballon, S., et al. (1982): Proceedings Am.Soc.Clin.Oncol. no.420.

47. Wijnen, J.A., and Aalders, J.G. (1983): In: Summaries ESSO Workshop. Farmitalia Carlo Erba, Amsterdam.

48. Wijnen, J.A., and Aalders, J.G. (1985): Surgical staging in endometrial cancer. In: New surgical trends and integrated therapies in gynecological malignancies, edited by A. Onnis, pp 91-94, Eur.J.Gynaecol. Oncol. series.

49. Young, P.C.M., Ehrlich, C.E., Cleary, R.E. (1976): Am.J. Obstet.Gynecol. 125:353.

Hormonal Manipulation of Cancer: Peptides,
Growth Factors, and New (Anti) Steroidal
Agents, edited by Jan G. M. Klijn et al.
Raven Press, New York © 1987.

ALTERNATING AND COMBINED TREATMENT WITH TAMOXIFEN AND
PROGESTINS IN POSTMENOPAUSAL BREAST CANCER

J. Alexieva-Figusch, F.H. de Jong, S.W.J. Lamberts,
A.S.Th. Planting, H.A. van Gilse, M.A. Blankenstein,
J. Blonk-v.d.Wijst and J.G.M. Klijn

Depts. of Int. Medicine and Clinical Endocrinology,
The Dr Daniel den Hoed Cancer Center, P.O.Box 5201, 3008 AE
Rotterdam, and Erasmus University, Rotterdam, The Netherlands

INTRODUCTION

Antiestrogens and progestins are extensively used as single
agent therapy in the treatment of metastatic breast cancer with
response rates of 20-40% and a median duration of response of
10-14 months in unselected groups of patients. Daily oral dosages of 1000 mg for medroxyprogesteron acetate (MPA) or 180 mg
for megestrol acetate (MA) produce therapeutical plasma levels
(> 100 ng/ml) and optimal endocrine effects (2,9). Better beneficial effects of higher doses have not been clearly observed
(29). Selection of patients for hormonal treatment on the basis
of the presence of estrogen and progesterone receptors (ER,
PgR) or disease-free interval (> 2 years) improves the response
rate up to 50-75%. At present these results appear to be the
best possible for hormonal treatment (5,10,18,27).

Although the mechanism of action for any modality of endocrine treatment is not completely understood, it apparently
involves alterations in plasma hormone concentrations and/or
biological effects of hormones through effects on hormone
receptors. In this way, both antiestrogens and progestins may
profoundly influence the hormonal milieu of the tumor cells.

The antiestrogen tamoxifen (TAM) and progestins have partly
synergistic, partly opposite effects on the secretion of different hormones. TAM may produce a decrease in plasma levels of
gonadotropins (LH,FSH) and prolactin (PRL), an increase of sex
hormone binding globulin (SHBG), while estradiol (E2) and testosterone remain unchanged in postmenopausal patients (3,26).
Progestins also produce a decrease of LH and FSH, but sometimes
an increase of PRL, as well as a decrease in plasma concentrations of ACTH, cortisol, sex hormones and SHBG (2,3,25).

It is difficult to separate the direct effects of (anti)hor-
mones on target tissues from indirect effects mediated by
alterations in plasma hormone concentrations. Both TAM and progestins influence also the ER and PgR availability in breast
tumors and may interfere with each other in this respect.
Horwitz et al. (16) demonstrated in vitro that short-term
administration of TAM induces PgR synthesis and proposed that

short pretreatment with antiestrogen may increase the sensitivity of ER positive tumors to subsequent progestin treatment (17). As suggested also by Baulieu et al. (7) this estrogen-progestin relationship may improve clinical results because of the clinical observation that hormonal treatment is most effective in patients with the highest PgR levels in their tumors.

In our previous work we studied the endocrine effects of MA alone (2) and combined with TAM (3). In the present study we compared these results with the endocrine effects of treatment with TAM, alternated with treatment with MPA in an equivalent dose as MA.

AIMS OF THE STUDY

On the basis of the different effects of antiestrogens and progestins on receptor synthesis and turnover and on the hormonal environment, three questions remain to be answered: 1) what are the endocrine effects of combined or alternating treatment with TAM and high dose progestin? 2) can combined or alternating treatment improve the clinical results? 3) cause such treatment less side effect than single treatment?

MATERIAL AND METHODS

In 3 consecutive studies the following selection criteria were used: postmenopausal patients with previously untreated progressive metastatic breast cancer who had a disease-free interval of more than 2 years. In the 3rd study also patients with a shorter disease-free interval were admitted when their tumors were ER or PgR positive.

The treatment schedules were as follows:
1. Single MA treatment (180 mg orally per day) was given during a period of 18 weeks (n=18)
2. Combination MA+TAM (180 and 40 mg respectively): responders to MA after 6 weeks of treatment received a combination of MA+TAM during the next 6-week period (n=6)
3. Alternating TAM/MPA: patients received at least 3 courses consisting of 1-week 2x10 mg TAM daily followed by 3 weeks of 1000 mg MPA orally per day (n=27)

Before and during the treatment period plasma levels of PRL, gonadotropins, E2, SHBG and 11-deoxy-cortisol were measured. The methods used have been described previously (21).

RESULTS

1. Endocrine effects

Prolactin

PRL levels were measured before and 30' after stimulation with TRH (200 µg i.v.). Single MA treatment increased mean basal plasma PRL significantly (from 7.1 to 13.9 ng/ml) after 6 weeks of treatment (2). There was also a hyperresponse of PRL to TRH. This effect was reproduced in a second study (3). However, addition of TAM to MA abolished the hyperresponse of PRL to TRH stimulation. In our third study concerning alternating therapy the initial lowering of plasma PRL after one week of treatment with TAM disappeared and PRL levels increased with time (Fig.1, p < 0.02) as observed during single progestin treatment.

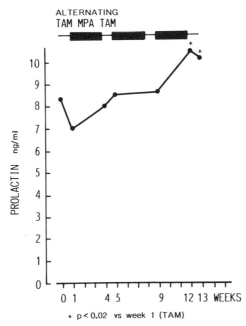

FIG.1. Mean basal prolactin levels before and during alternating therapy with tamoxifen and medroxyprogesterone acetate.

In preclinical studies PRL appeared to stimulate the growth of mammary tumor cells. Although in women hyperprolactinemia has not been proven to be related with an increased risk for developing manifest breast cancer, it appeared that hyperprolactinemia in patients with early or metastatic breast cancer is an unfavorable prognostic factor with respect to treatment response and survival (11,15).

There is no equivocal evidence, however, that lowering of plasma PRL concentrations in itself is of benefit in the treatment of metastatic breast cancer, although there are indications that lowering of plasma PRL might correspond with clinical improvement (13,15).

In our group of patients, treated with single MA therapy there was a tendency towards higher basal PRL levels at 0 and 6 weeks in patients who did not respond to progestin treatment compared to responding patients (Fig.2, p < 0.10) (2). This was more evident in the group of patients treated with the alternating scheme (Fig.2), where the difference in basal PRL between responders and non-responders at time 0 became significant (p < 0.05) confirming hyperprolactinemia as an unfavorable prognostic factor with respect to treatment response. However, in this latter study it was also found that after 12-13 weeks of treatment no difference in basal PRL was present between responders and non-responders.

Gonadotropins
The suppression of LH and FSH was more pronounced during combination or alternating treatment (about 80%) than during single progestin treatment (about 60%) (Fig.3).

Estradiol
Single treatment with MA caused a significant decrease of plasma estradiol (p < 0.001), which was not further influenced by addition of TAM in the combination scheme. However, if results were considered as % of the pretreatment value, alternating treatment resulted in a more pronounced suppression (37%) of mean plasma estradiol level at week 12-13, compared to that after 6 weeks (23%) and after 12 weeks (12%) of treatment with MA alone.

SHBG
While a significant decrease of SHBG (p < 0.001) (Fig.5) was found after 6 weeks of MA treatment, an increase in low SHBG levels during this treatment was found after addition of TAM to MA. In the alternating scheme of TAM/MPA treatment the SHBG increased during the TAM treatment period and decreased during the MPA period. This effect might be attributed to the (anti)-estrogenic properties of TAM as well as to the (anti-)androgenic properties of MPA.

11-deoxycortisol (compound S)
Chronic treatment with MA alone completely suppressed 11-deoxycortisol plasma concentrations before and after 6x750 mg metyrapone orally (p < 0.001) (Fig.6) (2). During combination treatment plasma cortisol remained unchanged in comparison to the results during single MA treatment (3); 11-deoxycortisol was not measured in this study. During alternating treatment partial reversibility of pituitary-adrenal function suppression appeared to be present after one week cessation of MPA treatment as measured by stimulated 11-deoxycortisol (metyrapone test) and basal androstenedione levels (Fig.6). This partial recovery of adrenal function decreased in time, i.e. after 3 months of treatment it was smaller than after one month.

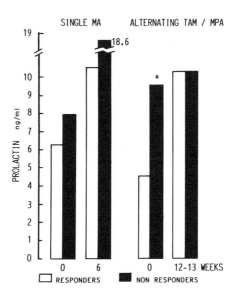

FIG.2. Basal plasma prolactin of responders versus non-responders is shown during MA therapy at time 0 and 6 weeks, and before and after 12-13 weeks of alternating TAM/MPA therapy.

* = $p < 0.05$

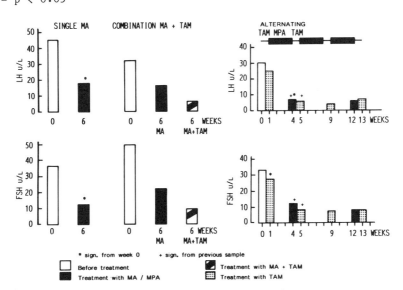

FIG.3. Gonadotropins LH/FSH were measured before and after 6 weeks of therapy with MA or combination MA+TAM, and during alternating TAM/MPA therapy at 1,4,5,9,12,13 weeks.

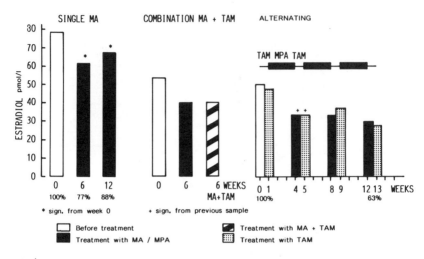

FIG.4. Plasma estradiol was measured before and after 6 weeks of therapy with MA or combination MA+TAM, and during alternating TAM/MPA therapy at 1,4,5,8,9,12 and 13 weeks.

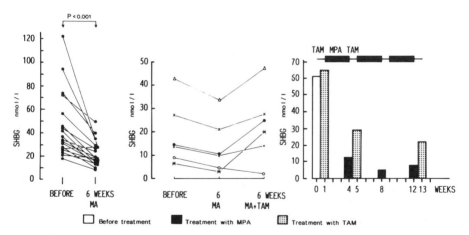

FIG.5. Plasma sex hormone binding globulin levels were measured before and after 6 weeks of therapy with MA or combination MA+TAM, and during alternating TAM/MPA therapy at 1,4,5,8,12 and 13 weeks.

2. Antitumor effects

In a previous study (1) we observed in 160 unselected patients with metastatic disease that the therapeutical results of single progestin treatment are the same as would be expected from any hormonal treatment, i.e. a response rate of circa 30%.

In our endocrine study during single MA treatment in 18

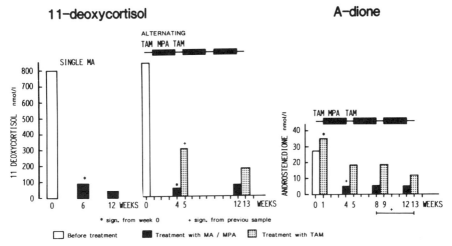

FIG.6.   Concentrations of stimulated plasma 11-deoxycortisol
were measured before, and after 6 and 12 weeks of MA therapy;
and during alternating TAM/MPA therapy at 4,5,12 and 13 weeks.
Further, during alternating TAM/MPA therapy also the concentrations of androstenedione were estimated at time 0,1,4,5,8,
9,12 and 13 weeks.

selected patients, complete and partial remission occurred in
55% (mean duration 10 months). No change was observed in 22% of
patients (20 months) (Table 1). The treatment was very well
tolerated; in one patient the drug was withdrawn because of
thromboembolism.

TABLE 1.   Clinical results of

	single therapy MA (N=18)	alternating TAM/MPA (N=26)
Complete + partial remission (mean duration in months)	55% (10)[*]	50% (15[+])[*]
No change	22% (20)[*]	34% (7[+])[*]
Failure	22%	16%

+   still on treatment
*   mean duration of response in months

    The clinical effect of combination treatment (MA+TAM) could
not be evaluated. Only 6 responders to MA were treated with the
combination, making the group too small to allow judgment of
response.
    The clinical results of alternating treatment (TAM/MPA)

permitted a preliminary analysis after 2 years of follow-up. Out of 27 treated patients 26 were evaluable. Complete and partial remissions were reached in 50% (mean duration 15+ months), and stable disease in 34% of patients (7+ months). Six patients are still under treatment with a maximal follow-up of 24 months.

3. Side effects

Progestins and TAM are very well tolerated drugs. Main side effects are weight gain and thromboembolism mainly during treatment with progestins. In the study concerning alternating treatment the side effects of the progestin treatment appeared to be predominant. In 5 patients we had to stop MPA treatment because of stomach perforation, gastric bleeding, disregulation of diabetes mellitus, angina pectoris, and a mental disorder with muscle cramps respectively. These side effects are probably caused by the glucocorticosteroid properties of high dose progestin treatment.

DISCUSSION

In a first report on single MA treatment in a large series of 160 patients with metastatic breast cancer we showed a response rate of 30% with a median duration of response of 9 months (1). Comparable results of high dose progestin treatment have been published by other groups using MA or MPA (review 18).

In a next study concerning sequential treatment with TAM and MA (and vice versa) it appeared that MA is more suitable as second line treatment because MA treatment is more effective after tamoxifen than tamoxifen treatment after MA (4). The same observation for sequential treatment with TAM and MPA has been described by others (18,22,32). Nevertheless, there was no difference in overall duration of response and in survival between the two sequences of endocrine therapy.

With regard to the endocrine effects in our study concerning combination therapy with simultaneous drug regimens it seemed that addition of TAM to MA could be more favourable than single progestin treatment; especially with respect to further lowering of plasma gonadotropins and estrogen concentrations and abolishment of the stimulatory effects of MA on PRL secretion. Trodella et al. (31) found an unexpected high response rate (44%) with combined TAM/progestin treatment in heavily pretreated patients. However, in a study comparing the efficacy of TAM with combined TAM plus (relatively low dose) MPA treatment in 101 patients with advanced breast cancer, Mouridson et al. (23) found that the drug combination provided no better results than treatment with TAM alone. Since both TAM and MPA influence the ER and PgR availability in a tumor (in sense of decrement during long-term treatment), the effects of the two drugs may have interfered with each other.

However, short-term TAM treatment of about 4-7 days stimulates PgR synthesis in vitro (7,16,24) and in about half of the patients with ER positive tumors in vivo (6) probably by its estrogenic properties. Iacobelli found an additive inhibition of CG-5 breast cancer cells proliferation in vitro by combined use of TAM and MPA (19,20). Furthermore, he showed an increase of the antiproliferative effect of MPA from 50 to 80% after pretreatment of the cells with TAM during 6 days (20). In a clinical study a rise in PgR content of tumors after one week TAM treatment appeared a reliable indication of hormone dependence i.e. 90% (6).

In our study we showed also a favorable effect of alternating TAM-MPA treatment on plasma hormone concentrations for LH, FSH, PRL and E2. Therefore the combined favourable effects both on the endocrine milieu and on receptor status during alternating treatment might improve therapeutical results. Efficient dose-schedule regimens with antiestrogens and progestin administration are yet to be established. On the basis of the studies mentioned above we have chosen for one week TAM followed by 3 weeks MPA trying to reach optimal PgR synthesis and less side effects of progestins. A number of variations in alternating TAM-progestin treatment schedules has been used by others especially with respect to the duration of "pretreatment" with TAM (1-8 weeks) and to application of a period without any treatment (8,12,14,28,30). In 27 patients we observed an objective response rate of 50% which is comparable with the 55% response reported by Bosset (8) who used a scheme of 30 mg TAM/day x 7 days followed by MPA 600 mg/day x 7 days. However, the duration of response appeared shorter in their study (5-12 months) than in our study ($\bar{x}$ = 15$^+$ months). Using another alternating treatment scheme Steindorfer (30) reported an objective response rate of 70% in 44 patients. In a preliminary comparative study Pouillart (28) found a significant higher response rate during alternating treatment when compared to effects of TAM alone (73% vs. 50%) but this significance disappeared (12) later on (60 vs. 48%). However, the mean duration of response remained significantly longer during alternating treatment (about 17 vs. 10 months). Finally, in another comparative study Gundersen (14) also found a higher response rate during alternating 8 weeks TAM/8 weeks MPA treatment (58%) than during single TAM treatment (39%) without difference in duration of response.

In conclusion: Hormonal manipulation of tumor cells by alternating treatment with TAM and high dose progestins seems attractive both on the basis of the influence on the endocrine milieu and on steroid receptor status as well as based on some phase II and small comparative studies. However, large randomized phase III studies are needed to prove whether such manipulation is indeed of clinical benefit for our patients.

REFERENCES

1. Alexieva-Figusch, J., Van Gilse, H.A., Hop, W.C.J., Phoa,
    C.H., Blonk-v.d.Wijst, J., and Treurniet, R.E. (1980):
    Cancer, 46:2369-2372.
2. Alexieva-Figusch, J., Blankenstein, M.A., Hop, W.C.J.,
    Klijn, J.G.M., Lamberts, S.W.J., De Jong, F.H., Docter,
    R., Adlercreutz, H., and Van Gilse, H.A. (1984): Eur.J.
    Cancer Clin.Oncol., 20:33-40.
3. Alexieva-Figusch, J., Blankenstein, M.A., De Jong, F.H.,
    and Lamberts, S.W.J. (1984): Eur.J.Cancer Clin.Oncol.,
    20: 1135-1140.
4. Alexieva-Figusch, J., van Putten, W.L.J. , van Gilse, H.A.,
    Blonk-v.d. Wijst, J., and Klijn, J.G.M. (1985): Med.
    Oncol. Tumor Pharmacother., 2:69-75.
5. Alexieva-Figusch, J., van Putten, W.L.J., Blankenstein,
    M.A., Blonk-van der Wijst, J., and Klijn, J.G.M. (1986):
    submitted.
6. Barnes, D.M., Howell, A., Harland, R.N.L., Baildam, A.D.,
    Suridell, R., and Sellwood, R.A. (1986): Eur. J. Cancer
    Clin. Oncol., 22:740.
7. Baulieu, E.E. (1983): In: Role of medroxyprogesterone in
    endocrine related tumors, vol.II, edited by L. Campio,
    G. Robustelli Dela Cuna, and R.W. Taylor, pp 15-19,
    Raven Press, New York.
8. Bosset, J.F., Pereal, M., Hurteloup, P., Altwegg, T.,
    Schraub, S., del Piano, F., and Colette, C. (1982):
    Bull. Cancer (Paris) 69:170-171.
9. Camaggi, C.M. (1982): In: Proceedings of the International
    Symposium on Medroxyprogesterone Acetate, edited by F.
    Cavalli, W.L. McGuire, F. Panutti, A. Pellegrini, and G.
    Robustelli Della Cuna, pp 185-189, Excerpta Medica,
    Amsterdam.
10. Cowan, K., and Lippman, M. (1982): Arch.Intern.Med., 142:
    363-366.
11. Dowsett,M., McGarrick,G.E., Harris,A.L., Coombes,R.C.,Smith
    I.E., and Jeffcoate,S.L.(1983): Br.J.Cancer,47:763-769.
12. Garcia-Giralt, E., Jouve, M., Palangie, T., Bretandeau, B.,
    Asselain, B., Magdelenat, H., Merle, S., Zajdela, A.,
    and Pouillart, P. (1984): In: Abstract book of 2nd Int.
    Symp. on Antihormones in Breast Cancer, edited by G.A.
    Nagel, p 116, ICI, Berlin, 21-24 October.
13. Grisoli, F., Vincentelli, F., Foa, J., Lavail, G., and
    Salamon, G. (1981): Lancet, 2:745-746.
14. Gundersen, S. (1984): In: Abstract book of 2nd Int.Symp. on
    Antihormones in Breast Cancer, edited by G.A. Nagel, p
    118, ICI, Berlin, 21-24 October.
15. Holtkamp, W., Wander, H.E., von Heyden, D., Rauschecker,
    and H.F., Nagel, G.A. (1983): J. Steroid Biochem.,
    19:153S.
16. Horwitz, K.B., Koseki, Y., and McGuire, W.L. (1978):

Endocrinol., 103:1742-1751.

17. Horwitz, K.B., and Freidenberg, G.R. (1985): Cancer Res., 45:167-173.

18. Horwitz, K.B., Wei, L.L., Sedlacek, S.M., and D'Arville, C.N. (1985): Recent Progress Horm. Res., 41:249-317.

19. Iacobelli, S., Natoli, C., Sica, G., and Marchetti, P. (1982): In: Proceedings Int. Symp. on Medroxyproges-terone Acetate, edited by F. Cavalli, W.L. McGuire, F. Panutti, A. Pellegrini, and G. Robustelli Della Cuna, pp 80-88, Excerpta Medica, Amsterdam.

20. Iacobelli, S., Natoli, C., and Scambia, G. (1983): J. Steroid Biochem. 19, suppl: 191 S.

21. Klijn, J.G.M., Lamberts, S.W.J., de Jong, F.H., Docter, R., van Dongen, K.J., and Birkenhäger, J.C. (1980): Clin. Endocrinol., 12:341-355.

22. Mattsson, W. (1980): In "Role of Medroxyprogesterone in Endocrine-Related Tumors" edited by S. Iacobelli and A. Di Marco, pp 65-71, Raven Press, New York.

23. Mouridsen, H.T., Ellemann, K., Mattsson, W., Palshof, T., Daehnfeldt, J.L., and Rose, C. (1979): Cancer Treat. Rep., 63:171-175.

24. Namer, M., Lalanne, C., Baulieu, E.E. (1980): Cancer Res., 40:1750-1752.

25. Pannuti, F., Martoni, A., Camaggi, C.M., Strocchi, E., Di Marco, A.R., Rossi, A.P., Tomasi, L., Giovannini, M., Cricca, A., Fruet, F., Lelli, G., Giambiasi, M.E. and Canova, N. (1982): In: Proceedings of the Int.Symp. on Medroxyprogesterone Acetate, edited by F. Cavalli, W.L. McGuire, F. Pannuti, A. Pellegrini, and G. Robustelli Della Cuna, pp 5-43, Excerpta Medica, Amsterdam.

26. Patterson, J.S. (1981): J. Endocr., 89:67P-75P.

27. Pearson, O.H., Hubay, C.A., Gordon, N.H., and McGuire, W.L. (1985): In: Hormonally Responsive Tumors, edited by V.P. Hollander, pp 487-506, Academic Press, New York.

28. Pouillart, P., Jouve, M., Palangie, T., Giralt, E., Bretandean, B., Asselain, B. and Magdelenat, H. (1983): J. Steroid Biochem., 19, Suppl.: 191 S.

29. Robustelli Della Cuna, G., Bernardo-Strada, M.R., and Ganzina, F. (1982): In: Proceedings of the Int.Symp. on Medroxyprogesterone Acetate, edited by F. Cavalli, W.L. McGuire, F. Panutti, A. Pellegrini, and G. Robustelli Della Cuna, pp 290-305, Excerpta Medica, Amsterdam.

30. Steindorfer, P., Neubauer, W. and Pierer, G. (1984): In: Abstract book of 2nd International Symposium on Anti-hormones in Breast Cancer, edited by G.A. Nagel, p 117, ICI, Berlin, 21-24 October.

31. Trodella, L., Ausilli-Cefaro, G.P., Turriziani, A., Saccheri, S., Venturo, I., and Minotti, G. (1982): Am. J. Clin. Oncol., 5:495-499.

32. Van Veelen, H., Willemse, P.H.B., Tjabbes, T., Schweitzer, M.J.H., and Sleijfer D.Th. (1986): Cancer, 58:7-13.

Hormonal Manipulation of Cancer: Peptides, Growth Factors, and New (Anti) Steroidal Agents, edited by Jan G. M. Klijn et al. Raven Press, New York © 1987.

PROLACTIN RECEPTORS IN BREAST CANCER :

IMPORTANCE OF THE MEMBRANE PREPARATION.

M. L'Hermite-Balériaux, S. Casteels, and M. L'Hermite.

Laboratoire de Recherche du Service de Gynécologie et Obstétrique, Université Libre de Bruxelles Hopital Brugmann, 4 place Van Gehuchten, 1020 Bruxelles, Belgium.

The role of pituitary hormones in the pathogenesis of human breast cancer remains still not fully elucidated. At the present time it is well known that, in mammals, prolactin (PRL) is primarily involved in the regulation of reproductive functions, especially in the development of the mammary gland and in the establishment and the maintenance of lactation. Following its binding to plasma membrane receptors, several effects within the cell can be observed, even at the nuclear level (10,15).

Prolactin-receptors (PRL R) have been identified not only in the target tissues where it exerts its biological action (mammary gland, ovary, testes) but also in other organs (liver, adrenals, brain, lungs, pancreas, kidney) and this in various animal species.

In animal species such as the rat and the mice, the prominent role played by PRL in the etiology and the physiopathology of mammary cancer is widely established (1, 4, 29). The regulation of PRL R in these circumstances was also investigated (13, 30).

In a number of established human breast cancer cell lines maintained in long term tissue culture, PRL R could be evidenced and characterized (43). Their modulation by steroid hormones, peptide hormones and new unknown factors is now largely investigated (8, 12, 33, 40). Also, since now about 10 years, the existence of PRL R in human mammary tumors has been demonstrated (14, 15, 24, 32) but, surprisingly, it is only recently that Malarkey et al. (20) demonstrated that physiological concentrations of PRL could promote the growth of some breast tumor cells in culture. An interrelationship between high levels of PRL and the incidence of breast cancer could be established in certain circumstances but not in others (reviewed in 18).

Several authors investigated in breast cancer the interrelationship between the presence of steroid hormone receptors and PRL levels as well as PRL R (5, 25, 34, 35, 45). While the clinical implications linked (28) to the presence of steroid receptors are now firmly established, the importance of the presence of PRL R remains to be confirmed, especially whether it could have some therapeutical consequences.

Since the first publication of Holdaway et al. (14) in 1977, several techniques have been proposed for the determination of PRL R in human breast tumors. Until now there is no general agreement about the methodology to be used : incubation conditions are sometimes quite different. The hormone used for label (hGH, hPRL or oPRL) seems to play a major role, as well as the labeling technique used.

The aim of the present study was to compare three different membrane preparation techniques, using always oPRL for PRL R determination, and to look if any correlation could be established between estrogen receptors (ER) and/or progesterone receptors (PgR) and PRL R.

MATERIAL AND METHODS.

Tumors.
Tumors of 199 patients were tested. One male patient was included in this group. The tumors were freed of fat and stored as soon as possible in liquid nitrogen.

Preparation of membranes.
Tumors were pulverised. The volume of buffer used for homogenation was always 5 times the weight of the tumor.
The membranes were then prepared according to one of the procedures detailed in Table 1.

TABLE 1. Conditions of membrane preparation : according to (a) Shiu et al. (42); (b) Martin et al. (22); (c) Bonneterre et al. (3)

	a	b	c
Buffer			
Tris (mM)	10	10	20
Sucrose (M)	0.3		
EDTA (mM)		1.5	3
Thioglycerol (mM)		12	
Glycerol %		10	
Dithiotreitol (mM)			1
pH	7.4	7.4	7.8
Centrifugations & time (min)			
600 - 800 g	10'	–	10'
10,000 - 15,000 g	30'	20'	
100,000 g	90'	60'	90'

Protocol a refers to the classic membrane preparation technique of Shiu et al. (42). The 100,000 g pellet is immediately resuspended in assay buffer (Tris 25 mM, 10 mM MgCl2, pH 7.6) and stored in liquid nitrogen until assay.

Protocol b refers to the membrane preparation technique used in our laboratory (22) for the determination of ER and PgR. After the 100,000 g centrifugation, the supernatant is immediately used for steroid receptor assay and the pellet is stored in liquid nitrogen without being resuspended in buffer. Resuspension is performed at the time the PRL R are determined.

Protocol c refers to the methodology of Bonneterre et al. (3).
In this case the 15,000 g centrifugation is omitted. The 100,000 g pellets are resuspended in the assay buffer and stored in liquid nitrogen until assayed for PRL R.

The membrane preparations were not stored longer than two months and never frozen twice.

Reference membrane preparation : Late pregnant rabbit mammary glands or female rat livers, treated according to protocol a, were used as reference in order to check the quality of the labeled hormone.

Protein concentrations were measured following the method of Lowry et al. (19), using serum albumin as standard.

Hormones.
oPRL (AFP-4328C) was a gift of the NIADDK. This same oPRL preparation was used for iodination and for displacement study. The hormone (5 µg oPRL) was iodinated with 1 µCi of 125I (IMS 300, Amersham), using low concentrations of chloramine T (16). The specific activities varied between 52 to 82 µCi/µg.

Binding assay.
Approximatively 100,000 cpm of 125I oPRL were incubated with tumor membrane preparations (+ 300 µg proteins) in a final volume of 0.5 ml buffer (Tris 25 mM, 10 mM MgCl2, 0.1 % BSA). The incubation was performed overnight at room temperature and it was stopped by the addition of 3 ml ice cold buffer. The tubes were centrifuged at 1,500 g for 30 min at 4 C. After decantation the pellets were counted in an LKB gamma spectrometer.

Specific binding (SpB) was calculated as the difference between the radioactivity bound in the absence (Total binding: TB) and in the presence of an excess of 1 ug oPRL (non specific binding: NSpB). These data were then expressed as the percentage of the total radioactivity added. The membrane preparation was tested in duplicate. Only at two occasions could displacement curves be set up : one case was a female patient with an infiltrating duct carcinoma, the other case was a male patient with a poorly differentiated infiltrating carcinoma. The affinity constant (Ka) and the binding capacity (N) were derived from Scatchard plots.

ER and PgR assays.

Tumors treated according to procedures a and b had their ER and PgR measured according to the dextran coated charcoal method used in this laboratory (22). For tumors treated according to procedure c, the ER and PgR were determined by the technique of Noel et al. (31). Tumors were considered positive if at least 10 fmol/mg protein could be detected.

RESULTS

The TB varied between 4.9 to 14.9 % and the NSpB ranged from 4.3 to 13.1 %. Taking into consideration a number of factors such as counting errors, experimental errors, variation of the quality of the labeled hormone, a tumor was only considered positive when the SpB was at least 0.8 %.

The overall results showed that ,out of the 199 human breast tumors analysed, 38 cases had a SpB between 0.8 and 3 %. The overall rate of positive cases thus is 19 %.

TABLE 2. PRL R in human breast tumors according to the membrane preparation used.

	a	b	c
Number of tumors investigated (n=199)	23	131	45
PRL R positive	8	19	11
(%)	34 %	14.5 %	24 %

From Table 2, it appears that procedure b, in which the largest number of cases were analysed (n = 131), reveals the smallest number of positive cases (n = 19; 14.5 %). A $\chi 2$ test performed between groups a and c, and between groups b and c, did not reveal any statistically significant difference. But statistical analyse shows that procedure a allows to detect significantly more positive cases than procedure b (p < 0.02).

In the two cases for which enough material was available the tumors were treated according to protocol a and displacement curves could be set up. The tumor of the female patient revealed to have a Ka of 1.1 10-9 M with N = 20.2 fmol/mg protein. In the case of the male patient the Ka was 4.16 10-9 M but N was only 4.1 fmol/mg protein. The Ka of these two tumors were in the range of those observed with pregnant rabbit mammary gland membrane preparations (18).

TABLE 3. Distribution of PRL R positive and negative tumors in 164 cases according to the presence or absence of the steroid receptors.

	ER+		ER-	
	PgR+	PgR-	PgR+	PgR-
PRL R+ n = 33	14(8.5%)	4(2.4%)	9(5.4%)	6(3.6%)
PRL R- n=131	60(36.5%)	17(10.3%)	18(10.9%)	36(21.9%)

Table 3 shows the distribution of the presence of PRL R positive and negative tumors in 164 tumors in which steroid receptors analyses were also available. The highest amount of PRL R+ tumors (8.5 %) was associated with ER+ and PgR+ tumors. But also the highest amount of PRL R- tumors was associated with ER+ and PgR+ tumors (36.5 %). In a few cases of ER- and PgR- tumors, PRL R could be detected (3.6 %). In 16.4 % of the PRL R+ tumors at least one steroid receptor was positive.

DISCUSSION

In the last few years several reports (7, 25, 46) confirmed the fact that human breast tumors contained low but measurable levels of PRL R. The results are rather controversial due to the different techniques used to evidence PRL R. As shown previously and confirmed in this report, several points are crucial : 1) the membrane preparation technique, 2) the label (oPRL, hGH, hPRL) used for the displacement and saturation studies, 3) the interpretation of the results.

Thus the results are quite different when the threshold limit for positive PRL R is put at 0.5 % (7), 0.8 % (3), 1 % (25) or 3 % (2). This remark is also valid for correlations established between the presence of ER, PgR and that of PRL R. If the threshold limit for positivity for ER is put at 3 fmol/mg protein (25) or at 50 fmol/mg protein (35), the interpretation of the data becomes quite different.

Di Carlo et al (7), using a membrane preparation technique similar to the one used by Shiu et al. (42) and by us (protocol a), reported a PRL SpB of 0.5 % or more in 49 % of their tumors and of 30 % in benign breast tumors. In their assay the label used was hPRL. These data are rather similar to ours, when considering that oPRL is not the optimal hormone to be used for such investigations (18).

Turcot-Lemay et al. (46), analysed more than 759 human breast tumors: they showed clearly that when oPRL was used as label, 13 % of the tumors had a SpB superior to 1 %, while with labeled hGH only 2 % of the tumors could be considered positive.   These authors were using the membrane pellet left over from the cytosolic preparation for ER and PgR.   Our data with a similar membrane preparation technique (protocol b) are identical.   It appears thus that this membrane preparation technique in not optimal since it gives the lowest percentage of PRL R positive tumors.

Considering the fact that human breast tumors are now detected when still very small, thus when very little material is available, the goal of this study was to investigate if one single method for cytosol and membrane preparation, could be set up and allow to detect ER, PgR and PRL R from the same initial tissue specimen.   At the light of the low percentage of PRL R positive tumors, it could be postulated that either the PRL R is degraded or   not isolated in sufficient amounts to be detected when this technique is used.

Peyrat et al. (35), using a cut off limit of 0.8 % between NSpB and SpB, reported that 49 % of their tumors where positive. The label used was hGH.   Our results with this membrane preparation technique (protocol c) but with oPRL as label, allowed us to detect only 24 % of positive tumors.

Murphy et al. (25) reported the highest incidence (65 %) so far published despite the use of hGH as label and a positive limit for SpB at 1 %.   Their membrane preparation technique is rather different than all previously published; it requires large amounts of tumoral tissue; but only 75 to 100 ug of membrane proteins as well as 30,000 cpm of hGH are used.   These data are rather conflicting with those of Peyrat et al. (36) who were using high amounts of label hGH (200,000 cpm) and 400 ug of purified membrane proteins in their study investigating the optimal conditions for characterization of human PRL R.

Only a single report by Murphy et al (25) demonstrated a clearly linear correlation between ER concentration and the SpB of PRL to membrane preparations of human breast cancer biopsies.   Such a correlation between ER and PRL R had been previously repeatedly reported (3, 38, 45), but several investigators failed to evidence such a correlation (14, 34).   These discrepencies could perhaps be related to the use of different labeled hormones and to the interpretation of the data.   That we could not find any statistically significant correlation can be due to the use of oPRL. Alternatively or in addition, it can be the result of different methods used to measure and the PRL R as well as the ER and PgR.

It should be mentioned that, out of 33 PRL R positive tumors, 27 were associated with at least one positive steroid receptor.   The striking detection of some PRL R positive tumors which lack of steroid receptors, could be explained by the fact that hGH or other peptides might also be involved in the regulation of PRL R.   In 1974, Costlow et al (5) reported already that, in some rat mammary tumors, PRL R could be detected but ER were absent.

Peyrat et al. (37) investigated whether the presence of PRL R could be considered as an index of mammary cancer cells sensitivity to PRL. They observed a stimulation of DNA synthesis by PRL in only 29 % of the cases with PRL R. Stimulation never occurred, however, in the absence of PRL R, and no correlation could be demonstrated between the response to PRL and the ER and PgR levels. Comparable results have been similarly reported by others (9, 23, 41, 47). Here also the amount of hormone put in the culture medium as well as the nature of the lactogenic hormone used, seemed to be essential. Since DNA synthesis could be induced by PRL in only 29 % of their 55 % PRL R positive tumors (37), it suggests that the presence of PRL R is mandatory but not sufficient for PRL to exhibit any effect.

Several growth factors have been isolated and characterized; their role in cancer is now largely established (see review in 12). They may act as autocrine and paracine factors, not only to stimulate but also to inhibit the growth of breast cancer cells, as reported in vitro (11, 40, 44, 48). Correlations between hormone dependency and the regulation of these growth factors in human mammary carcinoma cells is now under investigation (8, 26, 39). The role of the pituitary hormones in the growth of human breast cancer has been established for several years (33), but other novel pituitary factors might also be implicated in the etiology of human breast cancer (6, 17). The mechanisms of action of these factors on the regulation of PRL R remain to be established; it might lead to elucidate properly the role played by PRL in breast carcinogenesis (21, 27).

ACKNOWLEDGMENTS

We thank the NIAMDD (Bethesda, Md, USA) for generous gift of ovine PRL; the medical and nursing staff of the departement for the specimens of tumors; A. Vokaer and J.P. Lescrainier (ULB) as well as G. Noel (UCL) for Er and PgR determinations; Mrs. Cl. Bekaert for skilfull edition of the manuscript.

REFERENCES

1. Aylsworth, C.F., Van Vugt, D.A., Sylvester, P.W., and Meites, J., (1984) : Cancer Res., 44 : 2835-2840.
2. Bohnet H.G. (1980) : Arch. Gynecol., 229 : 333-344.
3. Bonneterre, J., Peyrat, J.Ph., Vandewalle, B., Beuscart, R., Vie, M.C., and Cappelaere, P. (1982) : Eur. J. Cancer Clin. Oncol., 18 : 1157-1162.
4. Briand, P., (1983) : Anticancer Res., 3 : 273-282.
5. Costlow, M.E., Bushow, R.A., and Mc Guire, W.L., (1974) : Science, 184 : 85-86.
6. Dembinski, Th.C., Leung, Cl.K.H., and Shiu, R.P.C., (1985) : Cancer Res., 45 : 3083-3089.
7. Di Carlo, R., Muccioli, G., and Di Carlo, F. (1983); in : Endo-

crinology of Cystic Breast Disease, edited by Angeli, A., Bradlow, H.L., and L. Dogliotti, pp. 211-218. Raven Press. New-York.

8. Dickson, R.B., Huff, K.K., Spencer, E.M., and Lippman M.E., (1985) : Endocrinology, 118 : 138-142.

9. Dilley, W.G., and Kister, S.J. (1975) : J. Natl. Cancer Inst., 55 : 35-36.

10. Djiane, J., Kelly, P.A., Katch, M. and Dusantes-Fourt, J., (1985) : Hormone Res., 22 : 179-188.

11. Furlanetto, R.W., and Di Carlo, J.N. (1984) : Cancer Res., 44 : 2122-2128.

12. Goustin, A.Sc., Leof, E.B., Shipley, G.D., and Moses, H., (1986) : Cancer Res., 46 : 1015-1029.

13. Holdaway, I.M., and Friesen, H.G. (1976) : Cancer Res., 36 : 1562-1567.

14. Holdaway, I.M., and Friesen, H.G. (1977) : Cancer Res., 37 : 1946-1952.

15. Houdebine, L.M. (1983) : Ann. Endocr., 44 : 85-100.

16. Kuo-Jang, and Ramirez, V.D. (1978) : J. Endocrinol. Invest., 1 : 233-238.

17. Leung, Cl.K.H., and Shiu, R.P.C. (1981) : Cancer Res., 41 : 546-551.

18. L'Hermite-Balériaux, M., Casteels, S., Vokaer,A., Loriaux,C., Noel, G., and L'Hermite, M., (1984) : In : Progress in Cancer Research and Therapy. Ed. Bresciani, F., King R.J.B., Lippman, M., Namer, M., Raynaud, J.P., vol. 31, pp. 325-3347.

19. Lowry, O.H., Rosebrough, N.J., Farr, A., and Randall, R.J. (1951) : J. Biol. Chem., 193 : 265-275.

20. Malarkey, W.B., Kennedy, M., Albred, L.E., and Milo, G. (1983) : J. Clin. Endocrinol. Metab., 56 : 673-677.

21. Manni, A., Pontari, M., and Wright, C., (1985) : Endocrinology, 117 : 2040-2043.

22. Martin, P.M., Rolland, P.H., Jacuemier, J., Rolland, A.M., and Toga, M. (1978) : Biomedecine, 28 : 278-287.

23. Masters, J.R.W., Sangster, K., Smith, H., and Forrest, A.P.M. (1976) : Br. J. Cancer, 33 : 564-566.

24. Morgan, L., Raggatt, P.R., de Souza, I., Salih, H., and Hobbs, J.R. (1977) : J. Endocrinol., 73 : 17P-18P.

25. Murphy, L.J., Murphy, L.C., Vrhovsek, E., Sutherland, H.L., and Lazarus, L., (1984) : Cancer Res., 44 : 1963-1968.

26. Murphy, L.J., Vrhovsek, E., Sutherland, R.L., and Lazarus, L. (1984) : J. Clin. Endocrinol. Metab., 58 : 149-155.

27. Murphy, L.J., Sutherland, R.L., Stead, B., Murphy, L.C., and Lazarus, L., (1986) : Cancer Res., 46 : 728-734.

28. Nagai, R., Kataoka, M., Kobayashi, S., Ishihara, K., Tobioka, N., Nakashima, K., Naruse, M., Saito, K., and sakuma, S., (1979) : Cancer Res., 39 : 1835-1840.

29. Nagasawa, H., (1983) : Life Sci., 33 : 1451-1455.

30. Nagasawa, H., Sakai, S., and Banerjee, M.R. (1979) : Life Sci., 24 : 193-208.

31. Noel, G., and Maisin, H. (1981) : Arch. Int. Phyiol. Biochem., 89 : B189-B190.

32. Partridge, R.K., and Hahnel, R. (1979) : Cancer, 43 : 643-646.

33. Pearson, O.H., Manni, A., Chambers, M., Brodkey, J., and Marshall, J.S. (1978) : Cancer Res., 38 : 4323-4326.
34. Pearson, O.H., Manni, A., Chambers, M., Brodkey, J., and Marshall, J.S. (1978) : Cancer Res., 38 : 4326-4328.
35. Peyrat, J.P., Dewailly, D., Djiane, J., Kelly, P.A., Vandewalle, B., Bonneterre, J., and Lefebvre J., (1982) : Breast Cancer Res. and Treat., 1 : 369-373.
36. Peyrat, J.P., Djiane, J., Kelly, P.A., Vandewalle, B., Bonneterre, J. and Demaille, A., (1984) : Breast Cancer Res. Treat., 4 : 275-281.
37. Peyrat, J.P., Djiane, J., Bonneterre, J., Vandewalle, B., Vennin, Ph., Delobelle, A., De Padt, G., and Lefebvre, J., (1984) : Anticancer Res., 4 : 257-262.
38. Rae-Ventor, B., Nemeto, T., Schneider, S.L., and Dao, T.L., (1981) : Breast Cancer Treat., 1 : 233-243.
39. Roos, W., Fabbro, D., Kung, W., Costa, S.D., andEppenberger, U. (1986) : Proc. Natl. Acad. Sci., 83 : 991-995.
40. Rowe, J.M., Kasper, S., Shiu, R.P.C., and Friesen, H.G., (1986) : Cancer Res., 46 : 1408-1412.
41. Salih, H., Flax, M., Brander, W., and Hobbs, J.R., (1972) Lancet, 25 : 1103-1105.
42. Shiu, R.P.C., Kelly, P.A., and Friesen, H.G., (1973) : Science, 180 : 968-973.
43. Shiu, R.P.C., (1980) : J. Biol. Chem., 255 :4278-4281.
44. Sporn, M.B., and Roberts, A., (1985) : Nature, 313 : 745-747.
45. Stagner, J.I., Jochimsen, P.R., and Sherman, B.M., (1977) : Clin. Res., 25 : 302A.
46. Turcot-Lemay, L., and Kelly, P.A. (1982) : J. Natl. Cancer Inst., 68 : 381-383.
47. Welsch, C.W., De Itturi, C., and Brennan, M., (1976) : Cancer, 38 : 1272-1281.
48. Yang, J., Elias, J.J., Petrakis, N.L., Wellings, S.R. and Nandi, S., (1981) : Cancer Res., 41 : 1020-1027.

Hormonal Manipulation of Cancer: Peptides,
Growth Factors, and New (Anti) Steroidal
Agents, edited by Jan G. M. Klijn et al.
Raven Press, New York © 1987.

PROLACTIN AND BREAST CANCER

P.F. Bruning

The Netherlands Cancer Institute
(Antoni van Leeuwenhoekhuis), 1066 CX Amsterdam

Animal experience

As early as 1916 it was observed that pregnancy related hormonal changes stimulated the development of mammary cancers in mice (16). Loeb and Kirtz (18) and later Mühlbock and Boot (22) published experimental evidence that mammary tumors could be induced in mouse strains with a low frequency of spontaneous breast cancer by long-lasting exposure to high blood levels of prolactin (PRL). Such sustained elevation of blood PRL could be established by pituitary isografts which persistently secrete PRL when placed under the renal capsule. The very small amount of growth hormone secreted by these isografts were thought to have no significant influence. Further experimental data from hypothalamic lesions, prolonged exogenous PRL administration and treatment with reserpine (a potent stimulator of PRL secretion) supported the notion that the elevated PRL blood levels were responsible for the increased mammary tumor incidence in mice. The development and growth of the hyperplastic alveolar nodules (HAN) of the mouse mammary gland, which have been established as the precursors of mammary cancer in certain strains (e.g. C_3H, BALB/c) were also PRL dependent.

Geyer et al (7) originally developed the experimental Sprague-Dawley rat mammary cancer model in which 7, 12 dimethyl-benz(a)anthracene (DMBA) was used as carcinogen. The model was subsequently perfected by Huggins (12) and is the most intensely studied rodent mammary tumor model. When female Sprague Dawley rats, 50 to 65 days of age, are treated with DMBA they will develop multiple mammary carcinomas within 3 to 4 months. These tumors are of ductal origin and mostly hormone responsive. Suppression of prolactin secretion by the administration of 2-bromo-α-ergocriptin (bromocriptin) early after DMBA administration significantly reduced the incidence of such mammary cancers. When low doses of DMBA are used, the animals could stay alive for a sufficiently long period to show that the development of benign mammary tumors, virtually all fibroadenomas, was also significantly reduced by the suppression of PRL. The bromocriptin dose used did not interfere with the estrous cycle, body weigth or endocrine

factors except blood PRL levels. Early bromocriptin-induced
sustained suppression of PRL secretion was also found to
reduce the incidence of spontaneous mammary tumors in
susceptible mouse strains. This effect was more pronounced in
nulliparous mice which, different from human females, tend to
develop mammary carcinoma less frequently than animals with
offspring.
It has been hypothesized that the reduction of mammary gland
DNA synthesis by suppression of PRL at the time of DMBA
treatment, renders the epithelium less sensitive to the
carcinogenic stimulus (23). PRL suppression shortly after DMBA
treatment would cause the reduction of an important growth
promoter (30).
Once advanced stages of mammary cancer had developed the
tumors in most strains of mice appeared to be PRL independent.
However, the growth of most established rat mammary cancers
still appeared to be regulated by PRL and ovarian hormones.
It thus appeared that:
1. PRL may be regarded as an additional important factor in
   rodent mammary cancerigenesis, acting mainly as a promoter;
2. most advanced stages of mouse mammary cancers have lost
   their PRL dependence, whereas most rat mammary tumors have
   not;
3. in the intact animal a thusfar only partially elucidated
   interaction of ovarian and adrenal steroid hormones with
   PRL may be superimposed on the role of PRL in rodent
   mammary carcinogenesis.

Human experience

Occasional regression of metastatic breast cancer has been
reported as the result of treatment with bromocriptin or L-
dopa. However, a phase II clinical trial with bromocriptin was
entirely negative (5), and the results of another dopamine
agonist, Lergotril, were equally disappointing (8). The
experience, that hyperprolactinemia induced by transsection of
the pituitary stalk or treatment with estrogens does not
prevent tumor regression seems consistent with these findings.
Also the fact that specific binding of lactogenic hormones to
breast cancer cell membrane receptors, which have been
demonstrated in 20 to 70 percent of cases, does not predict
clinical response to endocrine therapy fits the general idea
that PRL does not significantly stimulate the growth of
established human breast cancer. In contrast with the animal
data, which demonstrate a definite stimulatory role of PRL in
rodent mammary carcinogenesis, the human situation is less
clear. The measurement of PRL serum levels in breast cancer
patients has yielded conflicting results: a few groups found
elevated levels, but most investigators have not been able to
observe such correlation. However, when studying PRL serum
levels in breast cancer patients one is confronted with two
major difficulties. The first, rather technical problem is,

that PRL blood levels show considerable fluctuation due to diurnal variation, stress and a variety of other factors. The second and more fundamental problem is, that the development of human breast cancer takes many years. Epidemiological data on the influence of the age at menarche, or early first full term pregnancy, and the results of migration studies indicate that endocrine factors may act at a very young age, when the breast itself is still developing. Therefore, the endocrine situation at the stage of manifest breast cancer much later in life is even unlikely to be representative of what has happened during tumor development. The latter problem has been approached in various ways. In a prospective follow-up of an ostensibly healthy population on the Island of Guernsey urine and blood samples were collected yearly. When one of the 5000 participating females presented with breast cancer, her PRL and other data could be compared to matched controls. In this still ongoing study postmenopausal women who subsequently developed breast cancer had significantly elevated PRL plasma levels up to 5 yrs before the manifestation of their disease (15).

In the same study Kwa and Wang (13) had already looked into subpopulations considered to be at risk. They observed that when the time of day at which blood was collected was taken into account (because of the diurnal variation), the mean plasma PRL level at 7 P.M. was slightly, but significantly elevated in the unaffected premenopausal daughters of women with breast cancer. Nulliparous and women who were both tall and heavy showed a similar abnormality (14); all samples were collected from women in the luteal phase of their menstrual cycle. In a study of adolescent girls between 14 and 20 years of age with or without a family history of breast cancer no differences in serum PRL or steroid hormone levels were found (2), confirming the second report on adolescent daughters of breast cancer patients by Henderson et al (24). However, using hourly blood sampling during the luteal phase of the menstrual cycle, Levin and Malarkey (17) reported significantly elevated mean 24 h PRL serum levels and a diminished PRL suppression after dopamine administration in 13 daughters (mean age 28.8 $\pm$ 2 yrs) of affected mothers, compared with matched controls. Very few other investigators have studied nocturnal PRL abnormalities in women at risk of breast cancer, which could be most relevant since the circadian rhythm of human PRL secretion causes a plasma peak usually between 1 and 5 AM, which is considered to be sleep related.

Fishman et al (6) measured hormonal levels in the morning every other day throughout the menstrual cycle and observed no difference in PRL between women at familial risk and matched controls. Our own experience (3) has shown no significant differences in plasma PRL between premenopausal women at risk because of their family history (at least one sister and mother having breast cancer), histologically defined benign

breast lesions, a previous apparently cured $T_1N_0M_0$ breast
cancer and controls matched for age, body mass index, parity
and socio-economic factors. Blood sampling was performed
during day 18 to 24 of the luteal phase of the menstrual
cycle, only when plasma progesterone levels indicated active
secretion by the corpus luteum. To correct for the fluctuating
nature of plasma PRL levels a technique for continuous venous
blood withdrawal from 3 till 11 P.M. was used. We observed
that early evening elevation of PRL plasma levels do occur in
women at risk, but can be similarly found in matched controls.
When the ratios of average PRL level: average cortisol level
were compared to correct for the possible influence of stress,
again no significant differences could be found.
Hill et al (10) showed that high fat dietary intake was
associated with higher PRL serum levels compared to low fat
vegetarian diet. This finding seemed of interest as
vegetarians generally show a decreased risk of breast cancer.
However, in a large epidemiological survey of Caucasian, Bantu
and Japanese females having different dietary habits and
different breast cancer risks Hill et al (9) had not found
convincingly different serum PRL concentrations before
puberty, and before or after menopause. It may be concluded,
that no consistent relationship has as yet been demonstrated
between dietary or other life style factors which are thought
to be related to breast cancer risk and serum PRL.
Since various drugs are known to increase serum PRL levels,
the breast cancer incidence in long-term users of reserpine,
chlorpromazine and other neuroleptics has been studied by
various investigators. Although their results have not been
uniform the weight of evidence has been largely against any
association between long-lasting drug induced elevation of PRL
and increased risk of breast cancer. Whether the estrogen
related serum PRL elevation in users of the contraceptive
pill, which is counteracted by it's progesterone content has
any role to play with regard to the diminished incidence of
benign breast disease or the risk of breast cancer is entirely
unknown. Further collection of data on breast cancer risk in
long-term users of steriodal contraceptives has to be awaited.
So it seems that, notwithstanding the animal data, PRL has
little, if anything to do with human breast cancer.
However, two more issues require discussion.
The first is the recognition of the fact that what has been
measured as PRL immunologically may not be entirely relevant
to the growth of human breast epithelium. Heterogenous forms
of human PRL have been demonstrated to circulate in normal
plasma. Beside PRL a minor fraction of 2 to 3 x larger "big"
PRL, has been measured in normal serum, and in some normal
sera even some "big-big" PRL has been described (26). In
contrast to these two latter larger moieties which have very
low radioreceptor activity compared to PRL, physiologically
occurring fragments of PRL have been demonstrated (20,25).

Some of these fragments have greater mitogenic activity on
mammary epithelial cells compared with the intact hormone. The
existence of these so called cleaved 16K mol wt forms of PRL
was first shown in the rat pituitary gland (21). Cleaved 16K
PRL has now also been found in normal and tumor pituitary
tissue from a prolactinoma patient and in the plasma of
pregnant women.

Recently, Love and Rose (19) reported elevated levels of
bioactive lactogenic hormone in the plasma of 8 healthy
premenopausal women, who had at least two first-degree
relatives with breast cancer. Blood samples from these women
at risk and 19 control women were taken every other day
throughout one menstrual cycle, and additionally during TRH
stimulation tests performed with 500 µg at the mid-follicular
and mid-luteal phases. Compared with the control specimens
basal plasma growth hormone and PRL concentration determined
by radioimmunoassay were similar. Also the PRL response to
TRH, as measured immunologically, was unremarkable. However,
the women with a strongly positive family history had markedly
elevated levels of bioactive lactogenic hormone both basally
and after TRH stimulation compared with the controls. The
investigators concluded that a mitogenic form of PRL not
recognized by RIA is elevated in the serum of women at risk of
familial breast cancer. Emerman et al (4) reported elevated
serum levels of growth hormone in 40 percent and of PRL in 17
percent of breast cancer patients as determined by
radioimmunoassay. When in addition total lactogens were
measured in a bioassay the bioassay: radioimmunoassay ratio
was greater in the patients than the controls, indicating the
presence of variant forms of the hormones with greater than
control bioactivity in breast cancer patients. These findings
both in rats and humans seriously suggest that the question of
the role of bioactive PRL in breast cancerigenesis is still
open.

The second issue to be discussed is a very different one and
relates to what is known about PRL physiology. In humans the
regulation of PRL secretion seems to be dominated by estrogen
levels. After puberty PRL rises with estradiol to adult
levels. Postmenopausal PRL levels are lower than premenopausal
serum concentrations. We have demonstrated that, parous women
have significantly lower plasma PRL levels compared with
nulliparous women measured during the afternoon and evening
and that this effect of parity is still demonstrable after
more then 10 yrs since the delivery of the last child (3).
Wang et al found that average PRL levels measured during the
night decreased with increasing parity (29). Bernstein et al
(1) reported that the levels of PRL, but also of estrogens,
were lower in parous women compared with nulliparous women.
Sex hormone binding globulin showed the opposite trend.

The highest physiological PRL levels occur during pregnancy
and the first months of lactation with spurt increases during

suckling (9). Experimental data show that PRL satisfies the anterior pituitary requirements of both ductal and alveolar growth. However, physiologically growth hormone may be more important to ductal formation during adolescence, whereas placental lactogen may play a greater role in alveolar formation during the second half of pregnancy (28). Therefore, the major role of PRL seems to be its influence on differentiation required for lactogenesis.

So it remains possible that PRL or at least "bioactive PRL", contributes to breast cancer risk because of its stimulation of mammary epithelial growth. This may be especially important during puberty and adolescence. However, when it comes to full term pregnancy, high PRL levels in conjunction with various other hormones, strongly promote structural and functional differentiation of the mammary gland, which may just protect against the development of malignant growth. The protection of an early first full term pregnancy against breast cancer may thus at least partially be explained. Further pregnancies may further protect (27) by consolidation of differentiation, PRL and estrogen levels after pregnancies becoming gradually lower and lower, thereby contributing to a decrease of risk.

REFERENCES
1. Bernstein, L., Pike, M.C., Ross, R.K., Judd, H.L., Brown, J.B., Henderson B.E. (1985): J. Natl. Cancer Inst., 74:741-745.
2. Boffard, K., Clark, G.M.G., Irvine, J.B.D., Knyba, R.E., Bulbrook, R.D., Wang, D.Y., Kwa, H.G. (1981): Eur. J. Clin. Oncol., 17:1071-1077.
3. Bruning, P.F., Bonfrer, J.M.G., Hart, A.A.M., de Jong-Bakker, M., Kwa, H.G., Nooyen, W.J., Verstraeten, A.A. (1984): In: Progress in Cancer Research and Treatment, Vol. 31, edited by F. Bresciani, pp. 335-342. Raven Press, New York.
4. Emerman, J.T., Leahy, M., Gout, P.W., Bruchovsky, N. (1985): Horm. Metab. Res., 17:421-424.
5. European Breast Cancer Group, (1972): Eur. J. Cancer, 8:155-156.
6. Fishman, J., Fukushima, D., O'Connor, J., Rosenfeld, R.S., Lynch, H.T., Lynch J.F., Guirgis, H., Maloney, K. (1978): Cancer Res., 38:4006-4011.
7. Geyer, R.P., Bleisch, V.R., Bryant, J.E., Robbins, A.N., Saslaw, I.M., Stare, F.J. (1951): Cancer Res., 11:474-478.
8. Guerzon, P.G., and Pearson, O.H. (1974): Clin. Res., 22/2:632A.
9. Hill,P., Wynder, E.L., Helman, P., Hickman, R., Rona, G.,Kuno, K. (1976): Cancer Res., 36: 4102-4106.
10. Hill, P., Garbaczewski, L., Helman, P., Walker, A.R., Wynder, E.L. (1981): Cancer Res., 41:3817-3818.

11. Howie, P.W., McNeilly, A.S., Houston, M.J., Cook, A., Boyle, H. (1982): Clin. Endocrinol. (Oxf), 17:315-322.
12. Huggins, C., Grand, L.C., Brillantes, F.P. (1961): Nature, 189:204-209.
13. Kwa, H.G., and Wang, D.Y. (1977): Int. J. Cancer, 20:12-14.
14. Kwa, H.G., Bulbrook, R.D., Cleton, F.J., Verstraeten, A.A., Hayward, J.L., Wang, D.Y. (1978): Int. J. Cancer, 22:691-693.
15. Kwa, H.G., Cleton, F.J., Wang, D.Y., Bulbrook, R.D., Bulstrode, J.C., Hayward, J.L., Millis, R.R., Cuzick, J. (1981): Int. J. Cancer, 28:673-676.
16. Lathrop, A.E.C., and Loeb, L. (1916): Cancer Res., 1:1-19.
17. Levin, P.A., and Malarkey, W.B. (1981): J. Clin. Endocrinol. Metab., 53:179-183.
18. Loeb, L., and Kirtz, M.M. (1939): Am. J. Cancer, 36: 56-82.
19. Love, R.R., and Rose, D.P. (1985): Eur. J. Clin. Oncol., 21:1553-1554.
20. Meuris, S.,Svoboda, M., Vilamala, M., Christophe, J., Robyn, C. (1983): FEBS Letters, 154:111-115.
21. Mittra, I. (1980): Biochem. Biophys. Res. Commun., 95:1760-1767.
22. Mühlbock, O., and Boot, L.M. (1959): Cancer Res., 19:402-412.
23. Nagasawa, H. (1979): Med. Hypotheses, 5:499-510.
24. Pike, M.C., Casagrande, J.T., Brown, J.B., Gerkins, V., Henderson, B.E. (1977): J. Natl. Cancer Inst., 59:1351-1355.
25. Sinha, Y.N., Gilligan, T.A., Lee, D.W., Hollingsworth, D., Markoff, E. (1985): J. Clin. Endocrinol. Metab., 60:239-243.
26. Suh, H.K., Frantz, A.G. (1974): J. Clin. Endocrinol. Metab., 39:928-935.
27. Thein, H., Thein, M.M. (1978): Int. J. Cancer, 21:432-437.
28. Topper, Y.J., Freeman, C.S. (1980): Physiological Reviews, 80:1049-1106.
29. Wang, D.Y., Sturzaker, H.E., Kwa, H.G., Verhofstad, F., Hayward, J.L., Bulbrook, R.D. (1984): Int. J. Cancer, 33:629-632.
30. Welsch, C.W., and Nagasawa,H. (1977): Cancer Res., 37:951-963.

Hormonal Manipulation of Cancer: Peptides,
Growth Factors, and New (Anti) Steroidal
Agents, edited by Jan G. M. Klijn et al.
Raven Press, New York © 1987.

THE PROGNOSTIC SIGNIFICANCE OF HYPERPROLACTINAEMIA

IN BREAST CANCER

M. Dowsett[1], G.E. McGarrick[1], A.L. Harris[2], R.C. Coombes[3],
I.E. Smith[4], and S.L. Jeffcoate[1]

1. Endocrine Department
Chelsea Hospital for Women
London SW3 6LT, U.K.

2. Department of Radiotherapy and Clinical Oncology
Newcastle General Hospital
Newcastle NE4 6BE, U.K.

3. Ludwig Institute for Cancer Research
St. George's Hospital
London SW17 0QT, U.K.

4. Medical Breast Unit
Royal Marsden Hospital
London SW3 6LJ, U.K.

Numerous case control studies have failed to show a clear
relationship between prolactin and breast cancer (13,16). This
together with the lack of clinical benefit in advanced breast
cancer of therapy aimed solely at prolactin suppression (4,5)
has led to the widely-held view that prolactin has no major role
to play in the development or growth of human breast cancer. An
illustration of this is the inclusion of a prolactin suppressor
in only very few of the numerous combination therapies which have
been evaluated in breast cancer. Despite this there is continued
interest in a potential role for prolactin in breast cancer and
this interest has been increased by the demonstration of specific
binding sites for prolactin in breast carcinomas (1) and by the
finding that prolactin can promote the growth of human breast
cancer cells in vitro (10,11).

In this short review an assessment is made of evidence for a
possible relationship between plasma prolactin levels and
response to therapy or overall prognosis of breast cancer
patients. The following questions are addressed: (i) is there
evidence for such a relationship being causative? (ii) is plasma
prolactin level a useful prognostic marker? (iii) are there any
implications for the therapeutic manipulation of prolactin
secretion?

STUDIES

Our interest in a possible prognostic significance for
prolactin in breast cancer was stimulated by our observation that
during treatment with aminoglutethimide plus hydrocortisone 14/40
non-responders but only 2/35 responders had on-treatment
prolactin levels greater than 500 mIU/1 (6). Similar
observations were made by Willis et al (19) who found that after
6 weeks treatment with tamoxifen 2/17 patients in whom treatment
was successful and 9/23 in whom it was unsuccessful were
hyperprolactinaemic. Holtkamp et al (7) showed clearly that
there is a high incidence of hyperprolactinaemia in metastatic
breast cancer (values >500 mIU/1 occurred in 26%, compared with
7% in patients with primary disease). In the same study the
geometric mean level of prolactin was higher in non-responders
during treatment in all of six groups which differed according to
treatment received (both cytotoxic and endocrine).
    There would thus seen to be a clear relationship between
prolactin levels on treatment and response to therapy. It is,

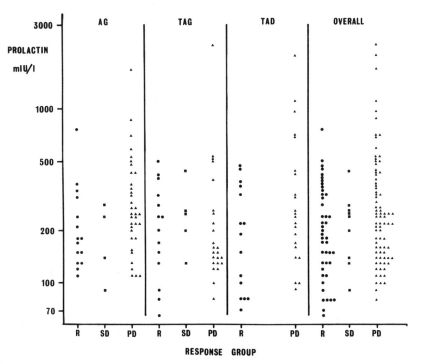

FIG. 1. Pretreatment prolactin level and response of patients
with advanced breast cancer. The prolactin levels are plotted
on a logarithmic scale. R = responders, SD = stable disease, PD
= progressive disease. The overall column shows the combined
data from all 3 treatment groups.

however, axiomatic that during treatment the responders will as a group be less diseased and the hyperprolactinaemia in the non-responders may be a result of disease-dependent stress. We therefore conducted 2 studies, one in advanced disease, the other in early disease to determine if pretreatment levels of prolactin would show a similar relationship. In each of these studies a single blood sample was drawn for each patient between 09.30 and 12.00 on the basis that (i) frequent sampling does not significantly improve the value of prolactin analyses (12,14) (ii) variation due to diurnal variation would be minimised and (iii) venepuncture rarely, if ever, induces prolactin release (2,8,14). All patients were postmenopausal and their response to therapy was assessed according to standard UICC criteria. No patient had received endocrine therapy for at least 4 weeks.

(i) <u>Advanced disease</u> (published in detail elsewhere, ref. 3). Samples were taken from patients about to start one of 3 treatment regimes: aminoglutethimide (AG, 55 patients), tamoxifen + AG (TAG, 43 patients) or TAG + danazol (TAD, 37 patients). Previous endocrine therapy had been received by 40 patients, all of whom were in the AG group. The pretreatment prolactin levels in all patients are shown in Figure 1 according to treatment group and response. When data for all groups were combined there was a significantly higher level of prolactin in the non-responders than the responders (p = 0.026) or the responders and stable disease patients combined (p = 0.021). Similarly there were significantly more patients with a prolactin level $\geqslant$ 500 mIU/l in the group that developed progressive disease (15/82) than in either the group who responded (2/44; chi-squared, p < 0.05) or those who responded or had stable disease (2/53, p < 0.02).

In those patients who progressed on treatment prolactin levels $\geqslant$ 500 mIU/l were associated with a shorter survival than those with lower levels (Figure 2). The median survival time for those patients with prolactin $\geqslant$ 500 mIU/l was 5.3 months whilst for those with prolactin < 500 mIU/l it was 10.0 months.

The possibility was examined that this relationship might have been a result of differing severity of disease at the start of treatment by assessing the number of sites and distribution of metastatic disease at that time in those patients who did not respond to treatment and who died within 6 months of starting. For those patients with < 500 mIU/l (n = 21) the mean number of involved sites was 2.24 ± 0.94 (SD), whilst in those with higher prolactin levels 2.45 ± 0.93 (n = 11) sites were involved (p > 0.2). Additionally, there was no significant difference in the distribution of sites of metastatic disease.

The results of this study indicate that advanced breast cancer patients with high prolactin levels prior to endocrine treatment have a reduced probability of response to therapy and a poor overall prognosis. There was no evidence to suggest that the hyperprolactinaemic patients carried a heavier load of disease

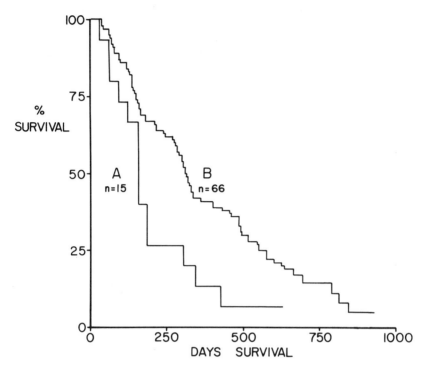

FIG. 2. Actuarial probability of survival of patients with advanced breast cancer according to pretreatment prolactin level. Only those patients who progressed on treatment are plotted. A: prolactin ⟩ 500 mIU/1, B: prolactin < 500 mIU/1. Log-rank p = 0.006.

but no account was taken of prolactin-stimulating drug administration in this study.

   Willis et al (19) also found that hyperprolactinaemia prior to tamoxifen therapy was more common in patients who subsequently failed to respond, but the number of patients was relatively small and the difference was not statistically significant. Sarfaty et al (15) found that the mean prolactin level before adrenalectomy was higher in non-responders than responders and although Holtkamp et al (7) found no difference in pretreatment prolactin levels between responders and non-responders to endocrine treatment, mean levels in non-responders to cytotoxic therapy were nearly double those in responders. All of these investigations support a poorer therapeutic response of patients with high prolactin levels, but there do not appear to be any data additional to ours on the overall prognosis of patients with advanced disease.

   (ii) <u>Early disease</u>. Blood samples were drawn from 152

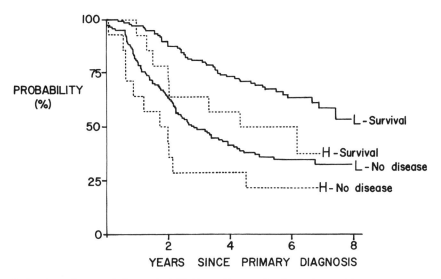

FIG. 3. Actuarial probability of survival and no disease
according to prolactin level in operable breast cancer patients.
L < 350 mIU/1, H > 350 mIU/1.

patients with primary breast cancer between 2 and 14 days before
mastectomy, and serum was stored in liquid nitrogen until
analysis between 5 and 9 years later. A record of concurrent
medical problems and of drugs being taken at the time of sampling
was made. Only 5 patients had prolactin levels greater than 500
mIU/1. Discrimination was therefore made at the upper 10th
centile (350 mIU/1) and the two groups thus formed were examined
to determine whether there was a relationship between prolactin
level and time to first relapse or length of survival. Actuarial
disease-free interval and survival curves are shown in Figure 3.
In both cases the group with higher prolactin levels apparently
performed worse but in neither case was the difference
statistically significant (for survival: $0.10 > p > 0.05$,
log-rank test). There was no difference in terms of age, tumour
grade or size, or node status at operation which would have
indicated a worse prognosis for the group with higher prolactin
levels but there was a higher incidence of concurrent medical
complaints in that group (7/14 compared with 32/138). Four of
the patients with prolactin > 350 mIU/1 were taking drugs which
might have been expected to be the cause of the high prolactin
levels. It was notable that only one of these 4 patients had
died whilst 7 of the other 10 patients with high prolactin levels
had died.
 Wang et al (18) have recently provided the only published
study of prolactin and prognosis in early breast cancer,
including 258 pre- and 357 post-menopausal subjects. The
disease-free interval was not examined but associations with

survival were sought between prolactin levels 1 day before and 10 days after operation (markedly higher) as well as the increment between the two measurements. No significant relationship was found in the groups as a whole between prolactin level and survival but five subgroups were identified in which pre-operative prolactin was related to survival and in all of these the group with higher prolactin levels fared worse. A further 4 such associations were found in subgroups for post-operative prolactin and the pre/post-operative increment.

Both our own study and that of Wang et al (18) have thus found no strong relationship between prolactin and prognosis in early breast cancer but the results suggest that a higher plasma prolactin level may be indicative of a poorer survival for some groups.

DISCUSSION AND CONCLUSIONS

There seems little doubt that a correlation does exist between prolactin and prognosis for advanced breast cancer and possibly for early breast cancer also. It is most unlikely, however, that prolactin could be a useful marker or index of prognosis since prolactin levels show a very wide, logarithmically-distributed normal range and there is also a broad overlap between responders and non-responders to treatment. Whether prolactin is an independent variable or is associated with other factors which are themselves related to prognosis is less certain. In our study in advanced disease we could find no evidence that extent of disease caused this relationship. It should also be noted that immunoassay of prolactin may not necessarily be an accurate measure of biologically active prolactin (17). Prognosis should be examined in relation to biologically active prolactin and/or total lactogenic stimuli. Love and Rose (9) have found that the ratio of biologically/immunologically active 'lactogenic hormone' is abnormally high in women with a strong family history of breast cancer.

From none of the studies cited can evidence be provided for prolactin causing the poorer prognosis by stimulation of tumour growth. However, the observations that many breast carcinomas show high-affinity binding of prolactin and that physiological concentrations of prolactin can lead to the growth of primary cultures of breast carcinomas in vitro suggest that prolactin might be significant in the support of breast cancer growth in vivo. Whilst clinical trials of bromocriptine and L-dopa alone have been disappointing it is possible that use of such agents in combination with oestrogen suppressive therapy may be more successful. There seems little rationale in such trials to treat only hyperprolactinaemic patients since basal levels of prolactin may also be supportive (there is no evidence to suggest that suppression of oestrogen levels is any more effective in patients with higher pre-treatment levels). Such combination of agents which have totally separate targets might be expected to have greater likelihood of benefit than the combination of agents which are targeted solely at oestrogen suppression.

Acknowledgement: Figures 1 and 2 were reproduced by permission of British Journal of Cancer.

REFERENCES

1. Bonneterre, J., Peyrat, J.Ph., Vandewalle, B., Beuscart, R., Vie, M.C., and Cappelaere, P. (1982): Eur. J. Cancer Clin. Oncol., 18:1157-1162.
2. Cowden, E.A., Ratcliffe, W.A., Beastall, G.H. and Ratcliffe, J.G. (1979): Ann. Clin. Biochem., 16:113-121.
3. Dowsett, M., McGarrick, G.E., Harris, A.L., Coombes, R.C., Smith, I.E. and Jeffcoate, S.L. (1983): Br. J. Cancer, 47:763-769.
4. Engelsman, E., Heuson, J.C., Blonk-van der Wijst, J., Drochmans, A., Maas, H., Cheix, F., Sobrinho, L.G. and Nowakowski, H. (1975): Br. Med. J., 2:714-715.
5. European Breast Cancer Group (1972): Europ. J. Cancer, 8:155-156.
6. Harris, A.L., Dowsett, M., Smith, I.E. and Jeffcoate, S. (1983): Br. J. Cancer, 48:585-594.
7. Holtkamp, W., Nagel, G.A., Wander, H-E., Rauschecker, H.F. and von Heyden, D. (1984): Int. J. Cancer, 34:323-328.
8. Koninckx, P. (1978): Lancet, i:273
9. Love, R.R. and Rose, D.P. (1985): Eur. J. Cancer Clin. Oncol., 21:1553-1554.
10. Malarkey, W.B., Kennedy, M., Allred, L.E. and Milo, G. (1983): J. Clin. Endocrinol. Metab., 56:673-677.
11. Manni, A., Wright, C., Davis, G., Glenn, J., Joehl, R. and Feil, P. (1986): Cancer Res., 46:1669-1672.
12. Moult, P.J.A., Dacie, J.E., Rees, L.J. and Besser, G.M. (1981): Clin. Endocrinol., 14:387-394.
13. Nagasawa, H. (1979): Europ. J. Cancer, 15:267-279.
14. Pearce, J.M., McGarrick, G., Chamberlain, G.V.P. and Jeffcoate, s.L. (1980): Br. J. Obstet. Gynaecol., 87:366-369.
15. Sarfaty, G., Tallis, G.M., Murray, R.M.L., Pitt, P., Garder, H. and Leppard, P. (1976): Excerpta Medica International Congress Series No. 403:399-404.
16. Smithline, F., Sherman, L. and Kolodny, H.D. (1975): New Eng. J. Med., 292:784-792.
17. Soong, Y.K., Ferguson, K.M., McGarrick, G., and Jeffcoate, S.L. (1982): Clin. Endocrinol., 16: 259-265.
18. Wang, D.Y., Hampson, S., Kwa, H.G., Moore, J.W., Bulbrook, R.D., Fentiman, I.S., Hayward, J.L., King, R.J.B., Millis, R.R., Rubens, R.D. and Allen, D.S. (1986): Eur. J. Cancer Clin. Oncol., 22:487-492.
19. Willis, K.J., London, D.R., Ward, H.C., Lynch, S.S. and Rudd, B.T. (1977): Br. Med. J., 1:425-428.

Hormonal Manipulation of Cancer: Peptides, Growth Factors, and New (Anti) Steroidal Agents, edited by Jan G. M. Klijn et al. Raven Press, New York © 1987.

MEDROXYPROGESTERONE ACETATE HIGH-DOSE (MPA-HD)

versus MPA-HD plus BROMOCRIPTINE IN ADVANCED BREAST CANCER:

PRELIMINARY RESULTS OF A MULTICENTER RANDOMIZED CLINICAL TRIAL.

L. Dogliotti, *G. Robustelli della Cuna and **F. Di Carlo, on behalf of BROMPA Italian Cooperative Group §.

Dipartimento di Biomedicina, Oncologia Clinica, Università di Torino, Strada San Vito 34, 10126 Torino, Italy; *Fondazione Clinica del Lavoro, Divisione di Oncologia, Università di Pavia, Italy, and **Istituto di Farmacologia, Università di Torino, Italy.

INTRODUCTION

It has been well known for a long time that Prolactin (PRL) is one of the most important hormones involved in the control of mammary growth and function (14).

A number of experimental data suggest that PRL plays a prominent role as a stimulating factor not only for normal mammary gland, but also for breast cancer growth. As recently reviewed by Nagasawa (15), this role is particularly evident in rodents. PRL or hyperprolactinemic drugs administered to mice or DMBA-tumors bearing rats increase the promotion and the number of mammary cancer, while PRL suppression by ergot-derivatives of hypophysectomy inhibits the development of breast neoplastic lesions (22).

The data obtained in rodents have not a similar counterpart in humans. However, recent clinical and esperimental findings suggest an important role for PRL also in human breast cancer (2,6). The detection and characterization of specific PRL receptors (PRL-R) in human breast cancer may indirectly support the importance of this hormone in breast neoplasia. Many Authors found a specific binding for PRL in 25-50% of cases, not correlated with the presence of steroid receptors (6). The clinical usefulness of PRL-R status is still unclear, although preliminary data coming from Waseda et al. (21) suggest that PRL-R positive patients have a significantly worse survival than PRL-R negative group, independently from steroid receptor status. Moreover, binding sites for Dopamine have been recently identified in normal and particularly in neoplastic human mammary tissue(1).

Accordingly, a series of clinical studies suggests that patients with advanced breast cancer who had hyperprolactinemia, even

if mild, at the beginning or during treatment, showed a significantly poor prognosis and increased resistance to both endocrine
and cytotoxic treatment, in comparison with patients with normal
PRL levels (7,16). Moreover, some evidence has been reported
that if hyperprolactinemia is found in patients during remission,
it usually precedes a tumor relapse (12). So, hyperprolactinemia
in advanced breast cancer might be considered a marker of progres
sive disease and bad prognosis.
    On these grounds, it is reasonable to state that treatment
with PRL-lowering drugs has to be revisited for potential therapeutic value. Some previous trials (always carried out in a little number of unselected patients) have failed to demonstrate a
significant therapeutic effect of PRL-inhibitors, like bromocriptine or L-DOPA, employed as a single drug in advanced breast cancer (8,9). However, a pilot study by Dogliotti et al. (5)
has shown that combination of medroxyprogesterone acetate at high
doses (MPA-HD) plus bromocriptine in 70 patients with advanced
breast cancer, resulted in a higher number of responses and
longer remissions, when historically compared to MPA-HD treatment
alone.
    On this basis, we started in March 1984 a controlled randomi-
zed multicenter study in order to evaluate the efficacy and tolerability of MPA-HD plus Bromocriptine versus MPA-HD alone in post
menopausal patients with advanced breast cancer (BROMPA trial).
    Here we wish to report the preliminary results of this study,
which is still ongoing. Patients accrual is expected to finish
by Autumn 1986. As it is usual for multicenter cooperative studies, many data both for quality and duration of responses, as
well as detailed information on treatment side-effects,will be
provided after a final extramural review of all evaluable cases.

PATIENTS and METHODS

Criteria of eligibility

    Postmenopausal women less than 75 years of age with measurable
metastatic breast cancer, at first recurrence, were eligible for
the study.
    Previous adjuvant cytotoxic or endocrine therapy (Tamoxifen)
did not exclude patients from the study, provided that the therapy had been discontinued for at least 3 months prior to entrance.
    A steroid receptor status positive (ER+ PgR+ / ER+ PgR- / ER-
PgR+; cut-off $>$ 6 femMol/mg/cytosol protein) or unknown was required. Patients with concomitant neoplasias, congestive heart

failure, severe hypertension, type I diabetes, peptic ulcera and endocrinopathies, somehow inferring with treatments were excluded. Were also excluded patients with brain metastatic lesions and those with a life expectancy minor than 3 months. Overall, a Karnofsky performance status > 40 was required for entering the trial.

Trial Design

After an informed consent was received, patients who fulfilled these criteria were stratified according to the site of dominant lesion (soft tissue, bone, viscera, mixed) and subsequently randomly alloccated to receive one of the following treatments:
Regimen A: MPA i.m./1 g daily for 4 weeks except Saturday and Sunday, then 500 mg. i.m. twice weekly.
Regimen B: MPA as in regimen A plus Bromocriptine 2.5 mg orally/ four times a day.

If positive responses or stabilization were achieved, the treatment was not discontinued until disease progression, unless occurrence of severe drug related side-effects. All patients were hospitalized during the initial week of treatment; then they were usually followed as outpatients. Strict emphasis was placed on punctual observance of the dose and the time of administration of drugs scheduled.

Pretreatment and follow-up investigations

Basal investigations included history and physical patient examination. TNM and histology of primary tumor was always recorded. Metastatic lesions had to be carefully measured and described, and skin lesions photographed.

Complete biochemical profile, ECG, X-ray of chest and skeleton, bone scintigraphy, echo-scans were done in all patients. When indicated, CT-scans and visceral lesions biopsies were performed. All baseline investigations were repeated after 3 months of treatment; afterwards according to a precise schedule of follow-up.

Plasma PRL evaluation (RIA-kit, Sorin, Saluggia, Italy) was done before treatment and every 3 months during treatment in all patients.

Definition of response and side-effects

Complete response (CR),partial response (PR), no change (NC) and progressive disease (PD) were assessed according to the UICC criteria (10). Patients were considered evaluable for response if they had received treatment at least for 3 months.

Duration of response was defined by the time from the beginning of the treatment until progression.

Side-effects were carefully assessed according to the WHO criteria (23)

Statistics

Age and performance status data were compared between groups by means of Student's t test for unpaired data, two tailed. For % performance status data, Student's t test was performed considering the arcsin transformed data. Disease free-interval was compared between groups by means of Mann Whitney's U test. Location of metastatic site was analyzed by chi-square test, two tailed. For all tests, significance level was set at $p < 0.05$.

Analysis of time response to treatment was performed by means of life-table actuarial method according to Cutler and Ederer.

RESULTS

From March 1984 to April 1986, 171 patients were entered in the study from 9 participating centers. As stated before, this is an interim report of the study, which is still ongoing.

Patient evaluability is shown in Table I.

Table I.   Patient evaluability

	Group A	Group B	Overall
Entered	83	88	171
Not eligible (protocol violation)	2	3	5
Eligible	81	85	166
Not evaluable	19	23	42
Early progressive disease	2	6	8
Early withdrawal	4	5	9
Too early to evaluate	13	12	25
Evaluable	62	62	124

Patients characteristics are given in Table II.

Table II.   Patient characteristics

		Group A	Group B
Age (yr)	Mean	58	60
	Range	34-75	35-75
Performance status (%)	Mean	86.5	87.3
	Range	40-100	40-100
Disease free interval	Median	32.5	25.5
(months)	Range	0-213	0-168
ER+ and/or PgR+ (No.patients)		25	19
Dominant site:			
soft tissue		16 (21%)	15 (20%)
bone		34 (45%)	34 (46%)
viscera		11 (15%)	9 (12%)
mixed		14 (19%)	16 (22%)
total		75	74

As shown in the table, the two groups of eligible patients
are well-balanced in terms of age, performance status, disease-
free interval and dominant site of metastatic lesions. All the
examined variables did not show any statistically significative
differences. Steroid receptor status is only known in about 30%
of patients, since most of the cases entered had mastectomy
before the determination of hormone receptors became a routine
procedure in all institutions involved in this study. So, this
variable will be considered only at the end of the study.

Response to treatment

Overall response to treatment in evaluable patients is shown
in Table III.

Table III. Overall response to treatment in evaluable patients

	Group A		Group B		
	No.	%	No.	%	
PD	16	26	6	10	*
NC	26	42	28	45	
PR	14	22 } 32	20	32 } 45 **	
CR	6	10	8	13	
total	62		62		

Chi-square two-tailed test
*   p < 0.02
** p = 0.13

A trend was apparent to respond better between patients treated with regimen B (MPA-HD + Bromocriptine) vs regimen A (MPA-HD),
although the difference is so far not significant (p = 0.13).
Stabilization of disease was superimposable between the two
groups, whereas failures are significantly more frequent in group
A vs group B (p < 0.02).

When considering responses according to dominant site of metastatic localizations (Table IV) no significant differences between the two groups were apparent in any subclasses of patients.

Table IV. Response according to dominant site of metastasis

Metastatic site	Group A				Group B			
	No.	PD	NC	PR + CR	No.	PD	NC	PR + CR
Soft tissue	12	1	3	6	2	13	1	4	4	4
		8%	25%	67%			8%	30%	62%
Bone	30	8	14	5	3	26	2	14	10	-
		27%	46%	27%			8%	54%	38%
Viscera	9	3	5	-	1	6	2	3	1	-
		33%	56%	11%			33%	50%	17%
Mixed	11	4	4	3	-	17	1	7	5	4
		36%	36%	28%			6%	41%	53%

As expected, soft tissue lesions had a very good response
rate, both in group A and B (67% and 63%, respectively).

In patients with bone lesions, frequently multiple, there is
a trend to better respond in group B vs group A (38% vs 27%),
whereas NC are superimposable. On the whole the number of failures is higher in group A vs group B (27% vs 8%), although not
significant.

Viscera lesions, the majority of them accounted for by liver
lesions, showed a discrete number of stabilization rate in both
arms (56% and 50%), whereas the number of positive responses is
disappointing.

Finally, a trend to a better response in favour of group B
patients (53% vs 28%) appears when considering patients bearing
mixed lesions, again without reaching a statistical significance.

As previously reported with MPA-HD treatment, most of patients
presenting with pain improved this symptom: however, a precise
evaluation of their performance status during treatment will be
considered only at the end of the study.

So far, the median duration of response from initiation of
treatment to progressive disease for all treated patients is 9
months, without any difference between the two groups. Patients

responding to treatment (CR + PR) have yet to reach the median value of duration of response at 23 months of observation, both for group A and B. It is still too early to analyze the impact of response on patient survival.

Side-effects

Side effects, assessed according to the WHO criteria, are reported in Table V.

Table V.   Side-effects

	Group A	Group B
No. of patients evaluable for side-effects on treatment arm	81	85
No. of patients with side-effects	34	42 *NS
No. of patients without side-effects	47	43
No. of reports for each effect		
Weight gain	53	43
Moderate hypertension	10	24
Cushing-like appearance	17	12
Hyperglycemia	5	19
Nausea	3	12
Glutea abscess	3	7
Vaginal bleeding	5	5
Skin reactions	7	-
Vertigo	1	4
Fluid retention	1	4
Thrombophlebitis	2	3
Orthostatic hypotension	2	2
Weakness	4	-
Hand tremor	2	2
Constipation	2	1
Vomiting	-	2
Sweating	2	-

* Chi-square two-tailed test

About 50% of patients did not experienced side-effects in both treatment groups. When considering the number of reports for each side-effect, our data are in agreement with those previously reported for MPA-HD treatment. Bromocriptine-related side-effects occurred in the initial stages of treatment: nausea and vertigo were the most common. To minimize these symptoms we usually started with a lower dose of the drug, taken with meals, gradually increasing every three days. On the whole both treatments were well tolerated with a little number of side-effects related drop-outs.

DISCUSSION

The reevaluation of endocrine therapy in the management of breast cancer during the last years has been largely dependent on the new biochemical understanding of the action of hormones in normal and neoplastic breast tissue. Accordingly, new drugs or more rational combination of drugs are actually under investigation in order to obtain, as much as possible, positive results with the lowest side-effects.

About ten years ago the administration of MPA in advanced breast cancer patients, employed at doses much higher than the previously used, was reevaluated by Pannuti et al.(17,18). The central and peripheral mechanisms accounting for by MPA activity in breast cancer have been many times reported (4,20). Nowadays, when considering the results coming from multicenter studies, MPA-HD gave an average response rate of 35%, and somewhat higher when the disease is localized mainly in soft tissue and bone (3,13). These results parallel those obtained with other endocrine treatments.

The optimum amount of MPA to be administered in advanced breast cancer is still debatable. However, the schedule of MPA administration we choosed, also in the light of our previous experience, is now recognized as one of the best in order to obtain stable high plasma MPA level (more than 60 ng/ml), which is considered rate-limiting for having good responses (11,19).

Bromocriptine, a well known long-acting dopaminergic drug, is actually the best drug to be employed for continuous PRL suppression, provided its regular assumption.

The rationale and the main effects on the hypothalamus-hypophysis-adrenal axis and on neoplastic breast cells of combining Bromocriptine and MPA-HD in the treatment of advanced breast cancer have been fully reported elsewhere (5). Apart from the anti-prolactin effect, Bromocriptine might be considered an antiproliferative drug with regard to breast cancer cells. In fact, we have very recently reported that Bromocriptine causes a strong inhibition of proliferation (>40% vs controls) of the CG-5 cells, a human mammary estrogen-sensitive cell line, variant of the MCF-7 cell line (6). So, the combination of Bromocriptine with other hormonal or cytotoxic drugs merits further consideration for future clinical trials.

The preliminary data coming from our randomized study, even if show only a trend toward a significant difference, with regard to complete and partial responses, between the groups A and B, appear already now of some interest when considering the overall success (CR+PR+NC) and the number of failures, which are significantly in favour of patients who received MPA-HD plus Bromocriptine.

Obviously, a more precise clinically definition of the place of Bromocriptine in the overall treatment strategy of breast cancer will come after the completion of our and other trials now ongoing in Europe.

ACKNOWLEDGMENT

The Authors wish to thank dr.R.Ferrara, Biometric Department, Sandoz s.p.a., Milan, Italy for help in the statistical evaluation of the data.

§ List of participating centers:

Oncologia Clinica, Università di Torino (L.Dogliotti, R.Faggiuolo) / Clinica Chirurgica I, Università di Torino (A.Mussa, O.Alabiso) / Divisione di Oncologia Medica, Ospedale S.Giovanni, Torino (C.Bumma, G.Gentile) / Fondazione Clinica del Lavoro, Divisione di Oncologia, Università di Pavia (G.Robustelli della Cuna, G.Bernardo) / Divisione Medica III, Ospedale Civile, Brescia (G.Marini, P.Marpicati) / Divisione di Oncologia Medica, Ospedale S.Maria Nuova, Reggio Emilia (F.Saccani, G.Becchi) / Divisione di Radioterapia Oncologica, Istituto di Clinica Ostetrica e Ginecologica, Università Cattolica, Roma (L.Trodella, S.Dell'Acqua) / Clinica Chirurgica e Clinica Ostetrica e Ginecologica, Università di Pisa (P.Miccoli, G.B.Melis) / Divisione Chirurgica II, Ospedale Civile, Cremona (A.Bottini, C.Andres).

REFERENCES

1. Angeli, A., Dogliotti, L., Orlandi, F., Muccioli, G., Bellussi, G., and Di Carlo, R. (1986): In: Endocrinology '85, edited by G.M.Molinatti and L.Martini, Excerpta Medica, Amsterdam, in press.
2. Bonneterre, J., Peyrat, J.P., and Demaille, A. (1985): Breast Disease.Senologia, 1: 3-26.
3. Cavalli, F., Goldhirsch, A., Jungi, F., Martz, G., Mermillod, B., Schäfer, P., and Alberto, P. (1984): In: Role of Medroxy-

progesterone in Endocrine-Related Tumors, vol.III, edited by A.
Pellegrini, G.Robustelli della Cuna, F.Pannuti, P.Pouillart
and W.Jonat, pp.79-89. Raven Press, New York.
4. Di Marco, A. (1980): In: Role of Medroxyprogesterone in Endocri
ne-Related Tumors, vol.I, edited by S.Iacobelli and A.Di Marco,
pp.1-20. Raven Press, New York.
5. Dogliotti, L., Mussa, A., and Di Carlo, F. (1983): In: Role of
Medroxyprogesterone Acetate in Endocrine-Related Tumors, vol.II
edited by L.Campio, G.Robustelli della Cuna and R.W.Taylor, pp.
115-129. Raven Press, New York.
6. Dogliotti, L., Faggiuolo, R., Muccioli, G., Natoli, V., Sica,
G., and Di Carlo, F. (1986): In: Endocrine and Malignancies,
edited by S.Iacobelli. Parthenon Press, in press.
7. Dowsett, W.M., McGarrick, G.E., Harris, A.L., Coombes, R.C.,
Smith, I.E., and Jeffcoate, S.L. (1983): Br.J.Cancer, 47: 763-
769.
8. Engelsman, E., and Heuson, J.C. (1975): Br.Med.J., 2: 155.
9. European Breast Cancer Group (1972): Europ.J.Cancer, 8: 155.
10. Hayward, J.L., Carbone, P.P., Heuson, J.C., Kumaoka, S., Segaloff, A., and Rubens, R.D. (1977): Cancer, 39: 1289-1294.
11. Hesselius, I. (1983): In: Role of Medroxyprogesterone in Endocrine-Related Tumors, vol.II, edited by L.Campio, G.Robustelli
della Cuna and R.W.Taylor, pp.25-34. Raven Press, New York.
12. Holtkamp, W., Nagel, G.E., Wander, H.E., Rauschecker, H.F.,and
Von Heyden, D. (1984): Int.J.Cancer, 34: 323-328.
13. Lober, J., Mouridsen, H.T., and Rose, C. (1983): In: Role of
Medroxyprogesterone in Endocrine-Related Tumors, vol.II, edited
by L.Campio, G.Robustelli della Cuna and R.W.Taylor, pp.105-114
Raven Press, New York.
14. Lyons, W.R., Li, C.H., and Johnson, R.E. (1958): Rec.Progr.
Horm.Res., 14: 219-248.
15. Nagasawa, H. (1983): J.Steroid Biochem., 19 (Suppl.): 1395.
16. Nagel, G.A., Wander, H.E., and Blossey, H.C. (1981): Schweiz.
Med.Wschr., 111: 1977-1981.
17. Pannuti, F., Martoni, A., Pollutri, E., Camera, P., Losinno, F.
and Giusti, H. (1976): Panmin.Med., 18: 129-136.
18. Pannuti, F., Martoni, A., Lenaz, G.R., Piana, E., and Nanni, P.
(1978): Cancer Treat.Rep., 62: 499-504.
19. Pannuti, F., Camaggi, G.M., Strocchi, E., Martoni, A., Beghelli
P., Biondi, S., Costanti, B., and Grieco, A. (1984): In: Role
of Medroxyprogesterone in Endocrine-Related Tumors, vol.III,
edited by A.Pellegrini, G.Robustelli della Cuna, F.Pannuti, P.
Pouillart and W.Jonat, pp.43-77. Raven Press, New York.

20.Robustelli della Cuna, G., Bernardo-Strada, M.R., and Ganzina, F. (1983): In: Proceedings of the International Symposium on Medroxyprogesterone acetate, edited by F.Cavalli, W.L.Mc Guire, F.Pannuti, A.Pellegrini and G.Robustelli della Cuna, pp.290-305. Excerpta Medica, Amsterdam.

21.Waseda, N., Kato, Y., Imura, H., and Kurata, M. (1985): Jpn.J. Cancer Res., 76: 517-523.

22.Welsch, C.W., and Nagasawa, H. (1977): Cancer Res., 37: 951-963.

23.WHO Handbook for Reporting Results of Cancer Treatment. (1979): WHO, Geneva.

Hormonal Manipulation of Cancer: Peptides, Growth Factors, and New (Anti) Steroidal Agents, edited by Jan G. M. Klijn et al. Raven Press, New York © 1987.

EFFECTS OF LONG TERM TREATMENT WITH THE LHRH-ANALOGUE BUSERELIN ON THE PITUITARY-TESTICULAR AXIS IN MEN WITH PROSTATIC CARCINOMA (PCA).

F.H. de Jong*, F.H. Schroeder[§], M.T.W.T. Lock[§], F.M.J. Debruyne[+], H.J. de Voogt[Δ], and J.G.M. Klijn[°]

Departments of *Biochemistry II, *Internal Medicine III, and [§]Urology, Erasmus University Rotterdam, departments of Urology, [+]University Nijmegen, and [Δ]Free University Amsterdam, and [°]Department of Internal Medicine, Rotterdam Radio-Therapeutic Institute, Rotterdam.

INTRODUCTION

Since Huggins & Hodges (4) discovered that the growth of prostate cancer (PCA) is androgen dependent, endocrine treatment of PCA has consisted of castration or administration of oestrogens. The observation of the paradoxical decrease of gonadotropin and androgen concentrations in peripheral blood after prolonged stimulation of the pituitary gland with long-acting, super-active LHRH-analogues in animals (9) and in men (8) indicated that this medication might also be useful in the treatment of PCA.

The aim of the present study was to assess the clinical efficacy of the daily administration of the LHRH-analogue Buserelin in the treatment of PCA-patients by confirming the rapid suppression of serum testosterone (T) concentrations and its long-term maintenance and by determining response rates and response duration. The present report describes the hormonal data obtained during this study.

Furthermore, data on the diurnal rhythms of T, cortisol and LH during Buserelin-therapy are provided. Data on the clinical response during this study are published elsewhere (11).

PATIENTS, MATERIALS AND METHODS

58 patients with histologically documented metastatic PCA were

treated with Buserelin (Hoe 766, Hoechst, Frankfurt, W-Germany)
During the first week, three daily injections of 500 µg were
given. Thereafter, the daily dose was 3 times 400 µg, administered
intranasally. After 1 year, 32 of these patients showed regression
of the PCA or had stable disease (Group I), while 26 patients had
progression of the disease (Group II).

During the first week of treatment, blood samples were
collected daily. Thereafter, weekly samples were obtained during
the first month of treatment, followed by monthly samples during
the first year. Subsequently, endocrine follow-up was continued by
collecting blood samples at 3-months intervals.

The following hormonal parameters were estimated: T (12), 5α-
dihydrotestosterone (DHT), using the same antibody after separation of DHT and T on microcolumns of silicagel (2), sex hormone
binding globulin (SHBG, 3) LH and FSH before and after i.v. administration of 100 µg LHRH (Relefact, Hoechst) (6), cortisol before
and after i.v. administration of 250 µg synthetic ACTH 1-24
(Synacthen, Organon, Oss, The Netherlands) using radioimmunoassay
(RIA)-kits provided by Clinical Assays Corporation (Cambridge, MA,
USA) and oestradiol (E_2), using the RIA-kit provided by EIR
(Würenlingen, Schweiz). Results are presented as means ± s.e.m.
Differences were considered significant when $p < 0.05$ (two
tailed).

RESULTS

Plasma gonadotropin concentrations

During therapy with Buserelin alone, plasma concentrations of both
LH and FSH gradually declined (data not shown). When the response
of LH and FSH to exogenous LHRH was estimated, a significant
increase of plasma gonadotropin levels was observed 30 min after
administration of the secretagogue at each time ($p < 0.05$ Student's
paired t-test), with the exeption of plasma FSH after 1 year of
treatment.

No significant differences between results for group I (no
progression) and group II (progression within 1 year) were
detected.

Steroid concentrations

Peripheral concentrations of T during the first year of treatment
in groups I and II are summarized in Fig. 1. Differences between T
concentrations in the 2 groups were not significant at any time
after the start of treatment. (Student's t-test).

After 2 months of treatment, between 80 and 90% of the
patients showed plasma T levels below 3 nmol/1, while between 50
and 60% had values below 2 nmol/1 (Fig. 2). Comparison with plasma
T concentrations in castrated men indicates that in the latter

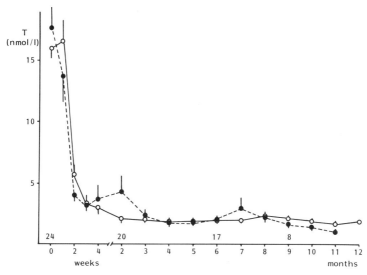

Fig 1. Plasma testosterone concentrations in 32 PCA patients
without progression (o——o) and in the indicated number of
PCA patients with progression within 1 year (● – ●) of
treatment with Buserelin (mean ± s.e.m.).

population T levels lower than 3 nmol/l were found in 47 out of 50
samples, and levels lower than 2 nmol/l in 33 out of 50 samples.
    Plasma concentrations of DHT, E_2 and SHBG during the first
year of treatment have been summarized in Table 1. DHT levels
before treatment were highly correlated with concentrations of T
in the same samples (n=44, r=0.73, DHT=-0.074 + 0.093T). After 3
months of treatment, the mean DHT concentration was 18% of the
pretreatment level; it did not change significantly after that
time. For the 141 samples, in which T and DHT were estimated
during treatment, the correlation coefficient for the relationship

Table 1. Plasma concentrations of 5α-dihydrotestosterone (DHT),
         oestradiol (E_2) and sex hormone binding globulin (SHBG)
         in PCA patients during treatment with Buserelin[a]

Time after start of treatment	n	DHT (nmol/1)	E_2 (pmol/1)	SHBG (nmol/1)
0 months	58	1.56 ± 0.11	67 ± 4	49 ± 3
3	54	0.27 ± 0.02	22 ± 2	61 ± 4
6	51	0.28 ± 0.04	22 ± 2	55 ± 4
9	42	0.27 ± 0.03	19 ± 2	53 ± 4
12	32	0.23 ± 0.02	20 ± 1	58 ± 5

[a]mean ± s.e.m.

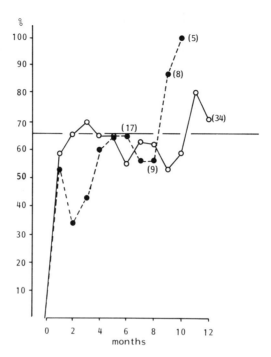

Fig 2. Percentage of PCA patients with plasma testosterone
        concentrations < 2 nmol/l in Group I (no progression within
        1 year, o——o) and in Group II (progression within 1 year,
        •--•) after various periods of treatment with Buserelin.

between plasma concentrations of these hormones was 0.66
(DHT=0.117 + 0.064T). Plasma E_2 was suppressed to 28% of
pretreatment values after 3 months. Thereafter, no further changes
of plasma E_2 levels occurred. The plasma concentration of SHBG
increased slightly, but significantly, during the first three
months of treatment (Student's paired t-test). Further changes in
the SHBG concentration were not observed. No significant
differences were found between plasma concentrations of DHT, E_2
and SHBG in patients in Groups I and II.

     Finally, no significant effects of treatment on plasma
cortisol levels before or after administration of synacthen were
found in groups I and II. However, basal levels of cortisol in
group II were significantly higher than those in group I before
treatment and after 3 and 6 months of treatment (Table 2).

Effects of time of blood sampling on concentrations of T, LH and cortisol in Buserelin-treated patients

In order to investigate if the intranasal administration of
Buserelin has acute effects on plasma concentrations of LH and/or

Table 2. Plasma cortisol concentrations (µmol/l) before (-) and after (+) i.v. administration of 250 µg Synacthen, in PCA patients during treatment with Buserelin[a]

Time after start of treatment	ACTH	Group I[b]	Group II[b]
0 months	-	0.37 ± 0.02 (30)	0.50 ± 0.03* (24)
	+	0.73 ± 0.04	0.75 ± 0.03
3 months	-	0.31 ± 0.02 (26)	0.43 ± 0.04* (19)
	+	0.73 ± 0.03	0.76 ± 0.04
6 months	-	0.35 ± 0.02 (31)	0.46 ± 0.06 (17)
	+	0.76 ± 0.04	0.81 ± 0.07
12 months	-	0.30 ± 0.02 (27)	
	+	0.72 ± 0.04	

[a] mean ± s.e.m.
[b] Group I: PCA patients, not showing progressive disease within one year of treatment .
   Group II: PCA patients, showing progressive disease within one year of treatment.
* significantly different from data in Group I (p<0.05, Student's t-test).

T, these hormones were estimated in blood samples obtained before and at 30, 60, 120 and 240 min after the 3 daily "sniffs" of Buserelin in 8 patients. Data for T are shown in Fig. 3: it is apparent that no acute increases occured after the administration of the LHRH-analogue, and that a diurnal rhythm was present. For this reason, cortisol concentrations were also estimated in the same plasma samples. No significant correlation was found between concentrations of LH and T (r=0.100, n=112), while the correlation between concentrations of cortisol and T was significant (r=0.392, n=112). This relationship between concentrations of cortisol and T was even more obvious, (r=0.587, n=88) when concentrations after the "sniff" were normalized by subtraction from the value before the administration of Buserelin in individual patients.

DISCUSSION

Gonadotropin concentrations

The steady decline of LH, as observed during this study, is comparable with the data presented by Santen et al. (10).

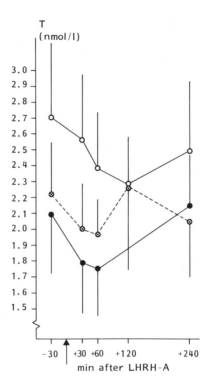

Fig 3. Plasma testosterone concentrations in 8 Buserelin-treated
       PCA patients at various times after the intranasal
       administration of the drug at 8.00 h (o), at 16.00 h (⊗)
       and at 23.00 h (●).

However, the present data for FSH contrast with those of Santen et
al. (10), who observed increasing concentrations of FSH after week
11 of treatment and suggested that this increase might be due to
lack of inhibin.
     The physiological significance of the increases of LH and FSH
which are observed 30 min after the i.v. administration of LHRH is
not clear. It might be that this immunologically active material
has no or little biological activity, as suggested by Warner et
al. (13). Furthermore, these increases contrast with the absence
of changes in LH concentrations after intranasal administration of
Buserelin as observed during the study of diurnal rhythms. This
difference may be explained on basis of the much larger dose of
LHRH, which was administered intravenously in the LHRH stimulation
tests.

Steroid concentrations

The concentrations of T as measured in the present study after the prolonged administration of Buserelin correspond to levels found in castrated men using the same method (Figure 2), but are higher than those reported earlier (7,10). This difference may be caused by the characteristics of the antibody used to measure T: cross-reaction with steroids from the adrenals - which are not suppressed as judged by the non-changing concentrations of cortisol - might play a role. These data do not indicate that progression of the disease is in any way related to failure to achieve the desired level of T: concentrations of T in groups I and II were not different at any time (Figure 1).

The decrease in the concentrations of DHT and E_2 is probably due to the decrease in the concentration of their main peripheral precursor: T. An increase of the ratio between the plasma concentrations of DHT and T was found after treatment with Buserelin, as was reported earlier (10,13). The increase in the concentration of SHBG can be explained on basis of the decreasing concentration of T, which normally has a suppressive effect on SHBG concentrations (1).

The difference between basal plasma cortisol concentrations in groups I and II cannot be explained yet; more data need to be collected before a causol role of the adrenal steroid production in the course of the disease may be postulated.

Diurnal rhythms of LH, T and cortisol

This part of the study was prompted by the publication of Kerle et al. (5), who described acute increases of both LH and T after injection of the LHRH-analogue ICI 118630, even after 6 or 12 months treatment with this analogue. The results of the present study indicate that no such phenomenon is observed after the administration of Buserelin in a 3-times per day scheme. This suggests that frequent administration of relatively low doses of LHRH analogues leads to a stronger suppression of the pituitary-testicular axis than the less frequent administration of higher doses.

Finally, the correlation between cortisol and T levels indicates that in these "chemically castrated" men adrenal function affects plasma T concentrations, as is the case in normal women. The lack of correlation between LH and T levels is another indication for altered bio/immuno ratios of LH after LHRH-analogue treatment.

REFERENCES

1. Anderson, D.C. (1974): Clin. Endocr., 3: 69-96.
2. Hämäläinen, E.K., Fotsis, T., and Adlercreutz, H. (1984): Clin. chim. Acta, 139: 173-177.
3. Hammond, G.L., and Lăteenmăki, P.L.A. (1983): Clin. Chim. Acta, 132: 101-110.
4. Huggins, C., and Hodges, C.V. (1941): Cancer Res., 1: 293-297.

5. Kerle, D., Williams, G., Ware, H., and Bloom, S.R. (1984): Br. Med. J., 289: 468–469.
6. Klijn, J.G.M., Lamberts, S.W.J., de Jong, F.H., Docter, R., Van Dongen, K.J., and Birkenhager, J.C. (1980): Clin. Endocr., 12: 341–355.
7. Leuprolide Study Group (LSG) (1984): New Engl. J. Med., 311: 1281–1286.
8. Pinto, H., Waschenberg, B.L., Linia, F.B., Goldman, J., Comaru-Schally, A.M., and Schally, A.V. (1979): Acta endocr., 91: 1–13.
9. Sandow, J., Van Rechenberg, W., Jerzabek, G., Engelbart, K., Kuhl, H., and Fraser, H.M. (1980): Acta endocr., 94: 489–497.
10. Santen, R.J., Demers, L.M., Max, D.T., Smith, J., Stein, B.S., and Glode, L.M. (1984): J. clin. Endocr. Metab., 58: 397–400.
11. Schroeder, F.H. et al., this volume.
12. Verjans, H.L., Cooke, B.A., de Jong, F.H., de Jong, C.M.M., and van der Molen, H.J. (1973): J. Steroid Biochem., 4: 665–676.
13. Warner, B., Worgul, T.J., Drago, J., Demers, L., Dufau, M., Max, D., Santen, R.J. (1983): J. clin. Invest., 71: 1842–1853.

Hormonal Manipulation of Cancer: Peptides, Growth Factors, and New (Anti) Steroidal Agents, edited by Jan G. M. Klijn et al. Raven Press, New York © 1987.

PHARMACOKINETICS OF LHRH AGONISTS IN DIFFERENT DELIVERY SYSTEMS

AND THE RELATION TO ENDOCRINE FUNCTION

J. Sandow, H.R. Seidel, B. Krauss and G. Jerabek-Sandow

Hoechst AG, D-6230 Frankfurt 80, Germany F.R.

INTRODUCTION

The use of LHRH agonists for transient or long-term inhibition of gonadal steroid secretion covers a wide spectrum of indications in contraception, oestrogen-dependent disorders (endometriosis and leiomyoma uteri), and hormone-dependent tumours (prostate and mammary carcinoma). The clinical indications require treatment by single or multiple daily doses administered by injection (26), nasal spray (8, 26), sustained release formulations such as microcapsules (32) or injectable implants (1, 16, 21), and other forms of administration, e.g. vaginal suppositories. In our studies, we have attempted to correlate the pharmacokinetic results of monitoring release from different formulations of LHRH agonists with the biological and clinical responses observed during treatment. The studies were mainly performed with the agonist D-Ser(Bu^t)^6-LHRH(1-9)nonapeptide-ethylamide (buserelin), because of the clinical use of this peptide in treatment of hormone-dependent prostate carcinoma and mammary carcinoma.

Mechanism of action

The suppression of pituitary-gonadal function by buserelin is achieved by different mechanisms (25), of which the most important one is a reduction of pituitary LHRH binding capacity by an induced receptor loss (20). LHRH agonists bind to pituitary membrane receptors with high affinity, forming stable hormone receptor complexes, which are subsequently internalized and degraded. This mechanism is highly effective during the sustained release of agonists from injectable microcapsules or implants, at a relatively constant daily rate. A common characteristic of the hormonal response to LHRH agonists is increased gonadotrophin release during the first days (transitory stimulation phase), followed by a consistent decline of gonadal steroid secretion due to inhibition of gonadotrophin release and synthesis (18). The extent of pituitary desensitization during the suppression phase is dose-dependent. During low daily doses by nasal spray, a partial LH response may be preserved, although steroidogenic capacity of the ovarian follicles or Leydig cells is already severely impaired. During high daily doses (injections or sustained release), gonadotrophins and gonadal steroids decrease to uniformly low levels.

Pharmacokinetic monitoring

The analytical task of measuring serum or plasma concentrations of LHRH agonists is considerably facilitated by their chemical and biochemical differences in comparison with luteinizing hormone-releasing hormone (LHRH). LHRH excretion has been measured in the plasma (10, 11) and in the urine (3) under physiological conditions and during therapy. Highly specific radioimmunoassays have been developed for LHRH-decapeptide-agonists (4, 15), and LHRH-nonapeptide-agonists (20, 24, 33). Our studies were performed with a method of separation of intact buserelin and buserelin metabolites by high performance liquid chromatography (HPLC), and radioimmunoassay (RIA) with specific buserelin antisera as the detection method.

In studies with single doses of buserelin (1-20/ug i.v. or s.c.), the biological response (LH release) was a suitable dose-related parameter for absorption, also in studies with buserelin nasal spray (single doses of 300 or 400/ug in different solvent formulations, equivalent to 10/ug s.c.). After multiple doses, the biological response decreases by desensitization of LH release and cannot be used for bioequivalence studies. After high single doses (50-500/ug s.c.), the LH release is not dose-related, but indicates the maximal capacity for gonadotrophin secretion. Plasma concentrations of gonadal steroids decrease in proportion to the dose and frequency of administration, but this response is variable, because maximum suppression may be achieved by individually different serum concentrations of agonists. Since the biological response during suppression cannot be evaluated as a function of the dose, it is desirable to have pharmacokinetic methods for measuring the concentrations of LHRH agonists in the serum or other body fluids (20, 22, 24). After injection, local release or topical administration (e.g. by nasal

TABLE 1. Pharmacokinetics of LHRH and buserelin in rats after injection of 60/ug/rat (s.c.) and infusion of 60/ug/24 h (s.c.)

parameter		LHRH	buserelin
plasma elimination	$T_{1/2}$ min	15-20	60-80
biliary excretion	% dose	0.004	12.8
urinary excretion	% dose	0.002	25-30

spray), buserelin is absorbed, the invasion and transport to the target organ (gonadotroph cells) can be monitored by measuring the serum concentration. Enzymes in liver and kidney degrade buserelin (20, 23), and peptide metabolites are excreted and eliminated with bile or urine. A fraction of the dose is excreted as intact buserelin in the urine. In a method for long-term monitoring, sample collection is of particular clinical relevance. The analytical problems are facilitated, because significantly higher concentrations of immunoreactive buserelin are found in the urine after treatment, than after a similar dose of LHRH (Table 1). Protein binding of buserelin was about 15 %, in accordance with estimates for other LHRH-nonapeptide-agonists (29). A higher protein binding has been reported for nafarelin (4).

Problems to be investigated during treatment are the rates of absorption from different drug formulations and sites of administration, the individual response to treatment, and the drug concentrations during long-term treatment (cumulation in the body, or accelerated degradation by enzyme induction). The clinical task is to correlate the individual response of gonadal steroids with the pharmacokinetic concentrations in serum, plasma or urine. In contraceptive studies with buserelin, and in studies on endometriosis, a wide range of oestrogen responses has been noted (12). The pharmacokinetic studies were performed to investigate individual differences in absorption or metabolism, which might contribute to these response patterns. Treatment of hormone-dependent tumours requires highly effective and reliable sustained release formulations. The pharmacokinetic monitoring of such preparations was of particular concern (26, 30).

METHODS

For the measurement of buserelin in serum, plasma and biological fluids (bile, urine), a specific radioimmunoassay was developed. Several antisera of different specificity are used. One antiserum (AS-14) is suitable for buserelin in unextracted serum, another antiserum (AS-639) is suitable for buserelin and buserelin metabolites after HPLC separation. The biological activity of buserelin in serum, plasma or urine is determined by the LH release induced in male rats after 2 h infusion of the buserelin-containing sample, and calculated from a standard curve of 3-4 doses of buserelin. For HPLC analysis, serum, plasma or urine samples are extracted on octadecasilyl (C_{18}) cartridges (SEP-PAK, Waters/Millipore). Intact buserelin and metabolites are separated by HPLC (Waters/Millipore), as reported previously (24). At present, two separation systems are used (RAD-PAK 10 x 0.8 cm column, Bondapak 10/u particles, isocratic system of KH_2PO_4 0.12 M, pH 6.2/acetonitrile 35:65, or RAD-PAK 10 x 0.8 cm column, Novapak 5/u particles, isocratic system KH_2PO_4 0.05 M, pH 6.2/acetonitrile 70:30). With these systems, complete separation of C-terminal buserelin metabolites is achieved using buserelin antiserum AS-639 for post column RIA detection.

Pharmacokinetic studies in rats, dogs and monkeys are performed in unrestrained animals, with implantations and blood sampling under light anaesthesia. Urine samples are collected in metabolism cages. In long-term experiments, Alzet$^{(TM)}$ minipumps are used in rats, monkeys, and in dogs. In clinical studies, an external infusion system is used (9, 28), containing an osmotic minipump (model 2ML1 or 2ML2), with a subcutaneous catheter.

RESULTS

Treatment by injections

Serum or plasma concentrations of buserelin and D-Trp^6-LHRH-ethylamide were measured during clinical studies. After buserelin 15/ug i.v., the initial plasma concentrations were 8-10 ng/ml, they decreased rapidly due to the large distribution volume. After buserelin 15/ug s.c., an initial plasma concentration of 1-2 ng/ml was detectable for a short time, but a plasma half-life could not be calculated. The pharmacokinetic differences observed are similar to those during LHRH therapy (11). After treatment with buserelin nasal spray 300/ug (equivalent to 10/ug s.c.), buserelin determination in unextracted serum was difficult and ambiguous. After high doses (500/ug s.c. in prostate carcinoma, or 1000/ug s.c. in endometriosis), the serum concentration reached a maximum after 30-60 min and buserelin remained detectable for 6-8 h. In all studies with LHRH agonists (i.v.), a rapid distribution phase is followed by a slower elimination phase (10). After s.c. injection, plasma elimination was prolonged, the half-life estimate in endometriosis from 1-8 h after injection was 75-85 min. This estimate is in agreement with that reached after termination of an infusion of another LHRH agonist (2). In the therapy of precocious puberty, the LHRH agonist D-Trp^6-ethylamide is used (19). Its serum concentration was determined with buserelin antiserum AS-639 in girls treated with doses of 4-16/ug/kg once daily (s.c.). A dose-dependent increase of D-Trp^6-ethylamide with a maximum after 30-60 min was detected.

The urinary excretion of immunoreactive buserelin after treatment by injection was dose-related, urinary buserelin decreased

TABLE 2. Pharmacokinetics of buserelin in patients with endometriosis treated with injections for 7 days, followed by nasal spray maintenance therapy

treatment	dose/day	urinary excretion /ug/24 hours
injections	2 x 1000/ug	439.0 + 49.8 (10)
nasal spray	3 x 400/ug	14.4 + 3.4 (22)

( ) No. of observations

markedly (22) after changing from injections to maintenance therapy with buserelin nasal spray (Table 2).

Treatment by nasal spray

The buserelin nasal spray (16) is a significant improvement for long-term therapy with peptides (21). Two bioequivalent formulations of buserelin nasal spray are available (300 or 400/ug single dose). The LH release was used for calculation of bioequivalence with regard to i.v. injection. A more practical parameter of absorption than the short-lasting elevation of plasma buserelin (17) was the cumulative excretion of immunoreactive buserelin in the urine (within 6 h after treatment). Maximum urinary concentrations were reached after 2 hours, the urinary excretion was dose-dependent over a range of 3 x 300 to 8 x 300/ug/day. In long-term treatment, the daily excretion remained stable. A disadvantage was the necessity to collect urine samples for 12-24 hours, to determine the cumulative excretion. The biological response to the buserelin nasal spray depends on the dose and dose interval. In contraception, a single daily dose administered from the beginning of the cycle reduces responsiveness of the pituitary, preventing the preovulatory LH surge (26). For the arrest of follicular maturation, multiple daily doses are necessary to maintain loss of pituitary LHRH receptors (12, 14). Daily doses of 3 x 300/ug are generally sufficient to ensure oestrogen suppression in endometriosis.

Treatment by infusions

A highly effective regimen for consistent oestrogen- or androgen-suppression is the sustained release of LHRH agonists. The effective dose range can be established by infusion studies, using pumps with a constant or intermittent mode of dispensing. In several studies, an external minipump system has been used to deliver daily doses of 25-400/ug buserelin (s.c.) in women (9), and in men (28). In one study on oestrogen suppression in leiomyoma uteri (fibroids), a pulsatile pump provided a daily dose of 200/ug in pulses of 6/ug every 45 min (26). In these studies, the urinary excretion (buserelin/creatinine ratio in urine) was monitored. This method provides a significant improvement in long-term therapy control, because no quantitative urine collections are required. The urinary buserelin/creatinine ratio was consistent in groups of patients treated with 200 or 400/ug per day. During infusion of 400/ug/day, the average serum concentration was 1.15 ± 0.1 ng buserelin/ml, and the urinary buserelin/creatinine ratio was 82.3 ± 5.5/ug/g creatinine.

The biological response to these infusions was consistent, during 118-230/ug/day in normal male test persons, testosterone decreased within one week and remained suppressed for 12 weeks (28). At the end of the infusion, serum testosterone returned to pretreatment levels within 2 weeks. In women with endometriosis,

200/ug/day reduced serum oestradiol to the castrate-like range
throughout the treatment period. The initial stimulation phase
at the beginning of treatment was curtailed by infusion (200/ug/
day) in comparison with injections (2 x 200/ug s.c. per day), or
nasal spray treatment (3 x 300/ug/day, equivalent to 30/ug s.c.).
No formation of neutralizing antibodies against buserelin or LHRH
was found during long-term injection or infusion therapy (6).

Treatment by sustained release

Long-acting preparations of steroid hormones have been available for a long time, consisting of non-degradable polymer materials (e.g. silicone elastomers), or of biodegradable copolymers
of polylactic acid and glycolic acid used in resorbable surgical
suture material (13). Such preparations may be easily administered by injection, either as pellets (31), small rods (8), or as a
suspension of microcapsules (32). Sustained release formulations
for several LHRH agonists are currently under preclinical and
clinical investigation (8, 16, 30, 32). They provide a relatively constant rate of release, gradually declining to a critical
lower limit of release, at which gonadal suppression is no longer
maintained. The pharmacokinetics of such buserelin preparations
are easily monitored by the serum concentrations of buserelin at
release rates of 200-400/ug/day, whereas release rates of 10-
100/ug/day are preferably determined by the urinary buserelin/
creatinine ratio.

Microcapsules

Treatment with microcapsule suspensions (i.m. or s.c.) is a
convenient clinical approach to long-term control of precocious
puberty, and hormone-dependent tumours (32). The release from
buserelin microcapsule formulations was monitored in dogs by the
urinary buserelin/creatinine ratio and serum testosterone. A buserelin excretion of 4/ug/g creatinine was compatible with full
suppression of testosterone secretion. The suppressive effect of
a single dose lasts for 8 weeks. The release from microcapsules
has also been monitored using other LHRH agonists, and the polymer composition of polylactide/glycolide copolymers was found to

TABLE 3. Metabolism of buserelin in different species, percent
excretion in urine of intact buserelin and of the main metabolite

species	intact buserelin	(5-9) pentapeptide
rat	22.5	44.2
dog	70.2	22.4
monkey	54.2	31.8
human	55.1	31.6

be an important parameter for the release profile, immediate or delayed onset of action, and the duration of suppression (32).

Implant treatment

We have developed a disk-shaped tablet of polyhydroxybutyric acid (PHB), containing a dose of 0.5-5 mg buserelin for surgical implantation (16, 27). The effect on serum testosterone was confirmed in rats, dogs and monkeys. The release rate was dependent on the polymer composition, and the surface area. Tissue tolerance is excellent. A coated implant provided a relatively constant release rate for more than 8 weeks. PHB implants containing 5 mg buserelin were administered in patients with prostate carcinoma at a dose interval of 28 days (30). An initial stimulation phase of 4-7 days was followed by a decline to castration-like serum concentrations of testosterone between 2 and 3 weeks after the first implantation. Testosterone suppression has been maintained for more than 12 months.

Biodegradable polylactide/glycolide (PLG) implants have also been tested containing a dose of 2.6-4 mg buserelin, in a matrix of PLG 75:25 or 50:50. This implant material is derived from resorbable surgical suture material with an excellent tissue tolerance (13). The release of buserelin in rats, dogs and monkeys lasted for 8-23 weeks, with full suppression of oestrogen or androgen secretion. Biodegradation was dependent on the polymer composition. In dogs, a single implant reduced serum testosterone to castrate-like levels for 15-23 weeks (Fig. 1), and a buserelin excretion of 10/ug/g creatinine ensured long-term suppression. In monkeys, the release from an implant containing 2.6 mg buserelin suppressed follicular maturation for more than 80 days, provided that treatment started during the luteal phase of the cycle to prevent initial oestrogen hyperstimulation (7). A high level of buserelin excretion in the urine was maintained for 70 days. Preliminary experience in prostate carcinoma confirms the suitability of this implant for long-term control of testosterone secretion.

The material circulating in serum identified by HPLC/RIA consists mainly of intact buserelin, together with a small fraction of the (5-9)pentapeptide and smaller C-terminal fragments (26). In the urine, intact buserelin is excreted together with the (5-9)pentapeptide as the main metabolite, and small amounts of the (6-9)tetrapeptide, and (7-9)tripeptide. The percentage of intact buserelin and the (5-9)pentapeptide depends on the species investigated (Table 3).

CONCLUSIONS

The use of LHRH agonists as antigonadotrophic agents requires a clear therapeutic concept for each clinical indication. Gonadal steroid secretion should be depressed rapidly, followed by an extended phase of reversible or permanent suppression. The ini-

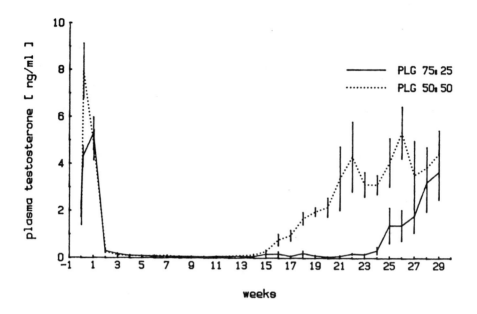

FIG. 1 Biological effect of buserelin implants in dogs on plasma concentrations of testosterone. Means and standard error of 6 dogs per group. Two different copolymer compositions of polylactic/glycolic acid were tested.

tial rise of androgens is neutralized by an androgen-receptor blocker, and pituitary suppression may be enhanced by a high dose progestagen. Pituitary inhibition is initiated with high doses, and maintained with lower doses. Selection of effective doses and dose intervals is facilitated by monitoring of the urinary buserelin/creatinine ratio. Analytical methods for the low concentrations of LHRH agonists in serum or plasma are specific radioimmunoassays, with or without extraction for sample concentration. A convenient non-invasive approach is monitoring of the daily urinary excretion (during treatment with injections or nasal spray), or the urinary buserelin/creatinine ratio (during infusions or implant treatment). Plasma elimination of buserelin after high dose injections is prolonged, and ensures therapeutic plasma concentrations for more than 8 h. In long-term maintenance with buserelin nasal spray in endometriosis and prostate carcinoma, urinary excretion is reproducible and consistent. Infusion studies with buserelin have established the release rates for implant treatment. Both the plasma concentration and the urinary buserelin/creatinine ratio are dose-related, reliable parameters for the effective use of sustained release formulations. Pharmacokinetics establish a correlation of the plasma concentration and/or urinary excretion with maintenance of steroid suppression. Clinically effective doses maintain pituitary desensitization by a progressive loss of LHRH receptors. Implant formulations of buserelin are active in rats, dogs and monkeys for 8-23 weeks after a single dose, and implant treatment in patients with prostate carcinoma is effective for more than 12 months, at dose intervals of 28 days. The numerous therapeutic indications for LHRH agonists require different regimens (19, 26). Thus, nasal spray formulations have their advantages for gynaecological indications which require reversibility of action, and sustained release formulations provide long-term control of gonadal steroid secretion in hormone-dependent tumours.

REFERENCES

1. Anik, S.T., McRae, G., Nerenberg, C., Worden, A., Foreman, J., Hwang, J.-Y., Kushinsky, S., Jones, R.E. & Vickery, B. (1983): J. Pharm. Sci., 73:684.
2. Barron, J., Millar, R.P. & Searle, D. (1982): J. Endocrinol. Metab., 54:1169.
3. Bourguignon, J.P., Hoyoux, C., Reuter, A., Franchimont, P., Leinartz-Dourcy, C. & Vrindts-Gevaert, Y. (1979): J. Clin. Endocrinol. Metab., 48:78-84.
4. Chan, R.L. & Chaplin, M.D. (1985): Biochem. Biophys. Res. Commun., 127:673.
5. Clayton, R.N., Bailey, L.C., Cottam, J., Arkell, D., Perren, T.J. & Blackledge, G.R.P. (1985): Clin. Endocrinol., 22:453.
6. Fraser, H.M., Sandow, J. & Krauss, B. (1983): Acta Endocrinol., 103:151-157.
7. Fraser, H.M. & Sandow, J. (1985): J. Clin. Endocrinol. Metab., 60:597-584.
8. Furr, B.J.A. & Hutchinson, F.G. (1985): In: EORTC Genitourinary Group Monograph 2, Part A: Therapeutic Principles in Metastatic Prostatic Cancer, pp. 143-153, Alan R. Liss, Inc.
9. Geisthövel, F., Rieger, B., Geyer, H., Peters, F. & Sandow, J. (1986): Acta Endocrinol., 111:80 (Suppl. 274).
10. Handelsman, D.J. & Swerdloff, R.S. (1986): Endocr. Reviews, 7:95-105.
11. Handelsman, D.J., Jansen, R.P.S., Boylan, L.M., Spaliviero, J.A. & Turtle, J.R. (1984): J. Clin. Endocrinol. Metab., 59:739.
12. Hardt, W. & Schmidt-Gollwitzer, M. (1983): Clin. Endocrinol., 19:613.
13. Jackanicz, T.M., Nash, H.A., Wise, D.L. & Gregory, J.B. (1973): Contraception, 9:227.
14. Lemay, A. & Quesnel, G. (1982): Fertil. Steril., 38:376-377.
15. Nerenberg, C., Foreman, J., Chu, N., Chaplin, M.D. & Kusninsky, S. (1984): Anal. Biochem., 141:10.
16. Petri, W., Seidel, R. & Sandow, J. (1984): In: LHRH and Its Analogues, edited by Labrie, F., Belanger, A. & Dupont, A., pp. 63-76, Elsevier Science Publishers B.V.

17. Saito, S., Saito, H. & Yamasaki, R. (1985): J. Immunol. Methods, 79:173-183
18. Sandow, J. (1982): In: Progress towards a male contraceptive, edited by S.L. Jeffcoate & M. Sandler, pp. 19-39, John Wiley & Sons Ltd., London.
19. Sandow, J. (1983): Clin. Endocrinol., 18:571-592.
20. Sandow, J. & Clayton, R.N. (1983): In: Hormone Biochemistry and Pharmacology, Vol. 2, edited by Briggs, M. & Corbin, A., pp. 63-106, Eden Press, Montreal.
21. Sandow, J. & Petri, W. (1985): In: Transnasal Systemic Medications, edited by Y.W. Chien, pp. 183-199, Elsevier Science Publishers B.V., Amsterdam.
22. Sandow, J., Jerabek-Sandow, G., Krauss, B. & Schmidt-Gollwitzer, M. (1984): In: LHRH and Its Analogues, edited by Labrie, F., Belanger, A., Dupont, A., pp. 123-137, Elsevier Science Publishers B.V.
23. Sandow, J., Jerabek-Sandow, G., Schmidt-Gollwitzer, M. (1985): In: LHRH and its Analogues, Fertility and Antifertility Aspects, edited by Schmidt-Gollwitzer, M. & Schley, R., pp. 105-121, Walter de Gruyter, Berlin.
24. Sandow, J., Jerabek-Sandow, G., Krauss, B. & von Rechenberg, W. (1985): In: Future Aspects in Contraception, Part 2, Female Contraception, edited by Runnebaum, B., Rabe, T., Kiesel, L., pp. 129-147, MTP Press Ltd., Boston.
25. Sandow, J., Engelbart, K. & von Rechenberg, W. (1985): Med. Biol., 63:192-200.
26. Sandow, J., Fraser, H.M. & Geisthövel, F. (1986): In: Symposium "Gonadotropin down-regulation in gynaecological practice", Nijmegen, April 25.-26., 1986, Alan Liss Inc. (in press).
27. Sandow, J., Seidel, H.R. & von Rechenberg, W. (1986): Acta Endocrinol., 111:77 (Suppl. 274).
28. Schürmeyer, Th., Knuth, U.A., Freischem, C.W., Sandow, J., Bint Akhtar, F. & Nieschlag, E. (1984): J. Clin. Endocr. Metab., 59:19-24.
29. Tharandt, L., Schulte, H., Benker, G., Hackenberg, K. & Reinwein, D. (1979): Horm. Metab. Res., 11:391.
30. Waxman, J. (1986): Behring Symposium "Neue Wege in der Therapie des fortgeschrittenen Prostatakarzinoms mit LHRH-Agonisten", Frankfurt/Main, 27.-28. September 1985, PMI Verlag, Frankfurt (in press).
31. Vickery, B.H. (1981): In: LHRH peptides as female and male contraceptives, edited by G.I. Zatuchni, J.D. Shelton & J.J. Sciarra, pp. 275-290, Harper & Row, Philadelphia.
32. Vickery, B.H. & Sanders, L.M. (1985): In: LHRH and its Analogues, Fertility and Antifertility Aspects, edited by Schmidt-Gollwitzer, M. & Schley, R., pp. 123-134, Walter de Gruyter, Berlin.
33. Yamazaki, I. & Okada, H. (1980): Endocrinol. Jpn., 27:593-605.

Hormonal Manipulation of Cancer: Peptides, Growth Factors, and New (Anti) Steroidal Agents, edited by Jan G. M. Klijn et al.
Raven Press, New York © 1987.

TREATMENT OF HORMONE-RESPONSIVE RAT MAMMARY AND PROSTATE TUMOURS WITH 'ZOLADEX'* DEPOT

B.J.A. Furr

Imperial Chemical Industries PLC, Pharmaceuticals Division, Mereside, Alderley Park, Macclesfield SK10 4TG, Cheshire, U.K.

Introduction

The properties of the clinically available luteinizing hormone releasing-hormone (LH-RH) agonists have been thoroughly reviewed recently (1,11). All of these LH-RH analogues appear to possess the same pharmacological properties and side-effects and have very similar potencies. To date, most attention has focussed clinically on the so called 'paradoxical' properties of LH-RH agonists, whereby chronic administration causes an inhibition of pituitary and gonadal hormone secretion to produce an effect akin to castration. In reality, this finding is not paradoxical but is a predictable consequence of the well-recognized phenomenon of tachyphylaxis alternatively called tissue desensitization or receptor down-regulation.

Since LH-RH agonists are peptides they all have poor oral potency and so are most effectively given by the parenteral route. Daily injection is inconvenient for the patient so alternative means of delivery have been developed. Multiple daily dosing from a nasal spray formulation has advantages over s.c. injection but in our experience gave low and variable absorption of drug. A decision was made, therefore, to produce a biodegradable depot formulation of the ICI LH-RH agonist, 'Zoladex' (ICI 118,630; D-Ser(Bu^t)^6,Azgly^{10}LH-RH). This depot is in the form of a rod approximately 1mm in diameter and from 5-12mm in length, depending on the dose of drug to be administered, and contains 'Zoladex' dispersed homogeneously throughout a matrix of 50:50 lactide-glycolide co-polymer. This preparation releases drug continuously for at least 28 days,

*Zoladex is a trade mark the property of Imperial Chemical Industries PLC.

is completely biodegradable and has shown no evidence of
toxicity in animal studies.

Pharmacological Studies

Although the primary objective was to develop a
formulation of 'Zoladex' which was more convenient to
administer and which would improve compliance, it was soon
appreciated that the depot formulation was also more
efficacious. For example, 'Zoladex' depot was more
effective at desensitizing the rat pituitary gland to a
bolus injection of 50μg 'Zoladex' than a comparable dose
delivered by daily s.c. aqueous injection; 'Zoladex' depot
was also able to induce a decrease in monkey serum
testosterone concentrations to castrate values, whereas
daily injection of a similar dose was incompletely effective
(3). There is also evidence that a depot containing 3.6mg
'Zoladex' given every 28 days to patients with prostate
cancer produces a superior endocrine effect to 250μg drug
given daily as an aqueous injection s.c. (12).

Because of its ability to induce a 'medical castration'
the efficacy of 'Zoladex' has been evaluated in two
hormone-responsive tumour models. The first was the
dimethylbenzanthracene (DMBA)-induced rat mammary carcinoma
(5), which is known to be dependent on both oestrogen and
prolactin (6). A single subcutaneous depot containing 300μg

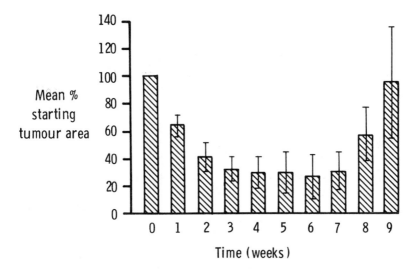

FIG. 1. Effect of a single subcutaneous depot containing
300μg 'Zoladex' given at time 0 on growth of DMBA-induced
rat mammary tumours. The values shown are means ± SEM for
10 rats.

'Zoladex caused an inhibition of oestrogen secretion, the disappearance of cornified cells from vaginal smears and the regression of DMBA-induced mammary tumours (Figure 1). Half of the tumours present at the start of the experiment were not palpable at 28 days but all save one of them reappeared between 40 and 60 days as the single 'Zoladex' depot became exhausted. In contrast, the DMBA-induced mammary tumours increased in size by more than 50% in control animals given a placebo depot.

Single depots of the drug given s.c. at weeks 0, 4 and 8 of the study caused more impressive tumour regression (Figure 2) and all of the tumours present at the start were non-palpable by week 11.

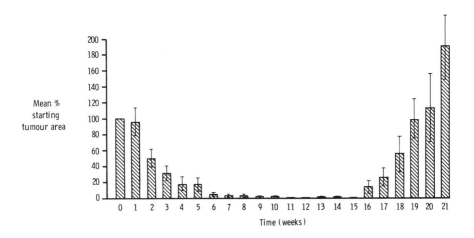

FIG. 2. Effect of single subcutaneous depots containing 300µg 'Zoladex' given at 0, 4 and 8 weeks on growth of DMBA-induced rat mammary tumours. The values shown are the means ± SEM for 10 rats.

Again, by week 16 regrowth of the tumours occurred because treatment stopped at week 8. By week 20 the tumours had reattained pretreatment size.

When given at days 30, 58 and 86 after administration of the carcinogen single depots containing 300µg 'Zoladex' delayed the appearance of tumours for a period of around 100 days i.e. the expected duration of action of such a treatment regimen (Figure 3).

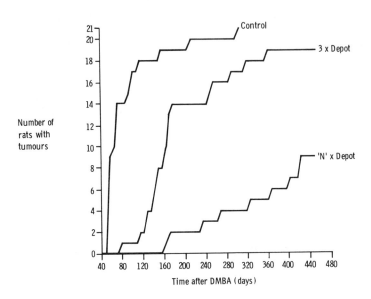

FIG. 3. Effect of depots containing 300µg 'Zoladex' on the
appearance of mammary tumours induced in rats by DMBA. The
number of rats with tumours in groups given placebo depots
(Control), single depots at day 30, 58 and 86 (3x Depot) or
single depots every 28 days starting at day 30 ('N' x Depot)
are shown. Each group comprised 21 rats.

When given at 28 day intervals, starting on day 30
after administration of the carcinogen, single subcutaneous
depots of 'Zoladex' caused a more profound inhibition of
tumour appearance and only 9 out of 21 rats had mammary
tumours at the end of the study on day 450. Those tumours
which were found did not regress following ovariectomy and
so were classified as non-hormone responsive. It is
concluded from this study, which approximates the adjuvant
therapy setting, that 'Zoladex' may be of benefit as a
treatment for primary breast cancer post-mastectomy in
premenopausal women.

The second tumour used is the Dunning R3327H rat
transplantable prostate adenocarcinoma, which is androgen
responsive and has been used extensively as a model for the
human disease (10). Single subcutaneous depots containing
1mg 'Zoladex' given every 28 days to rats bearing Dunning
R3327H prostate tumours implanted on each flank caused a

marked inhibition of tumour growth to values indistinguishable
from those in surgically castrated rats (Figure 4).

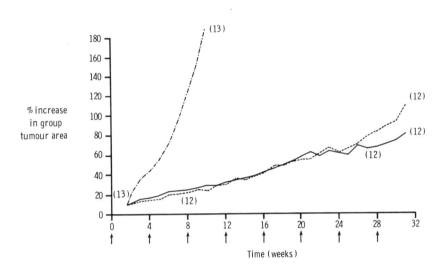

FIG. 4. Effect of single subcutaneous depots containing 1mg
'Zoladex' on the growth of Dunning R3327H transplantable rat
prostate tumours. The depots were given every 4 weeks as
shown by the arrows. The control group (.___.___.) had 13
animals and the 'Zoladex'-treated (----) and surgically
castrated (———) groups 12 animals each as shown by the
figures in parentheses.

Twenty-one days after the eighth depot was given the rats
were killed. The weights of the sex organs and serum
hormone concentrations measured by radioimmunoassay are
shown in Table 1.

Testes weights were about 10% those of control rats of a
similar age and weight and showed atrophic histological
changes; ventral prostate gland and seminal vesicle weights
were identical to those in the surgically castrated group
and histologically, were also completely atrophic. Serum
prolactin doubled in rats given 'Zoladex', as it did in
surgically castrated animals, probably as a consequence of
androgen withdrawal. This contrasts with the effect of
'Zoladex' in female rats where there is a significant
reduction in serum prolactin following oestrogen withdrawal
(4).

TABLE 1. Sex organ weights and serum hormone concentrations in 'Zoladex'-treated, and surgically castrated rats bearing Dunning R3327H prostate tumours. Control values for rats of a similar age and weight are shown for comparison

Parameter	'Zoladex'	Castrate	Control
Testes wt (mg)	366.5±10.2	-	∿3,500
Ventral prostate wt (mg)	21.3± 1.1	19.9±0.7	∿ 250
Seminal vesicle wt (mg)	54.3±1.0	53.8±0.8	∿ 350
Serum LH (ng/ml)	<0.2	12.9±1.0	∿ 1.5
Serum FSH (ng/ml)	174±6	1,413±24	∿ 400
Serum prolactin (ng/ml)	63.2±4.5	60.9±7.5	∿ 30
Serum testosterone (ng/ml)	<0.25	<0.26	∿ 3

    Because of interest in the concept of 'total androgen withdrawal' persuasively supported by Labrie and co-workers (7) a study of the effects of 'Zoladex' depot and a new antiandrogen, ICI 176,334, given alone and in combination, were evaluated. The results (Figure 5) clearly show that both 'Zoladex' depot and ICI 176,334 are effective at limiting tumour growth but that the combination offers no advantage over monotherapy with 'Zoladex'.

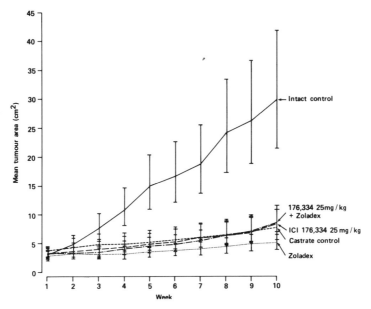

FIG. 5. Effect of single s.c. 1mg 'Zoladex' depots given every 28 days, daily oral administration of 25mg ICI 176,334/kg and the combination of both treatments on the growth of Dunning prostate tumours. The values shown are means ± SEM; n=8.

This finding is in agreement with a similar study by Redding and Schally (8) and the work of Ellis and Isaacs (2) who showed that antiandrogen failed to improve the effect of surgical castration in rats with Dunning tumours. It is possible that the rat secretes less androgen from the adrenal gland than man and that the rat may, therefore, not be the most suitable species in which to test the hypothesis. The results of the extensive, controlled, comparative clinical studies now being undertaken will, hopefully, soon answer this question.

At present, asymptomatic patients with prostate cancer usually remain untreated probably because of the unacceptability of the most widely used therapy, castration. This policy should be reconsidered now that LH-RH agonists and some newer antiandrogens have been introduced. It is important to know whether treatment early in the course of the disease reduces tumour growth rate and improves survival. Consequently, a study was made of the growth of Dunning tumours and the survival of rats given single 1mg 'Zoladex' depots every 28 days starting either 28 days after tumour implantation, when most tumours are not palpable, or when tumours had reached a size of $2 \geqslant cm^2$. Tumour growth was measured at weekly intervals and survival was assessed. In this experiment rats were killed for ethical reasons on the week the tumour burden exceeded 20 cm^2. The results shown in Figures 6 and 7 demonstrate that both treatment schedules reduce tumour growth rate and increase survival but that an early start of treatment produces the best result.

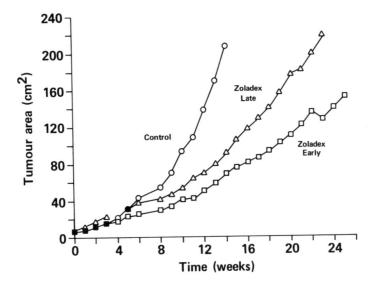

FIG. 6. Effect of single depots containing 1mg 'Zoladex' given every 28 days on growth of Dunning prostate tumours in rats. Control rats were untreated; early 'Zoladex' treatment started 28 days after tumour implantation; late 'Zoladex' treatment started when tumours measured 2 > cm^2. There were 14 rats in the control group and 13 rats in each 'Zoladex' treated group.

This finding is in accord with the work of Schally and Redding (9) who showed that combination of a LH-RH agonist with cytotoxic chemotherapy produced the most impressive response and increases in survival if started early post-transplantation of Dunning tumours. These results argue strongly that consideration should now be given to the treatment of patients with early stages of prostate cancer and it is hoped that clinical trials will soon confirm the animal data.

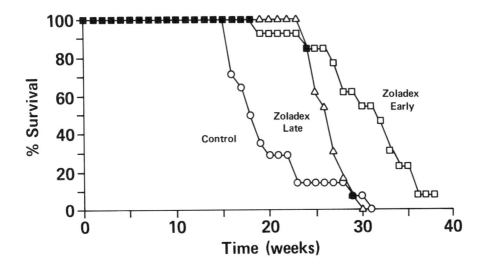

FIG. 7. Effect of single depots containing 1mg 'Zoladex' given every 28 days on survival of rats with Dunning prostate tumours. Control rats were untreated; early 'Zoladex' treatment started 28 days after tumour implantation; late 'Zoladex' treatment started when tumours measured $2 \geqslant cm^2$. There were 14 rats in the control group and 13 rats in each 'Zoladex' treated group.

Conclusions

'Zoladex' is a potent LH-RH agonist which can be released continuously from a biodegradable depot formulation over at least 28 days to give an effect which is similar to surgical castration. 'Zoladex' depot is more convenient than daily injections and the frequent use of a nasal spray, which should lead to improved compliance with treatment. An additional advantage of 'Zoladex' depot is that it is more effective at inducing pituitary desensitization than comparable daily aqueous s.c. injections. 'Zoladex' depot causes regression of DMBA-induced rat mammary tumours and prevents the appearance these mammary tumours when given in an adjuvant manner.

'Zoladex' depot also reduces the growth rate of Dunning prostate tumours in rats but combination with an anti-androgen fails to improve the response. Early treatment of rats with Dunning prostate tumours produces a superior reduction in growth rate and a better survival than if the drug treatment started later.

'Zoladex' depot should be effective in the treatment of advanced and primary breast cancer in pre-menopausal women and prostate cancer in men. The results provide no support for the concept that 'total androgen withdrawal' is superior to monotherapy but do argue that consideration should be given to beginning therapy for prostate cancer when the disease is first diagnosed.

Acknowledgements

NIAMADD, Professor L.E. Reichert and G.D. Niswender for reagents for FSH, LH and prolactin radioimmunoassays. The US National Prostate Cancer Agency for supplies of rats bearing Dunning R3327H tumours and F. Hutchinson, J. Tomenson, B. Valcaccia and J.R. Churchill for excellent support and criticism.

References

1. Dutta, A.S., and Furr, B.J.A. (1985): Ann. Rep. Med. Chem., 20:203-214.

2. Ellis, W.J., and Isaacs, J.T. (1985): Cancer Res., 45:6041-6050.

3. Furr, B.J.A., and Hutchinson, F.G. (1985): EORTC Genitourinary Group Monograph, 2, Part A. Therapeutic Principles in Metastatic Prostate Cancer, p.143-153. Alan R. Liss, New York.

4. Furr, B.J.A., and Nicholson, R.I. (1982): J. Reprod. Fert., 529-539.

5. Huggins, C., Briziarelli, G., and Sutton, H. (1959): J. exp. Med., 104:25.

6. Jordan, V.C. (1982): Clinics in Oncology, 1:21-40.

7. Labrie, F., Dupont, A., Belanger, A., Poyet, P., Giguere, M., Lacoursiere, Y., Edmond, J., Monfette, G., and Borsanyi, J.P. (1986). Lancet, i:48-49.

8. Redding, T.W., and Schally, A.V. (1985): The Prostate 6:219-232.

9. Schally, A.V., and Redding, T.W. (1985): Proc. Natl. Acad. Sci, U.S.A., 82:2498-25-2.

10. Smolev, J.K., Heston, W.D.W., Scott, W.W., and Coffey, D.S. (1977): Cancer Treat. Rep., 61:273-287.

11. Vickery, B.H., Nestor, J.J., and Hafez, E.S.E. (1984): LH-RH and its analogues, MTP Press, Lancaster.

12. Williams, G., Kerle, D.J., Roe, S.M., Yeo, T., and Bloom, S.R. (1985): EORTC Genitourinary Group Monograph 2, Part A 'Therapeutic Principles in Metastatic Prostate Cancer, p.287-295. Alan R. Liss, New York.

Hormonal Manipulation of Cancer: Peptides, Growth Factors, and New (Anti) Steroidal Agents, edited by Jan G. M. Klijn et al. Raven Press, New York © 1987.

LONG TERM TREATMENT WITH THE LHRH AGONIST BUSERELIN IN METASTATIC PROSTATIC CANCER. TWO PHASE II STUDIES INCLUDING BUSERELIN PLUS CYPROTERONE ACETATE.[a]

Fritz H. Schroeder[1], Tycho M.T.W. Lock[1], Paul J. Carpentier[1], Dev R. Chadha[2], Frans M.J. Debruyne[3], Frank H. de Jong[4], Jan G.M. Klijn[5], Ans W. Matroos[2] and Herman J. de Voogt[6].

Department of Urology[1] and Department of Biochemistry II and Internal Medicine III[4], Erasmus University, P.O. Box 1738, 3000 DR Rotterdam. Clinical Research Department, Hoechst Holland, P.O. Box 12987, 1100 AZ Amsterdam[2]. Department of Urology, Catholic University, P.O. Box 9101, 6500 HB Nijmegen[3]. Rotterdam Radiotherapeutic Institute, P.O. Box 5201, 3008 AE Rotterdam[5]. Department of Urology, Free University, P.O. Box 7057, 1007 MB, Amsterdam[6], The Netherlands.

LHRH agonists have become a new alternative in the management of hormone-responsive prostatic carcinoma patients. A number of early reports have shown the effectiveness of LHRH agonists in suppressing plasma testosterone to castration levels (11, 3, 1). More recently, it has been shown that management of metastatic prostatic cancer patients with LHRH analogues is clinically equally effective as standard forms of treatment (7, 8, 10). Labrie and his cooperators have claimed that management of prostatic carcinoma by means of "total androgen suppression" achieved by combining an LHRH analogue with a potent anti-androgen produces results that are far superior to standard treatment (5, 6).

The present study was undertaken to assess the clinical efficacy, safety and tolerability of Buserelin (HOE 766) in the treatment of metastatic prostatic carcinoma in a phase I-II study. A second, subsequent phase II study, carried out according to the same protocol and by the same investigators, aimed at determining the rate and duration of response and the progression rate in similar patients managed by total androgen blockade achieved by the use of Buserelin and Cyproterone Acetate (CPA). Preliminary results of the study have been reported by Debruyne (2), a complete report of the study will appear elsewhere (9).

A summary of the clinical results obtained are reported within this chapter. The endocrine data are reported in a separate chapter by De Jong and co-authors.

[a] This study was sponsored by Hoechst, The Netherlands.

MATERIAL AND METHODS

The objectives of the study are summarized in Table 1.

TABLE 1.   Objective of the study

Study 1.	To assess the clinical efficacy, safety and tolerability of Buserelin (HOE 766) in the treatment of metastatic prostatic carcinoma patients by:
a.	confirming the rapid progression of plasma testosterone and its maintenance on castration level
b.	determining the rate and duration of response and the rate of progression.
Study 2.	To determine the rate and duration of response and the progression rate in similar patients managed by total androgen blockade, according to the same protocol.

Criteria for inclusion. All patients had histologically proven prostatic carcinoma and clinically proven M1 or N4 disease. Plasma testosterone levels at entry were above 8 nmol/l. Patients with a WHO performance index of more than 2 were unacceptable. Patients had to be in an appropriate mental condition to be able to administer their medication. Only patients who gave an informed consent were eligible to the study. Patients with a second neoplasm except squamous cell carcinoma of the skin, or with rapidly fatal progressing illness were not eligible to the study. Also, patients with a history of alcohol or drug abuse were excluded. All patients were previously untreated.

Treatment schemes. The treatment regimens used in this study are indicated in Table 2.

TABLE 2.   Treatment regimens and evaluation

Study 1:	Buserelin 0.5 mg s.c./t.i.d. during 1 week, then 0.4 mg/t.i.d. intranasally
Study 2:	Buserelin, same as study 1, plus Cyproterone Acetate (CPA) 50 mg t.i.d. per os.

All patients were evaluated in monthly intervals. X-ray studies and bone scans were repeated whenever progression was suspected and 3-monthly.

Response criteria: modified NPCP criteria.

Patient population and follow-up. Fifty-eight patients were recruited to study 1, from March 1, 1983 to March 30, 1984. To study 2, 13 patients were recruited from June 1 to November 30,

1984. Both studies were carried out according to the same protocol and by the same investigators. For entry into study 2, in addition to M1 or N4 status, an elevated acid phosphatase had to be present. Patients were evaluated at entry and after 1 and 3 months and subsequently in 3-monthly intervals. All endocrine parameters were studied in one laboratory. No patients were lost to follow-up.

Response and progression. For the evaluation of response and progression, a combination of the criteria of the World Health Organisation and the National Prostatic Cancer Project was used.

Progression was present if the product of the two largest perpendicular diameters of a measurable lesion increased by more than 50%, when new bone lesions developed and persisted on a subsequent bone scan, when new palpable lymph node metastases were found and confirmed by biopsy, when new pulmonary metastases were seen on chest x-ray, when acid or alkaline phosphatase increased and this was combined with other progressive changes, with a decrease of performance by two scores and/or an increase of pain by two scores.

All patients were followed for at least 12 months and the results reported are limited to the 12 months' period in all patients. Recruitment of patients and periods of time are summarized in Table 3.

TABLE 3. Two consecutive phase II studies of previously untreated patients with metastatic prostatic carcinoma

	Study 1	Study 2
Treatment	Buserelin (LHRH agonist)	Buserelin + CPA
Number of patients	58	13
Study period	1.3.1983-30.5.1984	1.6.1984-30.11.1984
Period of follow-up	12 months	12 months

RESULTS

Study 1.

Fifty-eight patients were entered into study 1. The median age group was 65-69 years old. Table 4 shows the characteristics of these patients at entry. 82.8% had bone metastases, 79.5% were found to have either pelvic or abdominal lymph node metastases. 44.8% complained of pain at entry. Alkaline and/or acid phosphatase were elevated in a large proportion of patients.

TABLE 4. Characteristics at entry I

		PATIENTS	
		number	%
I.	Bone metastases		
	pelvis	24	41.4
	cervical spine	15	25.9
	thoracic spine	23	39.7
	lumbar spine	21	36.2
	thorax (ribs)	23	39.7
	scapula + clavicula	3	5.2
	skull	5	8.6
	upper extremities	2	3.4
	lower extremities	4	6.9
	total with abnormal bone scan	48	82.8
II.	Soft tissue metastases		
	lung	1	1.7
	pelvic lymph nodes	28	48.3
	abdominal lymph nodes	16	27.6
	liver	5	8.6
	brain	-	-
III.	Tumor pain	26	44.8
	performance status WHO 0	17	29.3
IV.	alkaline phosphatase 2x normal	14	24.1
	total acid phosphatase 2x normal	16	27.6
	prostatic acid phosphatase 2x normal	24	41.6
V.	Biopsy results		
	no malignancy	3	5.2
	well-differentiated	3	5.2
	moderately differentiated	31	53.4
	poorly differentiated	21	36.2

In study 1, three early deaths occurred within the first two months of treatment. The possibility of acute exacerbation of prostatic carcinoma during the initial rise of plasma testosterone cannot be excluded as contributing to the cause of death of these 3 men. All 3 patients suffered from heavy metastases but also from serious concomitant disease, such as coronary insufficiency, cardiac insufficiency, diabetes mellitus and uraemia.

Response rates seen during study 1 are summarized in Table 5. In agreement with WHO rules, stable disease is not accounted for as a response.

The protocol included a careful evaluation of pain and the use

TABLE 5. <u>Cummulative response and progression rates of 55 pa-</u>
<u>tients treated by Buserelin. All patients were</u>
<u>followed for 12 months.</u>

 6 (10.3%) patients achieved complete regression after
    3-10 months (mean 6.2 months).

23 (39.6%) achieved partial regression after 1-12 months
    (mean 4.2 months) which lasted from 1-11 months (mean
    6.5 months).

22 (37.9%) developed progression after 2-12 months
    (mean 7.6 months).

 3 (5.2%) patients died early.

of analgesics according to 4. scores. The results of this evaluation are shown in Table 6.

TABLE 6. <u>Pain and the use of analgesics in 58 patients treated</u>
<u>by Buserelin</u>

Pain/ analgesics	Entry N=58 %	1 month N=55 %	3 months N=54 %	6 months N=50 %	12 months N=34 %
No pain	53.4	69.1	72.2	74.0	82.4
Mild pain	17.2	10.9	18.5	6.0	14.7
Moderate pain and analgesics[a]	12.1	16.4	7.4	14.0	3.0
Severe pain and analgesics[a]	3.4	-	-	-	-

[a] Some patients with moderate and severe pain used no analgesics;
    percentages not mentioned.

It is evident, that more than half of the patients suffered
from pain at entry and that, after one year, more than 80% of all
living patients were free of pain. This stresses once again, the
palliative value of endocrine management of this disease.

Progression occurred in this study in 22 patients or 37.9%.
The 3 patients suffering early deaths are excluded from this evaluation. There was no documentation of progression.
The criteria that were fulfilled in the 22 patients showing
progression are shown in Table 7.

Side effects of Buserelin were studied in all patients and
were found to be mild. One patient went off study because of hot
flushes. It is remarkable that 44 of the 58 patients were sexually

inactive at entry of the study. At the end of the study, only 34 patients complained of a reduced sexual drive. Besides indicating that many patients were not impotent under Buserelin treatment, the improvement of sexual drive may be indicative of the general improvement of the health of these men. The other side effects included rhinitis, hot flushes and others. Their occurrence is indicated in a time-course fashion in Table 8.

TABLE 7. Criteria used for the determination of progressive disease in 22 patients treated by Buserelin

	number	%
increase of prostate volume	5	22.7
new bone lesions	17	77.3
lymph node metastases	2	9.1
alkaline phosphatase	5	22.7
total acid phosphatase	6	27.3
prostatic acid phosphatase	3	13.6
pain	11	50.0
miscellaneous[a]	4	18.2

[a] includes: liver metastases, general deterioration, paraparesis and retroperitoneal bleeding.

TABLE 8. Side effects of Buserelin, 58 patients

Patients with	at start	month 1	2	3	4	5	6	7	8	9	10	11	12
none	13	4	2	2	-	1	2	-	-	-	-	-	-
rhinitis		5	3	3	3	4	2	5	3	3	1	1	1
reduced sex drive	44	46	50	49	51	51	48	45	41	41	38	34	34
hot flushes	1	31	34	39	40	36	37	36	31	29	25	25	24
other[a]	4*	4	2	2	1	1	1	-	-	-	-	-	-

[a] includes: dry mouth, fever, gynaecomastia, headache (*), abdominal pain, back pain (*), thorax pain, sore throat, chest pain, paresthesia, thrombosis (*) and twitching.

Study 2.

Concerning study 2, this report will be limited to response and progression rates. Some of the biochemical and endocrine data have been reported elsewhere (4). The determination of acid phosphatase revealed in these 13 patients that the addition of

Cyproterone Acetate was suitable to suppress the initial rise that was observed in patients treated by Buserelin alone. The data on response and progression are summarized in Table 9 and compared with similar data of study 1.

TABLE 9. Clinical results

	Buserelin (Study 1)	Buserelin + CPA (Study 2)
Number of patients	58	13
Early deaths	3 (5.2)	0
Response, overall		
CR (%)	5 (8.6)	0
PR (%)	24 (41.4)	8 (61.5)
Response after 12 months		
CR (%)	5 (8.6)	0
PR (%)	12 (20.7)	6/12 (50.0)[a]
SD (%)	15 (25.9)	1/12 (8.3)
Progression	22 (37.9)	5/12 (41.7)

[a] One intercurrent death.

It is evident that progression rates are identical in both studies. Figure 1 and Figure 2 indicate the time to progression in months for study 1 and study 2. Statistical comparison of these data reveals no significant difference. The time to progression curves show the Kaplan-Meier estimation for both studies.

DISCUSSION

The data presented in this study confirm the observation of others, that the LHRH analogue Buserelin is safe and effective in treating patients with hormone-responsive prostatic carcinoma. Although no progressive disease has been documented, the early death of 3 patients in study 1 may be due to exacerbation (flare-up) resulting from the initial stimulation of plasma testosterone levels.

On the basis of testosterone determinations, poor compliance was documented in one patient. This patient was re-admitted for one week of subcutaneous injections. After that, he never showed rising plasma testosterone values again.

Response and progression rates in both studies were similar. The results of study 2 do not reproduce the favourable results

reported by Labrie and co-workers. The authors, after having
carefully analysed the mechanism of action of Cyproterone Acetate, feel that total androgen suppression is achieved effectively by the use of 150 mg of CPA a day.

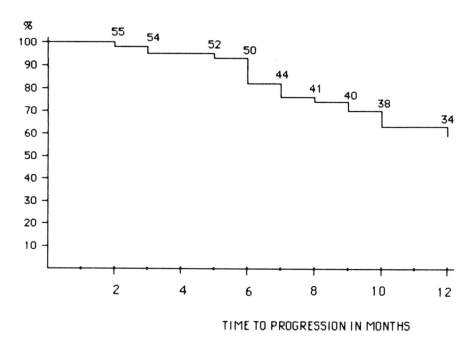

TIME TO PROGRESSION IN MONTHS

FIG. 1. Time to progression of 55 patients with M1 prostatic
carcinoma treated by Buserelin alone (study 1).

SUMMARY

During the years of 1983-1984, two simultaneous studies of
previously untreated M1 prostatic carcinoma patients were carried
out. A total of 71 patients were treated, 58 with an LHRH agonist
(Buserelin) alone, 13 with Buserelin and the anti-androgen Cyproterone Acetate (CPA). These latter patients, in addition to having M1 status, were required to have an elevated acid phosphatase. Buserelin was given in a dosis of 3 times 400 µgram/24
hours subcutaneously during the first week and later on intranasally. The dosis of CPA was 50 mg p.o./t.i.d. Duration of response and time to progression were evaluated according to
slightly modified response criteria of the National Prostatic
Cancer Project of the U.S.A. The endocrine effects of the drugs
on plasma testosterone and other parameters were followed by an
independent, central laboratory. All patients were studied in a
prospective, non-randomized fashion according to the same protocol.

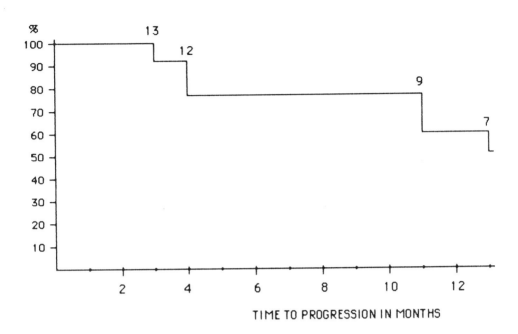

FIG. 2. Time to progression of 13 patients with M1 prostatic
carcinoma treated by Buserelin and Cyproterone Acetate (CPA)
(Study 2).

The following results were obtained: in the Buserelin part of
the study, 5 (8.6%) CR and 24 (41.4%) PR were achieved; 22 patients (38%) showed progression after 2-12 months. In the group
of patients treated with Buserelin and CPA, progression occurred
in 5 of 12 patients (41.7%) after 3-11 months (mean 7.0). The
addition of CPA resulted in a faster decrease of the initially
elevated acid phosphatase values during the first 3 weeks of
treatment. The results are comparable to those obtained by standard treatment. The equal progression rates in both parts of the
study suggest that there is no advantage of the long-term use of
CPA in addition to Buserelin.

REFERENCES

1. Borgmann, V., Nagel, R., Schmidt-Gollwitzer, M. and Hardt, W.
   (1982): Akt. Urol., 13: 200-203.
2. Debruyne, F.M.J., Karthaus, H.F.M., Schroeder, F.H., De Voogt,
   H.J., De Jong, F.H. and Klijn, J.G.M. (1985): In: Therapeutic Principles in Metastatic Prostatic Cancer, edited
   by F.H. Schroeder and B. Richards, pp 251-270. Alan Liss,
   New York.
3. Jacobi, G.H. and Wenderoth, I.K. (1982): Eur. Urol.8: 129-134.

4. Klijn, J.G.M, De Voogt, H.J., Schroeder, F.H. and De Jong, F. H. (1985): Lancet, August 31: 493 (Letter to the Editor).
5. Labrie, F., Dupont, A., Belanger, A., Lacoursière, Y., Raynaud, J.P., Husson, J.M., Gareau, J., Fazekas, A.T., Sandow, J., Monfette, G., Girard, J.G., Emond, J. and Houle, J.G. (1983): The Prostate, 4: 579-594.
6. Labrie, F., Dupont, A., Belanger, A., Emond, J. and Monfette, G. (1984): Proc. Natl. Acad. Sci. USA, Vol. 81: 3861-3863.
7. The Leuprolide Study Group (1984): N. Engl. J. Med., 311: 1281-1286.
8. Parmar, H., Lightman, S.L., Allen, L., Phillips, R.H., Edwards, L. and Schally, A.V. (1985): Lancet, November 30: 1201-1205.
9. Schroeder, F.H., Lock, M.T.W.T., Chadha, D.R., Debruyne, F.M. J., De Jong, F.H., Klijn, J.G.M., Matroos, A.W. and De Voogt, H.J. (1986): submitted for publication.
10. Sharifi, R., Lee, M., Ojeda, L., Ray, F., Stobnicki, M. and Guinan, P. (1985): Urology, Vol. XXVI, no. 2: 117-124.
11. Tolis, G., Ackman, D., Stellos, A., Mehta, A., Labrie, F., Fazekas, A.T.A., Comaru-Schally, A.M. and Schally, A.V. (1982): Proc. Natl. Acad. Sci. USA, Vol. 79: 1658-1662.

Hormonal Manipulation of Cancer: Peptides, Growth Factors, and New (Anti) Steroidal Agents, edited by Jan G. M. Klijn et al. Raven Press, New York © 1987.

ENDOCRINE AND CLINICAL EVALUATION OF 107 PATIENTS WITH ADVANCED PROSTATIC CARCINOMA UNDER LONG TERM PERNASAL BUSERELIN OR INTRAMUSCULAR DECAPEPTYL DEPOT TREATMENT

G.H. Jacobi, U.K. Wenderoth, W. Ehrenthal, H. v.Wallenberg
H.-W. Spindler, U. Engelmann, and R. Hohenfellner

Department of Urology, Johannes Gutenberg-University
Medical School, Langenbeckstraße 1, D-6500 Mainz,
Federal Republic of Germany

During the last five years a large number of publications emerged in the literature on the palliative effect of LHRH analogues given to patients with prostate cancer who would have otherwise been treated by either orchiectomy or oestrogens (1,2,4-7). The various hormone analogues used are almost equally effective and similar to surgical castration in withdrawing peripheral testosterone and achieving clinical response. However, the routes of either daily application (by subcutaneous injection as well as pernasally) or depot application (as intramuscular injection or implantation of microcapsules) differ among the various agents.

In recent years we have used the subcutaneously and pernasally applicable LHRH analogue Buserelin in 122 patients with advanced prostatic carcinoma (3,8-10). In the last two years we have also gained experience with patients treated by intramuscular injections of a depot formulation of another analogue, i.e. Decapeptyl, the D-Trp 6-LHRH.

We herein report our endocrine and clinical follow-up results accumulated over a clinically relevant period of time.

Patients and Tumor Characteristics

From October 1981 to May 1986 a total of 151 patients with advanced prostatic adenocarcinoma were treated, 122 in the Buserelin-group and 29 in the Decapeptyl-group. The following analysis is based only on patients fully evaluable endocrinologically as well as clinically.

Buserelin – October 1981 – May 1986: 85 patients

Decapeptyl – April 1984 – May 1986: 22 patients

These 107 patients had all newly diagnosed untreated tumors proven by biopsy.

Grade of tumor differentiation was assessed by using the W.H.O. grading system: 6.5 % grade I, 21.5 % grade II, and 72 % grade III.

Before treatment tumors were classified in stages after investigating their extention by sonography, computer tomography, chest x-ray, bone scan, bone survey if necessary, prostate specific acid phosphatase (PAP-EIA, ABBOTT), as well as prostate specific antigen (PSA-RIA, Diagnostic Products Corp.) in the majority of cases.

Using the TNM-system 76 patients (71 %) had bone metastases with or without lymph node involvement (M1), 31 patients (29 %) had locally advanced lesions of categories T3-4 N0 M0.

Treament Evaluation

All patients had measurable lesions in order to objectively assess treatment response. This was achieved by using the criteria of the E.O.R.T.C. as well as those of the American National Prostatic Cancer Treatment Group (NPCTG).

A total of 40 patients (31 in the Buserelin-group and 9 in the Decapeptyl-group) suffered from metastatic bone pain suitable for the assessment of subjective treatment response. Hormone monitoring was different in the two treatment groups.

Buserelin-group: Serum testosterone was measured before treatment, weekly during the first month, and 3-monthly thereafter for up to 42 months. Serum-LH was determined under basal conditions and one hour after stimulation with 25 µg of native LHRH. These LHRH-stimulation tests were performed in 14 patients before treatment, and every 6 months for the following 3 years.

Other hormone investigations consisted of sereal measurements of the adrenal steroids Delta-4-androstenedione and DHEA-S, Cortisol, Thyroxine, and Prolaktin in serum.

Decapeptyl-group: Serum testosterone and LH were measured in all patients initially and at the following treatment intervals: 6,12,24,48 hours; 1,2,3,4,5 weeks, and in 5-weekly intervals thereafter over 65 weeks, corresponding to 13 injections.

Treatment

Buserelin (Suprefact[R], Behringwerke) was either used subcutaneously for the initial 6-14 days and continued pernasally, or given per nasal spray from the beginning. The majority of patients received 3x500 µg per day s.c., the detailed dose regimen is summarized in Table 1. All different doses have proved equi-effective in achieving castrate levels of serum testosterone 4 weeks after treatment.

Dose Regimen

Buserelin
- 2 x 200 µg/d s.c. 14 days ⎤ and 3 x 400 µg/d
- 3 x 1000 µg/d s.c. 6 days ⎬ p.n.
- 3 x 500 µg/d s.c. 6 days   ⎦ thereafter
- 3 x 300 µg/d p.n. contineously

Decapeptyl
- D-Trp 6-LHRH 3.2 mg microencapsulated in 119 mg Lyophilisate injected i.m. every 5 weeks

Table 1:   Dose regimen used in 85 patients under Buserelin and 22 patients under Decapeptyl depot treatment.

D-Trp-6-LHRH (Decapeptyl[R] Depot, Ferring) was used as slow – release formulation of 3 mg in about 170 mg microcapsules. This dose was injected intramuscularly every 5 weeks.

Endocrine Data

Buserelin-group (fig. 1): Serum testosterone increased from initially 4.8 + 2.2 ng/ml to 5.6 + 2.4 ng/ml after 2 weeks of treatment. This was followed by an abrupt fall into the castrate range (0.5 ng/ml) after 4 weeks of treatment. Serum testosterone measured in 3-monthly intervals showed average values ranging between 0.4 + 0.1 and 0.2 + 0.1 ng/ml.

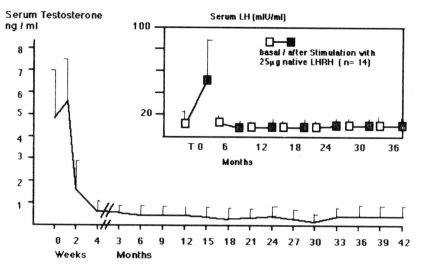

Figure 1: Serum testosterone (mean value + standard deviation) of serum testosterone in 85 patients treated with Buserelin; the inset depicts the LHRH stimulation results (for details see text!).

Serum-LH was initially 13 + 9 mlU/ml and reached by the stimulation with native LHRH 53 + 34 mlU/ml.

After initiation of treatment the stimulation tests were repeated every 6 months and showed basal levels ranging from 2 + 0.5 to 5 + 2 mlU/ml, the stimulatory LH levels ranged from 2 + 0.5 to 6 + 8 mlU/ml.

FSH was also determined during these stimulation tests with virtually the same pattern.

Pretreatment values of Delta-4-androstenedione and DHEA-S were 4.8 + 1 nMol/l and 1.2 + 0.5 mg/l, respectively, and did not change significantly throughout the study.

Initial values for serum thyroxine was 8 + 1 µg/dl, for

serum cortisol 15 ± 3 μg/dl, and for serum prolactin 7 ± 3 μg/l. All three hormones remained virtually identical over 36 months of treatment.

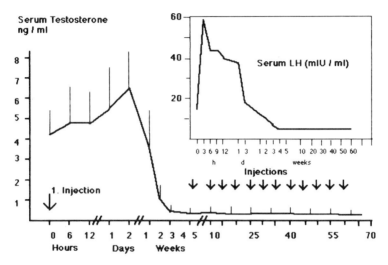

Figure 2: Serum testosterone (mean value ± standard deviation) of 22 patients treated with Decapeptyl; the inset shows the mean values of serum LH for the
same patients.

Decapeptyl-group (fig. 2): Compared to the Buserelin-group testosterone reached the peak stimulation level already at day 3, from initially 4.5 ± 1.2 ng/ml to 6.3 ± 1.8 ng/ml. Down-regulation was fully in progress after one week of treatment and castrate levels were universally reached at 3 weeks. During following 5-weekly injections testosterone levels changed between 0.2 and 0.3 ng/ml and this castrate range was maintained in all but one patients. In this particular individual (fig. 3) was at the second and fifth application the solvent injected by accident without the D-Trp 6-LHRH micro-capsules, resulting in an increase of testosterone after day 35 and day 140, respectively. In all properly treated patients, serum LH preceded testosterone in the stimulation peak about 40 hours, the state of down-regulation was achieved 3 weeks after treatment (fig. 2).

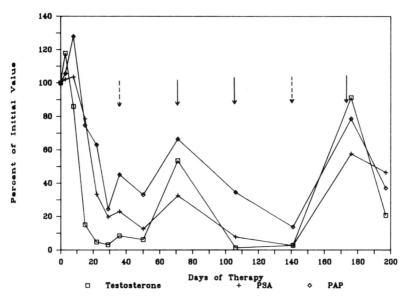

Figure 3: Testosterone and tumor marker profile of one patient inadequately treated with Decapeptyl depot
(for details see text!).

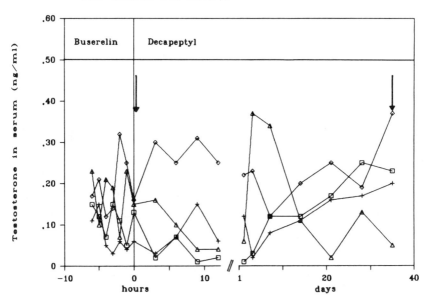

Figure 4: Testosterone levels of 4 patients who changed from
long term pernasal Buserelin treatment to intramuscular Decapeptyl treatment (for details see text!).

Change from Buserelin to Decapeptyl: A group of 4 patients treated pernasally with Buserelin for 11 to 26 months and responding objectively asked for a change to the depot form of Decapeptyl because of the inconvenience of the nasal spray. These cases are not included in the 2 aforementioned groups. After their last pernasal Buserelin application serum testosterone was determined in hourly intervals for 6 hours, and the first Decapeptyl injection was given intramuscularly. Testosterone was determined in 3-hourly intervals for up to 12 hours, and weekly thereafter (fig. 4). During this therapy change testosterone remained within the castrate range of 0.5 ng/ml.

Clinical Data

In all patients objective clinical response was first assess 6 months after initiation of treatment. Patients under Buserelin therapy have a follow-up ranging from 2 to 4.5 years, patients under Decapeptyl ranging from 15 to 24 months. For both treament groups rates for objective and subjective response are given in table 2. The average duration of response is 23 months in the Buserelin-group, and 14 months in the Decapeptyl-group. Subjective response was assessed after 2 months of therapy and in 32 of 40 patients a significant relief of metastatic bone pain was encountered.

Clinical Response
(E.O.R.T.C. Criteria)

Objective	Buserelin (n= 85)	Decapeptyl (n=22)
Partial and complete response	54 %	51 %
No Change	25 %	33 %
Progression	21 %	16 %
Subjective	25/31 (81%)	7/9 (78%)

Table 2: Response rates of the two treatment groups assessed 6 months after initiation of treatment.

Table 3 summarizes objective responses comparing data according to the E.O.R.T.C. and NPCTG criteria. Over all response is 52 % using E.O.R.T.C. criteria, and 81 % according
to the less rigid NPCTG criteria, in which the "stable
disease"- category is keyed as objective response.

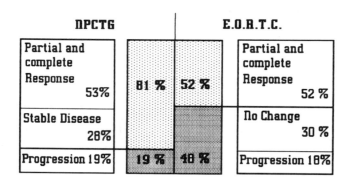

Different Response Criteria
Mainz June 1986 (n = 107)

Table 3:   Comparison of clinical response based on different
response criteria of the National Prostatic Cancer
Treatment Group (NPCTG) and the E.O.R.T.C.;
note, that the "no-change"-category of the
E.O.R.T.C. is named "stable disease" by the
NPCTG.

Follow-Up by the Use of Serum Tumor Markers

In the Decapeptyl treated group all patients had measurements of serum PAP and PSA at each interval of hormone
determination. If the initial values are taken as 100 %, all
patients responded to the treatment with an initial increase
and subsequent abrupt fall of PAP and PSA paralleling the
corresponding testosterone level (fig. 5). During the time of
clinical response PAP and PSA values remain below the 20 %
margin of initial pretreatment values. Patients who experienced clinical relapse showed, however, a steadily increase
of both tumor markers, while testosterone remain within the
castrate range (fig. 6). This early sign of progression was
observed 3 months before the first clinical evidence of relapse
was demonstrable.

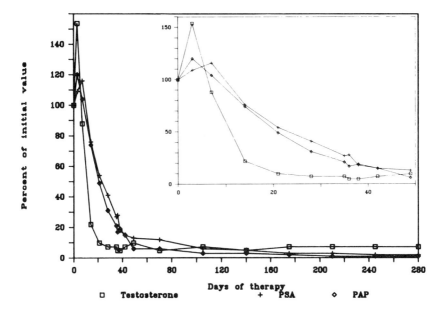

Figure 5: Mean values of serum testosterone, PSA and PAP
        in 22 patients treated with intramuscular injections
        of Decapeptyl depot; the inset shows the course of
        PSA and PAP in good correlation to testosterone; all
        values are expressed as percentage of initial pre-
        treatment values.

If PAP or PSA were plotted against serum testosterone
for the time up to clinical relapse, clear-cut logarithmic
correlations between either tumor marker and the individual
testosterone level could be computed (figs. 7 and 8). There
is an excellent linear correlation between PAP and PSA as
depicted in fig. 9.

Side Effects

There were two sudden deaths of unknown cause
2 weeks after initiation of Buserelin therapy. Despite close
clinical follow-up there was no case of satisfactorally documented so-called "flair-up" based on objective clinical
parameters. Five primarily symptomatic patients reported
continuity of symptoms during the first 3 weeks of treatment
with pain relief thereafter. Vice versa, however, 4 patients
reported a significant relief of bone pain while still in the
phase of testosterone as well as tumor marker stimulation

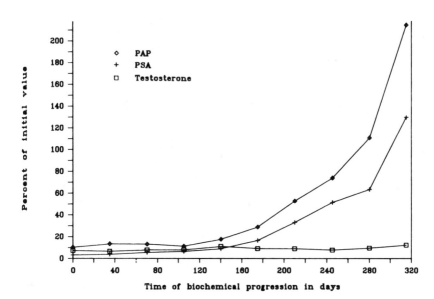

Figure 6: Mean values of serum testosterone, PSA and PAP in 5 patients under Decapeptyl depot treatment, who experienced clinical relapse. Time To is the standardized starting point of increasing PAP and PSA values, while serum testosterone remains within the castrate range.

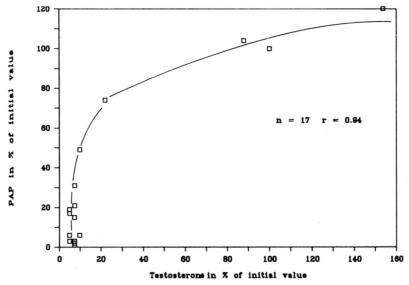

Figure 7: Logarithmic correlation of PAP versus testosterone in 22 patients under Decapeptyl depot treatment up to the time to progression; n=17 represents pairs of mean %-values of PAP and testosterone.

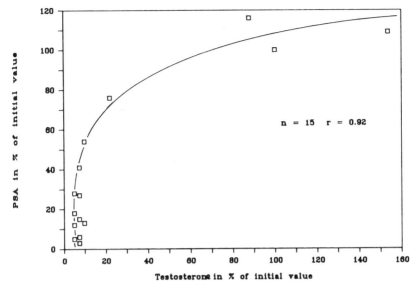

Figure 8: Logarithmic correlation of PSA versus testosterone in 22 patients under Decapeptyl depot treatment up to the time to progression; n=15 represents pairs of mean %-valus of PSA and testosterone.

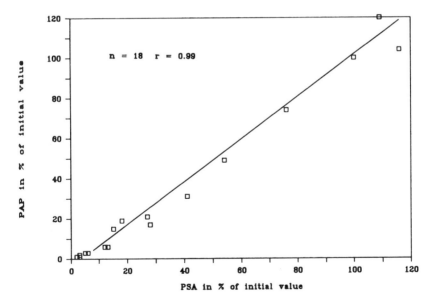

Figure 9: Demonstration of a linear correlation between PSA and PAP; n=18 represents pairs of mean %-values of PSA and PAP in 16 patients.

during the first 2 weeks. Bone pain alone as well as PAP or PSA increase are certainly insufficient parameters to characterize the dubious term of "flair-up".

Both LHRH-analogues were equally well tolerated, with hot flashes as the only unexpected untoward reactions in about 3/4 of all patients.

Critical Comment and Summary

Three major assumptions emerged from these clinical and endocrine long term studies.

First, Buserelin given pernasally in the conventional doses and Decapeptyl microcapsules administered intramuscularly in 5-week intervals are equally effective in terms of their long term castration effect in previously untreated patients with prostatic carcinoma. However, Decapeptyl causes complete LH and subsequent testosterone down-regulation one week earlier as compared to Buserelin. Furthermore this treatment is more convenient, and the compliance is better.

The somewhat superior rates of objective response of Buserelin over Decapeptyl – although without statistical significant difference – are most likely due to the longer follow-up of Buserelin treated patients. This is also underlined by the different duration of response in the two treatment groups. Both LHRH-analogues are equally well tolerated.

Second, in groups of prostate cancer patients with far advanced disease treated with palliative intention only true subjective or objective remission should by considered as a positive treatment response. No change in tumor burden or in the severe symptomatology of such patients must be rated as therapy failure and evaluated equal to progression. This modus of evaluation of treatment response is used by the E.O.R.T.C. In all well documented studies of patients treated with LHRH-analogues as monotherapy rates of partial plus complete remission between 50 % and almost 60 % are found, leaving the remainder 25 – 30 % for the "no-change"- category and about 20 % for progression. The National Prostatic Cancer Treatment Group (NPCTG), however, adds patients without change in tumor burden or symptomatology (so-called stable disease) to the group of objective remission and calls this entire group "objective response". Under such circumstances LABRIE and coworkers (4) have repeatedly reported response rates well above 90 % by using an LHRH-analogue in combination with an antiandrogen. The comparison of our monotreatment data using both E.O.R.T.C. as well as NPCTG criteria shows an improvement of the objective response category from 52 % (E.O.R.T.C.) to 81 % (NPCTG). Thus such a modus of reporting treatment data minimizes markedly the high response rate calculated after the combination therapy.

Third, our results comparing PAP und PSA as the two most useful tumor markers with the corresponding testosterone levels suggest a close correlation. It is tempting to conclude that during the initial phase of testosterone stimulation, the phase of down-regulation and the subsequent period of treatment response, peripheral testosterone has some unknown regulatory effect on the formation of these prostate specific products PAP and PSA and on their release from the cancer cells. It is conceivable that not all prostate cancer cells behave uniformly in this regard. Relapsing cell clons, however, which escape from testosterone deprivation and cause clinical tumor progression also escape from this tumor marker/androgen interrelationship.

Our data on five relapsing patients show that PAP and PSA concentrations increased while serum testosterone remained in the castrate range. Thus, PAP and PSA acquire under such circumstances true tumor marker function. Initial increase and subsequent decrease of PAP and PSA during the early phase of LHRH-treatment are of no prognostic value, since such changes are uniformly seen in all patients and only reflect their interrelation to the change in serum testosterone.

References

1. Borgmann, V., Hardt, W., Schmidt-Gollwitzer, M., Adenauer, H., and Nagel, R. (1982): Lancet, i:1097-1099

2. Happ, J., Schultheiss, H., Jacobi, G.H., Wenderoth, U.K., Buttenschön, K., Miesel, R., Spahn, H., and Hör, G. (1986) Rotterdamm: Int. Symp. Hormonal Manipulation of Cancer, Abstr. 108

3. Jacobi, G.H. and Wenderoth, U.K. (1982): Eur. Urol. 8:129-134

4. Labrie, F., Dupont, A., Bélanger, A., Lacoursiere, Y., Raynaud, J.P., Husson, J.M., Gareau, J., Fazekas, A.T.A., Sandow, J., Monfette, G., Girard, J.G., Emond, J., and Houle, J.G. (1983): Prostate, 4:579-594

5. Papadopoulos, I., Kleinschmidt, K., and Weißbach, L. (1986): Akt. Urol., 17:(in press)

6. Parmar, H., Lightman, S.L., Allen, L., Phillips, R.H., Edwards, L., and Schally, A.V. (1985): Lancet, ii:1201-1205

7. Roger, M., Duchier, J., Lahlou, N., Nahoul, K., and Schally, A.V. (1985): Prostate, 7:271-282

8. Wenderoth, U.K., Happ, J., Krause, U., Adenauer, H., and Jacobi, G.H. (1982): Eur. Urol. 8:343-347

9. Wenderoth, U.K., and Jacobi, G.H. (1983): World J. Urol. 1:40-48

10. Wenderoth, U.K. and Jacobi, G.H. (1985): Akt. Urol., 16:58-63

Hormonal Manipulation of Cancer: Peptides, Growth Factors, and New (Anti) Steroidal Agents, edited by Jan G. M. Klijn et al. Raven Press, New York © 1987.

PHARMACODYNAMICS, PHARMACOKINETICS AND BIOAVAILABILITY

OF THE PROLONGED LH-RH AGONIST DECAPEPTYL-SR

J. Happ[1], H. Schultheiß[3], G.H. Jacobi[4],
U.K. Wenderoth[4], K. Buttenschön[1], K. Miesel[1],
H. Spahn[2], and G. Hör[1]

Departments of [1]Radiology and [2]Pharmacology,
University of Frankfurt, 6000 Frankfurt on Main,
[3]Department of Pharmacology, Ferring GmbH, 2300 Kiel,
and [4]Department of Urology, University of Mainz,
6500 Mainz, Fed. Rep. of Germany

Supraphysiologic long-term stimulation of LH release by LH-RH or its potent agonist analogs leads to desensitization of the gonadotrophs which is followed by secretory deficiency of the Leydig cells (3). This phenomenon is the basis of "medical castration" in treatment of prostatic carcinoma (4). In order to avoid frequent parenteral or intranasal administration, a long-acting formulation (poly (DL-lactide-co-glycolide) microcapsules) of a long-acting LH-RH agonist (D-Trp[6] LH-RH) has been tested in rats (1). The same formulation has successfully been applied in patients with prostatic carcinoma (5). The purpose of the present study was the pharmacologic characterization of this formulation.

METHODS

Serum drug concentrations were measured in healthy male volunteers to whom Decapeptyl (DP) (D-Trp[6] LH-RH, kindly provided by Ferring, Kiel, FRG) was infused intravenously (i.v.) at rates of 4, 8, and 16 µg/h for 90 minutes (n=5) and a rate of 16 µg/h for 180 minutes (n=1).
During a therapeutic study on palliative treatment of prostatic carcinoma with a sustained release (SR)

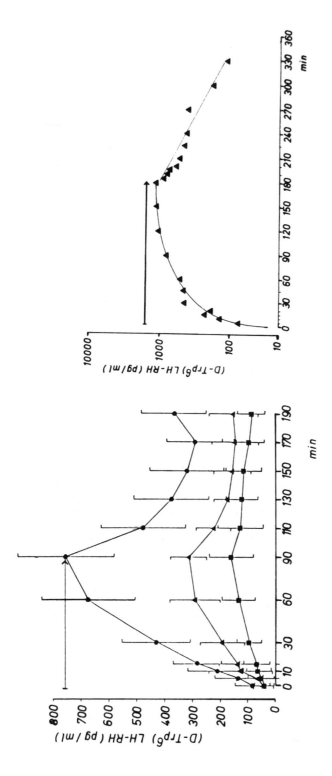

FIG. 1: Drug concentrations in serum during infusions of Decapeptyl (D-Trp⁶ LH-RH) in normal men (left: ■ 4, ▲ 8 and ● 16 μg/h for 90 min.; right: ▲ 16 μg/h for 180 min.)

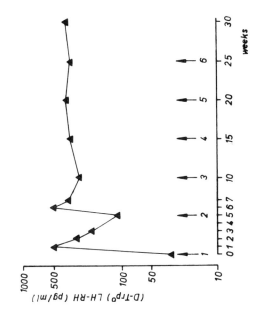

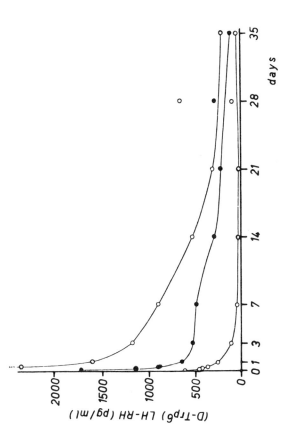

FIG. 2: Drug concentrations in serum after injection of Decapeptyl-SR (4 mg i.m.) in 8 patients with prostatic carcinoma; the measurements were done after the administration of the 1st dose (left) and before every subsequent dose (right); ● mean values, ○ extreme values, ↑ injections

formulation of DP (DP-SR) (Ferring, Kiel, FRG) (5), serum concentrations of LH, testosterone (T) and DP were measured by radioimmunoassay (RIA) in 8 patients who received 4 mg DP-SR intramusculary (i.m.) every 5 weeks for 7.5 months. DP-SR is D-Trp LH-RH in poly (D-lactide glycolide copolymere) microcapsules. Commercial kits were used for determination of LH and T; DP was measured by a RIA developed in the laboratories of Ferring, Kiel.

RESULTS

Dose-related DP serum levels were found after 90-minute infusions of DP in 5 normal men, a plateau, however, was not reached before 120 to 180 minutes of infusion as shown in 1 volunteer (Fig. 1). After termination of the infusions in normal men, the peptide was eliminated at a rate of 0.8 h corresponding to a biological half-life of 51.7 minutes.

In the 8 patients with prostatic carcinoma, serum LH decreased below 10 mU/ml within 2 to 3 weeks after the 1st injection of DP-SR; during the same time, serum T reached castration levels. This effect was maintained by repeating the injections every 5 weeks.

Highest DP serum levels (mean 1700 pg/ml) were measured 3 hours after the injection of DP-SR (Fig. 2). Thereafter, serum DP decreased quickly (t1/2α = 4.8 h). This was followed by a slow decrease of serum DP from about 500 pg/ml during the 1st week after the injection to 50 pg/ml after 5 weeks. A comparison of the DP concentrations recorded throughout the 1st week with the concentrations found with the infusion studies resulted in an inital rate of DP release from the microcapsules of about 10 µg/h. During repeated application of DP-SR, a slight accumulation was found (Fig. 2, right); minimum serum concentration of DP as measured before the 3rd to the 6th injection was about 400 pg/ml.

A comparison of the areas under the curves of serum DP after the injection of DP-SR with extrapolated data of the infusion studies resulted in a bioavailability of about 1 for DP-SR.

CONCLUSIONS

Decapeptyl-SR presents itself as an effective and convenient tool for "medical castration". Serum half-life of DP was found to be the same as reported by others (2). Injection of 4 mg DP-SR every 5 weeks leads to sufficient suppression of T secretion and causes only slight cumulation of DP.

REFERENCES

1. Asch, R.H., F.J. Rojas, A. Bartke, A.V. Schally, T.R. Tice, H.G. Klemcke, T.M. Siler-Khodr, R.E. Bray, M.P. Hogan (1985): J. Androl., 6: 83-88
2. Barron, J.C., R.P. Millar, D. Searle (1982): J. Clin. Endocrinol. Metab., 54: 1169-1173
3. Sandow, J. (1982): In: Neuroendocrine Perspectives, Vol. 1, edited by F.E. Mueller and R.M. McLeod, pp.339-391, Elsevier Biomed. Press, Amsterdam
4. Wenderoth, U.K., J. Happ, U. Krause, H. Adenauer, G.H. Jacobi (1982): Eur. Urol., 8: 343-347
5. Wenderoth, U.K., H.W. Spindler, W. Ehrenthal, H.v. Wallenberg, J. Happ, G.H. Jacobi (1986): In: S. Khoury and H.P. Murphy, Recent Advances in Treatment of Prostatic Carcinoma, Allen Liss, New York (in press)

*Hormonal Manipulation of Cancer: Peptides,
Growth Factors, and New (Anti) Steroidal
Agents,* edited by Jan G. M. Klijn et al.
Raven Press, New York © 1987.

CLINICAL RESULTS WITH THE DEPOT PREPARATION
OF ZOLADEX IN PROSTATE CANCER

F.M.J. Debruyne, E.H.J. Weil, P. Fernandez del Moral
and the Dutch South-Eastern Cooperative Urological Group

Department of Urology, Sint Radboud University Hospital,
P.O. Box 9101, 6500 HB Nijmegen, The Netherlands

Superactive analogues of luteneizing-hormone releasing hormone (LHRH) have become a well experienced method for reducing testicular androgen production. Hence, the use of these analogues has now been widely advocated as a valuable alternative to surgical castration or to other forms of testicular androgen suppression in the management of metastatic prostate cancer.

Different forms of LHRH-analogues are now available. Several reports on the effectiveness of chronic application of a nasal-spray (3, 7, 9, 18) as well as reports on the succesfull application of daily subcutaneous injections (1, 15, 21, 24) of LHRH have been published. These data show that an effective medical castration can be achieved with all different forms of LHRH-analogues.

Problems with patient compliance, however, are more likely to occur with these forms of administration. The intranasal application of a spray as well as the subcutaneous injection of the drug, both three times daily on an exact 8 hours regimen, could cause difficulties in patient's acceptance and compliance. Furthermore, the transnasal resorption of the drug can be hampered by rhinitis, atrophy of the nasal mucosa as well as by an intercurrent common cold.

Therefore, the development of a depot preparation of LHRH-analogue is a logical subsequent step, provided identical endocrinological and clinical results can be obtained in the management of these patients. Such depot formulation has recently been developed (ICI 118-630 Zoladex).

In the present study this depot formulation has been used. The aim of the study is to investigate the endocrinological and clinical efficacy and safety of this depot LHRH-analogue in patients with previously untreated metastatic prostate cancer.

PATIENTS AND METHODS

75 Patients between 50 and 86 years old (mean age 68.4 years) with previously untreated histologically documented metastatic prostate cancer were entered in this study between 21-08-1984 and 19-06-1985.

Table 1 gives the details of the TNM classification of the patients. Two patients were entered only on the base of elevated prostatic acid phosphatase. 73 Other patients had metastatic disease. 62 Patients had bone-metastases and 24 patients demonstrated extraskeletal metastases (lymph nodes 22 - lung 2). In some patients a combination of bone and extraskeletal metastases was present.

TABLE 1. TNM classification of the patients

PRIMARY TUMOR	LYMPH NODES METASTASES	NO		N+		TOTAL
		M0	M+	M0	M+	
TX			2			2
T0			2		2	4
T1			2			2
T2			10	2	1	13
T3		2	18	1	8	29
T4		7	11	1	6	25
TOTAL		9	45	4	17	75

The diagnosis was made by transrectal or perineal puncture biopsy or by the examination of specimens obtained during transurethral resection.

All histological specimens were reviewed by a referee pathologist and judged by the Mostofi (16) grading system. 13 Patients (17.3%) belonged to group I (well differentiated), 28 patients (37.3%) to group II (moderately differentiated) and 34 patients (45.5%) to the poorly differentiated group III.

The WHO-performance scale of the patients before treatment is documented in table 2. The majority of the patients showed a normal activity without severe symptoms related to their metastases (WHO 0-1). Only 11 patients had an impairment of their performance (WHO 2-3), whereas according to the inclusion criteria of this study no patients were completely bedridden (WHO 4).

TABLE 2. W.H.O. performance scale

SCALE		PATIENTS	
		NO.	%
0	NORMAL ACTIVITY NO SYMPTOMS	41	54.7
1	AMBULANT WITH SYMPTOMS	23	30.7
2	IN BED 50% DURING DAY	8	10.6
3	IN BED 50% DURING DAY	3	4.0
4	BEDRIDDEN	0	0.0
	TOTAL	75	100.0

Before the initiation of the therapy all patients were carefully examined including disease history, physical examination with detailed recording of the characteristic signs and clinical symptoms of carcinoma of the prostate and complete haematological and biochemical survey including blood count, liver and kidney function, alkaline and acid phosphatase, prostatic acid phosphatase. Endocrine test include measurements of testosterone (T), dehydrotestosterone (DHT) luteinizing hormone (LH) and follicle stimulating hormone (FSH) levels.

Treatment consisted of a four weekly injection of the depot preparation of the LHRH-analogue D-Ser(Bu^1)^6-Argly^{10}-LH-RH (ICI 118.630, Zoladex). The drug is dispersed in a cylindric rod of a biodegradable and biocompatible copolymer of d$_1$l-lactide and glycolide, and is released continuously over at least 28 days when injected subcutaneously. The depot is supplied in a purpose-designed applicator with a 16 gauche needle, and is injected subcutaneously in the anterior abdominal wall, with the use of local anaesthesia when necessary. A 3.6 mgr dose was used in each depot injection.

Patients were followed weekly during the fisrt month of therapy and monthly for the next 11 months. After 1 year, follow-up was continued with 3 monthly intervals. Each follow-up examination consisted of careful registration of tumor related signs and symptoms, clinical examination and haematological (blood counts) biochemical (liver and kidney function, alkaline and acid phosphatase) and endocrinological (T, DHT, LH and FSH) parameters. Bone scans and x-ray were repeated after 6 months and then at 6 monthly intervals. Subjective and objective response as well as side effects were carefully monitored.

RESULTS

All patients have been followed for a minimum of 12 months unless an earlier objective progression of the disease was evident. No patients have been lost to follow-up. The mean follow-up was 11.9 months with a maximun follow-up of 21 months. The patients compliance was 100%.

Haematological, biochemical and endocrinological response

All haematological and biochemical measurements remained within normal values, except for alkaline and acid phosphatase and for the serum levels of T, DHT, LH, and FSH. Before treatment an elevated level of prostatic acid phosphatase (PAP) was observed in 57 patients. Table 3 shows the evolution of PAP during the Zoladex therapy. Although a decrease in PAP was noticed in almost all responding patients complete normal values were obtained in only 69.1% of the evaluable patients at 6 months and in 58.5% at 12 months follow-up.

The endocrinological response of T and DHT is shown in fig. 1 and 2. After an initial raise in testosterone (and DHT) during the first week after the injection of the depot preparation, a gradual decrease of T, (DHT) is evident, with castrate levels obtained in all patients within 28 days. Castrate levels of T (DHT) were maintained during the whole follow-up period up to 21 months. 24 Hour endocrine-profiles of testosterone (and DHT) studied in 5 patients after 1, 3 and 6 months of therapy on day 28 (before the next depot injection) showed a constant daily castrate level without any flucturation (fig. 3).

Fig. 4 shows the levels of LH and FSH during follow-up. Again an initial raise of both hormones is noted in the first week followed by a sharp decrease to constant low values.

Subjective response

Subjective response was determined by asessing the effect of the treatment on each patient's need for analgesics and by the patients's own appraisal of the interference of the disease with his daily life, determined with the WHO scoring system.

In responding symptomatic patients, pain relief usually was

TABLE 3. PAP evolution during therapy

	START	3 MONTHS	6 MONTHS	12 MONTHS
ELEVATED	57 (81.4%)	32 (46.4%)	21 (30.9%)	24 (36.6%)
NORMAL	13 (18.6%)	37 (53.6%)	47 (69.1%)	38 (63.7%)
	70	69	68	62
NOT EVALUABLE	5	5	5	5
OFF STUDY		1	1	5

TABLE 4. Subjective response during zoladex therapy symptomatic patients

	3 MONTHS	6 MONTHS	12 MONTHS
SUBJECTIVE IMPROVEMENT	23 (79.4%)	22 (75.9%)	15 (60.0%)
SUBJECTIVE STABLE	4 (13.8%)	3 (10.3%)	2 (8.0%)
SUBJECTIVE PROGRESSION	2 (6.8%)	4 (13.8%)	8 (32.0%)
TOTAL EVALUABLE PATIENTS	29	29	25
NOT EVALUABLE	5	5	8
OFF STUDY			1
TOTAL	34 PATIENTS	34 PATIENTS	34 PATIENTS

a.   Testosterone levels during the therapy

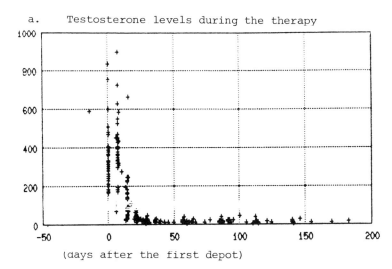

fig. 1

b.   Dihydrotestosterone levels   during the therapy

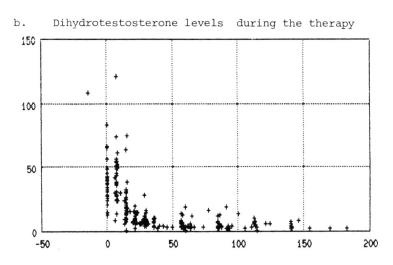

(days after the first depot)

fig. 2

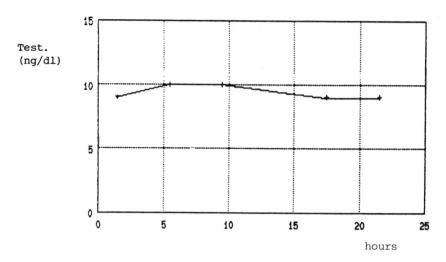

fig. 3: 24-hours profile of testosterone after 4 months

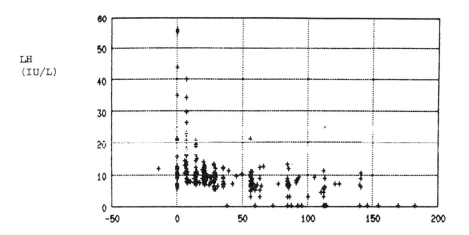

Days after first depot

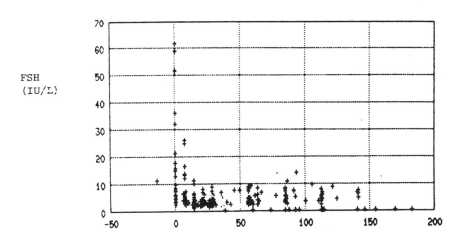

Days after first depot

Fig. 4: LH and FSH levels during ZOLADEX therapy

observed after a 2-6 weeks period. The subjective response of the symptomatic patients after 3 - 6 and 12 months is shown in table 4. Of the 34 symptomatic patients 79.4% experienced improvement of their symptoms at 3 months, 75.9% at 6 months and 60% after 12 months of therapy.

Objective response

Objective response was assessed according to the criteria used by the
British Prostate Group (5). The objective results after 3 - 6 and 12 months are shown in table 5.

TABLE 5. Objective response during follow-up

	3 MONTHS	6 MONTHS	12 MONTHS
CR	--	1.5%	4.8%
PR	62.9%	76.5%	54.8%
SD	32.9%	5.9%	1.7%
PD	4.2%	16.1%	38.7%

A gradual decrease in the number of responding patients (LR-PR-SD) can be observed, in accordance with the escape to hormonal treatment usually noticed in patients with metastatic prostate cancer. After 6 months 78% of the patients showed a remission and 16.1% progressive disease, whereas the remission rate at 12 months of follow-up is 59.6% with progression in 38.7%, despite the fact that testosterone levels remained at castrate level in all patients.
The correlation between objective response at 6 and 12 months and histological grade of the tumor is shown in table 6 and 7.
A tendency to escape from the hormonal therapy is noted in all grades, without significant differences between the three groups.

Side effects

Serial determination of complete blood counts and blood biochemistry did not reveal any evidence of drug related toxicity. Local side effects consisted of painful injection in two patients and a local haematoma in two others. The decrease in testosterone obtained in all patients, caused impotence in all previously sexually active patients. 7 Patients demonstrated moderate breast swelling and tenderness. Hot flushes as a symptom of testosterone reduction was seen in 54 patients (72%). In 1 patient a transient general allergic reaction was noticed, which prompted to withdrawal of the study.

TABLE 6. Correlation grading and objective response of patients with follow-up of 12 months

NO. EVALUABLE PAT. 62

	NO. PAT.	%	P.R. + C.R.		S.D.		P.D.	
			NO.	%	NO.	%	NO.	%
Gr I	11	(17.7)	7	63.6	--	--	4	36.4
Gr II	22	(35.5)	12	54.6	1	4.5	9	40.9
Gr III	29	(46.8)	18	62.1	--	--	11	37.9
TOTAL	62		37		1		24	

TABLE 7. Correlation grading and objective response of patients with follow-up of 6 months.

NO. EVALUABLE PAT. 68

	NO. PAT.	%	P.R. + C.R.		S.D.		P.D.	
			NO.	%	NO.	%	NO.	%
Gr I	13	(19.1)	11	84.6	--	--	2	15.4
Gr II	26	(38.2)	21	80.8	2	7.7	3	11.5
Gr III	29	(42.7)	21	72.4	2	6.9	6	20.7
TOTAL	68		53		4		11	

Flare-up of the symptoms was noticed is 6 patients (8.1%). This flare-up occured during the first two weeks of therapy and never forced to additonal measurements.

DISCUSSION

The availability of LHRH-analogues for the treatment of patients with metastatic prostate cancer is a major improvement with respect to the side effects and toxicity of the so-called standard hormonal manipulation such as bilateral orchiectomy and (or) estrogens. Estrogen administration is accompanied by a significant number of cardio-vascular and trombo-embolic, incidentically letal, accidents (2, 10). Although no clear-cut information is available, it is likely that some patients will find orchiectomy psychologically unacceptable.

Superactive LHRH-analogues reduce effectively plasma testosterone to castrate levels and these drugs can therefore be considered as the first choice alternative to estrogens or orchiectomy.

Although the mechanism of action of the LHRH-analogues is not completely understood it is assumed that these drugs act competitively on the level of LH and FSH receptors in the pituitary (22). Furthermore a direct effect on the gonads (6) and on the target organs of the sex steroids (17) is mentioned.

The first data of LHRH-analogues treatment in patients with metastatic prostate cancer indicated that a sustained suppression of testosterone is obtained with favourable effects on the local prostate tumor as wel as its metastases (1, 4, 14, 23, 26). Series of different LHRH-analogues have been used in these studies and if administered in appropriate dossage, all were usable to achieve castrate levels of testosterone.

Depot formulation have, however, major advantages. Administration of LHRH-analogues by intranasal spray or by daily subcutaneous injection is likely to be associated with poor compliance in the eldery patients in whom prostate cancer occurs. A depot preparation overcomes the compliance problem. Our study proves that the depot formulation ICI 118.630 (Zoladex) administered subcutaneously every 4 weeks reduces continuously testosterone and dihydrotestosterone to castrate levels and has benificial effect on both the local tumor growth and its metastases in patients with hormonal sensitive prostate cancer. These testosterone castrate levels could be maintained during a long-term follow-up of more than 20 months. Furthermore 24 hours endocrine profiles demonstrate no fluctuations in the levels of testosterone. These fluctuations have been described with other forms of LHRH-analogues (13).

The results obtained with this preparation are similar to those achieved with orchiectomy, estrogens or other LHRH-analogues. This means that initially 70 to 80% of the patients will respond to the therapy whereas another 10-20% will become hormone resistent during the first year of LHRH treatment. This phenomenon is due to the overgrowth of non-sensitive cell cloni which persist after killing of the hormone-responsive part of the tumor (11).

It has been suggested that poorly differentiated prostate cancers tend to be more resistent to hormonal manipulation (20). Although our study does not demonstrate significant differences between GI, GII and GIII tumors it is however possible that such differences will become obvious after a longer period of follow-up.

Flare-up of symptoms attributed to the initial stimulation of testosterone have not been a problem in our study. It has been noted in 8% of our patients. This figure is comparable with observations on the flare-up phenomenon in other studies where even serious consequenses have been described (8, 12, 25). As other authors do (19), we advise not to apply this treatment to patients with extensive metastatic disease in an impaired condition and that, in general, it is preferable to combine at least during the first 4 weeks of therapy, the depot-LHRH therapy with an anti-androgen.

Side effects were minimal in our study and no haematological toxicity has been observed. This, together with a 100% patient compliance demonstrate the safety of the LHRH depot formulation. The only adverse reactions experienced by our patients were impotence, due to testosterone suppression and a relatively high incidence of hot flushes. The reason for this phenomenon, that occurs with a much lower incidence after castration or estrogen therapy, is unclear.

So far no definitive results are available of studies in which LHRH-analogue therapy has been compared, in a randomized way, with estrogens, orchiectomy or other forms of anti-androgen therapy. It is, however, likely to accept that the results will be similar, since the endocrine response obtained by all these therapeutic regimens is similar. It remains however, necessary that such controlled clinical randomized trials will be completed. Similarly it is necessary to investigate whether total androgen suppression as proposed by Labrie et al (1983) is superior to LHRH therapy (and other forms of anti- androgen treatment). Such clinical trials are now under way (EORTC GU group).

From our study it can be concluded that LHRH depot therapy using a monthly subcutaneous injection of Zoladex is effective in reaching castrate levels of testosterone and dihydrotestosterone in all patients. These castrate levels are maintained during a long-term follow-up, and result is a favourable effect both on the local tumor and on its metastases in patients with hormone responsive prostate cancers. Side effects are minimal and compliance is optimal.

Therefore this depot formulation is a valuable and applicable alternative to other forms of hormonal treatment such as orchiectomy or estrogens. It is, however, advisable to combine the first depot injection with an effective anti-androgen to prevent flare-up in symptomatic patients or in patients with a larger tumor burden. It remains, however, to be proven if continuous total androgen suppression is necessary in patients with metastatic prostate cancer.

REFERENCES

1. Ahmed, S.R., Brooman, P.J.C., Shalet, S.M., Howell, A., Blacklock, N.J., Rickards, D. (1983): Treatment of advanced prostatic cancer with LHRH analogue ICI 118630: clinical response and hormonal mechanisms. The Lancet, II: 415.

2. Blackard, C.E. (1975): The veterans administration cooperative Urological Research Group Study of carcinoma of the prostate: a review. Cancer Chemother. Rep., 59: 225.

3. Borgmann, V., Hardt, W., Schmidt-Gollwitzer, M., Adenauer, H., Nagel, R. (1982): Sustained suppression of testosterone production by the luteneising-hormone releasinghormone agonist buselerin in patients with advanced prostate carcinoma. A new therapeutic approach. The Lancet, II: 1097.

4. Borgmann, V., Nagel, R., Schmidt-Golwitzer, M., Hardt, W. (1982): Langzeitsuppression der gonadalen testosteroneproduktion durch den LHRH-agonisten (Buserelinacetat: HOE 766) beim fortgeschrittenen Prostatakarzinom-eine neue Therapieform? Akt. Urol., 13: 200.

5. Chisholm, E.D. (1980): Prostate. In: Tutorials in postgraduate medicine: Urology, pp. 243. Heineman, London

6. Clayton, R.N., Katikineni, M., Chan, V., Dufau, M.L., Catt, K.J. (1980): Direct inhibition of testicular function by gonadotropin releasing-hormone: mediation by specific gonadotropin releasing-hormone receptors in interstitial cells. Proc. Natl. Acad. Sci., 77: 4459.

7. Debruyne, F.M.J., Karthaus, H.F.M., Schröder, F.H., De Voogt, H.J., De Jong, F.H., Klijn, J.G.M. (1985): Results of a Dutch phase II trial with the LHRH agonist Buserelin in patients with metastatic prostatic cancer. In: Therapeutic principles in metastatic prostatic cancer. Edited by FH Schröder and B Richards. pp. 251. Alan R. Liss, Inc., New York.

8. Faure, I., Lemay, A., Laroche, B., Robert, G., Plante, R., Jean, C., Thabet, M., Roy, R., Fazekas, A.T.A. (1983): Preliminary results on the clinical efficacy and safety of androgen inhibition by an LHRH agonist alone or combined with an antiandrogen in the treatment of prostatic carcinoma. The Prostate, 4: 601.

9. Faure, N., Lemay, A., Laroche, B., Robert, G., Thabet, M., Roy, R., Jean, C., Fazekas, A.T.A. (1984): Clinical response and safety of LHRH agonist treatment in prostatic carcinoma. J. Steroid. Biochem., 20: 1379 (A28).

10. Glashan, R.W., Robinson, M.R.G. (1981): Cardiovascular complications in the treatment of prostatic carcinoma. Brit. J. Urol., 53: 624.

11. Isaacs, J.T. (1985): New principles in the management of prostatic cancer. In: Therapeutic Principles in metastatic prostate cancer. Schröder FH, Richards, E.D., pp. 383. Alan R. Liss Inc. New York.

12. Kahan, A., Delrieu, F., Amor, B., Chiche, R., Steg, A. (1984): Disease flare induced by D-Trp6-LHRH analogue in patients with metastatic prostatic cancer. Lancet, 1: 971.

13. Kerle, D., Williams, G., Ware, H., Bloom, S.R. (1984): Failure of long term luteinizing hormone treatment for prostatic cancer to suppress serum luteinising hormone and testosterone. Brit. Med. J., 289: 468.

14. Klijn, J.G.M., De Jong, F.H., Lamberts, S.J.W., Blankenstein, M.A. (1984): LHRH agonist treatment in metastatic prostatic carcinoma. Eur. J. Cancer Clin. Oncol., 20: 483.

15. Mathé, G., Vo Van, M.L., Duchier, J., Misset, J.L., Morin, P., Keiling, R., Schwarzenberg, L., Kerbrat, P., Achille, E., Tronc, J.C., Mochover, D., Fendler, J.P., Pappo, E., Metz, R., Prevot, G., Comaru-Schally, A.M., Schally, A.V. (1984): Med. Oncol. Tum. Pharmacoth., 1: 119.

16. Mostofi, F.K., Price, E.B. Jr. (1973): Tumors of the male genital system. In: Atlas of Tumor Pathology Second Series fascicle 8 Armed force institute of pathology, p. 177. Washington DC.

17. Pedroza, E., Vilchez-Martinez, J.A., Coy, D.H., Arinura, A., Schally, A.V. (1980): Reduction of LHRH pituitary and estradiol uterine binding sites by a superactive analog of luteneising-hormone releasing hormone. Biochem. Biophys. Res. Comm., 95: 1056.

18. Presant, C.A., Soloway, M.S., klioze, S.S., Kosola, J.W., Yakabow, A.L, Mendez, R.G., Kennedy, P.S., Wyres, M.R., Neassig, V.L., Ford, K.S. (1985): Buserelin as rpimary therapy in advanced prostatic carcinoma. Cancer, 56: 2416-2419.

19. Schroeder, F.H., Lock, T.M.T.W., Chadha, D.R., Debruyne, F.M.J., De Jong, F.H., Klijn, J.G.M., Matroos, A.W., De Voogt, H.J. Metastatic cancer of the prostate managed by Buserelin (HOE 766) versus Buserelin plus cyproterone acetate (CPA). Submitted for publication.

20. Di Silverio, F. (1975): Histological type of tumor and hormone dependence. In: Bracci U and Di Silverio F (Eds): Hormone therapy of prostatic cancer, pp. 47. Cofese, Rome.

21. Smith, J.A. jr. (1984): Androgen suppression by a gonadotropin releasing hormone analogue in patients with metastatic carcinoma of the prostate. J. Urol., 131: 1110.

22. Swift, A.D., Crighton, D.B. (1978): Release activity plasma elimination and pituitary degradation of synthetic luteinizing hormonal releasing hormone and its analogues. J. Endocrin., 77: 35.

23. Tollis, G., Ackman, D., Stellos, A., Metha, A., Labrie, F., Fazekas, A.T.A., Comaru-Schally, A.M., Schally, A.V. (1982): Tumor growth inhibition in patients with luteinizing hormone-releasing hormone agonists. Proc. Natl. Acad. Sci., 79: 1658.

24. Walker, K.J., Nicholson, R.I., Turkes, A.O., Griffiths, K., Robinson, M., Crispin, Z., Dris, S. (1983): Therapeutic potential of the LHRH agonist ICI 118630 in the treatment of advanced prostatic carcinoma. The Lancet, II: 413.

25. Warner, B., Worgul, T.J., Drago, J., Demers, L., Dufau, M., Max, D., Santen, R.J. and members of the Abbott Study Group (1983). Effect of very high dose d-leucine[6]-gonadotropin-releasing hormone proethylamide on the hypothalamic-pituiatary testicular ascis in patients with prostatic cancer. J. Clin. Invest., 71: 1842.

26. Waxman, J.H., Wass, J.A.H., Hendry, W.F., Whitfield, H.N., Besser, G.M., Malpas, J.S., Oliver, R.T.D. (1983): Treatment with gonadotrophin releasing hormone analogue in advanced prostatic cancer. Brit. Med. J., 286: 1309.

ACKNOWLEGEMENTS

The authors wish to thank all participants of the Dutch South-Eastern Cooperative Urological Group, Prof.Dr. C.J. Herman, Loyolla University of Chicago (Ill.), referee pathologist and Mrs. D.M. Litjens-de Heus and Miss D.G.M. Berris for their secretarial assistance. We also thank Dr. J.P. van Laarhoven from the laboratory of experimental endocrinology for all endocrinological measurements.

Hormonal Manipulation of Cancer: Peptides,
Growth Factors, and New (Anti) Steroidal
Agents, edited by Jan G. M. Klijn et al.
Raven Press, New York © 1987.

USE OF LH–RH ANALOGS FOR THE TREATMENT OF
PROSTATE CANCER: COMBINATION THERAPY
AND DIRECT EFFECTS

A.V. Schally and T.W. Redding

VA Medical Center and Tulane University School of Medicine
Endocrine, Polypeptide, and Cancer Institute
1601 Perdido Street, New Orleans, LA 70146 U.S.A.

The finding that prolonged treatment with agonistic analogs
of LH–RH can result in testicular inhibition and chemical
castration (4,7,8,12,15,35,37,45), led us to try this method to
induce the regression of androgen-dependent prostate tumors in
rat models. Rats bearing the Dunning R-3327H prostate
adenocarcinoma were treated with D-Trp^6-LH–RH. The percentage
increase in tumor volume and actual tumor weight were reduced as
compared with untreated controls (30). Serum testosterone
levels in rats were significantly reduced after treatment with
D-Trp^6-LH–RH. This study demonstrated for the first time the
potential efficacy of D-Trp^6--and other LH–RH superagonists--in
the treatment of prostate carcinoma and other hormone-sensitive
tumors in man (30).

The finding that D-Trp^6-LH–RH inhibits the growth of prostate
tumors in rats led to clinical trials (46). The first
successful palliation of advanced prostatic carcinoma by
agonistic analogs of LH–RH was shown in a collaborative trial
carried out at the Royal Victoria Hospital in Montreal (46).
Ten patients with stage C and D prostatic carcinoma were treated
for 6 weeks to 12 months with agonistic analogs of LH–RH (46).
D-Trp^6-LH–RH was given subcutaneously and H-766 (buserelin) was
also given subcutaneously, or intranasally. In all patients,
mean plasma testosterone levels fell by 75% by the third week of
treatment and remained at castration values thereafter (46).
This was followed by a decrease or normalization of serum acid
phosphatase levels by the second month of treatment. In
patients presenting with urinary obstruction, there was a
noticeable clinical improvement and a decrease in the size of
the prostate was confirmed by ultrasonography. In patients with
stage D disease, there was relief of bone pain, and in one
patient improvement was documented by radioisotope bone imaging
(46). The only side effects were a decrease in libido and
climacteric-like "hot flashes" (46). This trial demonstrated
for the first time that superactive agonistic LH–RH analogs may
be efficacious therapeutic agents in patients with
androgen-sensitive prostatic adenocarcinoma. Persistent
suppression of Leydig cell function, manifested by significant

decreases in plasma testosterone and estradiol levels, suggests
that prolonged admininstration of D-Trp[6]-LH-RH, HOE 766 or other
agonists produces "medical" castration (46). Our findings have
been confirmed and extended by other clinical trials in Europe,
the United States, Canada, Mexico, and Brazil
(1,2,5,6,10,16,19,22,47,49,50).

Effects of LH-RH Antagonists

Successful suppression of rat prostate tumors by chronic
administration of the agonist D-Trp[6]-LH-RH prompted us to
compare its effects to those of LH-RH antagonists (29,40). A
modern antagonist, N-Ac-D-p-Cl-Phe[1,2]-D-Trp[3]-D-Arg[6]-
D-Ala[10]-LH-RH, at a dose of 25µg bid for 3 weeks significantly
inhibited the growth of the Dunning prostate tumor with similar
effectiveness to that of D-Trp[6]-LH-RH. Tumor weights, tumor
volumes and serum testosterone levels were greatly reduced by
both compounds as compared to controls (40). The use of
antagonistic analogs of LH-RH for the treatment of prostate
cancer would avoid the transient stimulation of the release of
gonadotropins and testosterone that occurs initially in response
to LH-RH agonists, thus preventing the occasional temporary
clinical flare-up of the disease. In the field of cancer,
however, no clinical studies have been performed with LH-RH
antagonists. A clinical evaluation in the treatment of prostate
cancer and a comparison of their therapeutic efficacy with
D-Trp[6]-LH-RH and other agonists is required.

Development of Long Acting Delivery Systems

The therapy for prostate cancer and other sex-steroid-
dependent tumors based on agonists of LH-RH was made more
practical and efficacious by the development of a long-acting
formulation of microcapsules of D-Trp[6]-LH-RH for controlled
release (3,21,32). Our studies showed that D-Trp[6]-LH-RH given
once a month in the form of continuous-release microcapsules
inhibits the growth of Dunning prostate tumors in rats (32).
Intramuscular injection of D-Trp[6]-LH-RH in microcapsules of poly
(DL-lactide-co-glycolide), designed to release a controlled dose
of the peptide over a 30-day period, decreased the weights of
the androgen-dependent Dunning prostate tumors in rats and
suppressed serum testosterone levels more effectively than daily
subcutaneous administration of unencapsulated D-Trp[6]-LH-RH (32).
The microcapsules or daily injections of D-Trp[6]-LH-RH also
significantly decreased tumor volumes. The once-a-month use of
microcapsules will make therapy with D-Trp[6]-LH-RH more practical
and convenient and should also better ensure patient compliance.

Study of the Combination of LH-RH Agonists with Antiandrogens

Antiandrogens, which neutralize the effect of endogenous
androgens, have been used in the management of prostate cancer

in man (9,23,26,28,34,42,43,44,48). In some clinical trials, a combination of the agonists HOE 766 with antiandrogens RU-23908 or Flutamide was used for treatment of patients with stage C and D_2 prostate carcinoma (17,18,19,20). It was stated that the combined treatment with the LH-RH analog and antiandrogen is more effective than the analog alone (17). We therefore decided to investigate the effects of a simultaneous administration of the antiandrogen flutamide and microcapsules of D-Trp[6]-LH-RH in the Dunning R-3327H rat prostate adenocarcinoma model to determine whether the combination of these two drugs might inhibit tumor growth more effectively than single agents (31). Microcapsules of D-Trp[6]-LH-RH, calculated to release a controlled dose of 25µg/day for a period of 30 days, were injected intramuscularly once a month. Flutamide was administered SC at a daily dose of 25 mg/kg. The therapy was started 100 days after the tumor transplantation and continued for 60 days (31). Tumor weights and volumes were significantly reduced in rats treated with microcapsules or flutamide alone, but the former drug inhibited tumor growth more than the latter. The combined treatment of flutamide and microcapsules significantly decreased tumor weight and volume, but did not exert a synergistic effect on tumor growth, the reduction being smaller for the combination than for the microcapsules alone (31). A significant elevation of serum testosterone, LH, and prolactin was seen in rats treated with flutamide. On the other hand, in rats given microcapsules of D-Trp[6]-LH-RH, testosterone fell to castration levels within 7 days and remained at nondetectable values; serum LH and prolactin levels were also suppressed in this group. The combined administration of microcapsules and flutamide also significantly decreased testosterone to nondetectable levels by day 7 and suppressed serum LH and prolactin (31). Our findings raise doubts of whether the daily administration of the combination of LH-RH agonist with an antiandrogen offers an advantage over the use of microcapsules of an agonist like D-Trp[6]-LH-RH alone in the treatment of prostatic carcinoma (31).

Combination of LH-RH Agonists with Chemotherapy

It is well established for other hormonal approaches that, in the majority of patients, the duration of remission is limited and a relapse to androgenablation therapy eventually occurs (9,13,14,24,25,41). The mechanism responsible for the relapse of prostate cancer is attributed to a selective proliferation of clones of androgen-independent cancer cells (13,14,25). Thus, the aim of combining hormonal therapy with chemotherapy would be to delay or prevent this situation and to prolong survival (24,25,41).

The effect of combining hormonal treatment consisting of long-acting microcapsules of the agonist D-Trp[6]-LH-RH with the chemotherapeutic agent cyclophosphamide was investigated in the Dunning R-3327H rat prostate cancer model (38). Microcapsules of D-Trp[6]-LH-RH formulated from poly (DL-lactide-co-glycolide) and calculated to release a controlled dose of 25μg/day were injected intramuscularly once a month. Cyclophosphamide (Cytoxan) (5 mg/kg of body weight) was injected intraperitoneally twice a week. When the therapy was started 90 days after tumor transplantation--at the time that the cancers were well developed and the therapy was continued for 2 months--tumor volume was significantly reduced by the microcapsules or Cytoxan given alone. The combination of these two agents similarly inhibited tumor growth, but did not show a synergistic effect (38). In another study, the treatment was started 60 days after transplantation, when the developing tumors measured 60-70 mm^3. Throughout the treatment period of 100 days the microcapsules of D-Trp[6]-LH-RH reduced tumor volume more than Cytoxan, and the combination of the two drugs appeared to completely arrest tumor growth (38). Tumor weights were diminished significantly in all experimental groups, the decrease in weight being smaller in the Cytoxan-treated group than in rats receiving the microcapsules. The combination of Cytoxan plus the microcapsules was 10-100 times more effective than the single agents in reducing tumor weights (38). In both experiments, testes and ventral prostate weights were significantly diminished, serum testosterone was suppressed to undetectable levels and prolactin values were reduced by administration of microcapsules of D-Trp[6]-LH-RH alone or in combination with Cytoxan (38). An experiment in which Novantrone (Mitoxantrone) was used in combination with microcapsules of D-Trp[6]-LH-RH produced similar results. Again, the combination with Novantrone led to a better inhibition of prostate cancer than D-Trp[6]LH-RH alone and in fact, arrested tumor growth. These results in rats suggest that combined administration of long-acting microcapsules of D-Trp[6]-LH-RH with a chemotherapeutic agent, started soon after the diagnosis of prostate cancer is made, might inhibit the proliferation of androgen-dependent and independent cells, further improve the therapeutic response and increase the survival rate.

Direct Effects of LH-RH Agonists on Prostate Tumors

Apart from its main antitumor activity, which is mediated by the pituitary, and a possible action on the gonads, D-Trp[6]-LH-RH may also act directly on prostate tumors. We have previously observed the binding of D-Trp[6]-LH-RH to plasma membranes isolated from Dunning R-3327H prostate tumors but not from normal prostate tissue (11). These data suggest that D-Trp[6]-LH-RH can act directly at prostate cell level but only after carcinogenic transformation induces changes in membrane structure and composition (11,36).

Recently we have shown that D-Trp^6-LH-RH, in a tissue culture system, can inhibit the growth of the Dunning R-3327H-G8-A1 clonal prostate adenocarcinoma cell line at doses as low as 10^{-8} Molar as based on the suppression of the uptake of tritiated thymidine. Three human prostate cancer cell lines--LNLCAP, DU-145 and PC-3--were also tested. Although they appeared to be somewhat less sensitive to the inhibitory action of this agonist in this culture system, an inhibition of growth could be demonstrated at higher concentrations ($10^{-7} - 10^{-6}$M).

Somatostatin Analogs

The use of superactive somatostatin analogs in combination with D-Trp^6-LH-RH for suppressing prostate cancers is described in our second article in this book (39).

Acknowledgements

We thank the National Hormone and Pituitary Program (NHPP) for the gifts of materials used in radioimmunoassays. The experimental work described in this paper was supported by National Institutes of Health Grants AM07467 and CA 40003, and by the Medical Research Service of the Veterans Administration.

References

1. Ahmed, S.R., Brooman, P.J.C., Shalmet, S.M., Howell, A., Blacklock, N.J., and Rickards, D. (1983): Lancet, ii:415-518.
2. Allen, J.M., O'Shea, J.P., Mashiter, K., Williams, G., and Bloom, S.R. (1983): Br. Med. J., 286:1607-1609.
3. Asch, R.H., Rojas, F.J., Bartke, A., Schally, A.V., Tice, T., Siler-Khodr, T.M., Klemcke, H.G., Bray, R.E., and Hogan, M.P. (1985): J. Androl., 6:83-88.
4. Auclair, C., Kelly, P.A., Coy, D.H., Schally, A.V., and Labrie, F. (1977): Endocrinology, 101:1890-1893.
5. Borgmann, V., Nagel, R, Al-Abadi, H., and Schmidt-Gollwitzer, M. (1983): Prostate, 4:553-568.
6. Comaru-Schally, A.M., Ramalho, A., Leitao, P.R., and Schally, A.V. (1984): Lancet, ii:281-282.
7. Corbin, A. (1982): Yale J. Biol. Med., 55:27-47.
8. Corbin, A., Beattie, C.W., Tracy, J., Jones, R., Foell, T.J., Yardley, J., and Rees, R.W.A. (1978): Int. J. Fertil., 23:81-92.
9. Geller, J., and Albert, J.D., (1983): Sem. Oncol., 10:34-41.
10. Gonzalez-Barcena, D., Perez-Sanchez, P., Ureta-Sanchez, S., Dominguez, H.B., Graef-Sanchez, A., Morales, M.B., Comaru-Schally, A.M. and Schally, A.V. (1985): Prostate, 7:21-30.
11. Hierowski, M.T., Altamirano, P., Redding, T.W., and Schally, A.V. (1983): FEBS Lett., 154:92-96.

12. Hsueh, A.J.W., and Erickson, G.F. (1979): Nature, 281:66-67.
13. Isaacs, J.T. (1984): Prostate, 5:1-7.
14. Isaacs, J.T., and Coffey, D.S. (1981): Cancer Res.,
      41:5070-5075.
15. Johnson, B., Gendrich R.L., and White, W.F. (1976): Fertil.
      Steril., 27:853-860.
16. Koutsilieris, M., and Tolis, G. (1983): Prostate, 4:569-577.
17. Labrie, F., Belanger, A., Dupont, A., Emond, J., Lacoursiere,
      Y., and Monfette, G. (1984): Lancet, ii:1090.
18. Labrie, F., Dupont, A., Belanger, A., Emond, J., and Monfette,
      G. (1984): Proc. Natl. Acad. Sci. U.S.A., 81:3861-3863.
19. Labrie, F., Dupont, A., Belanger, A., Lacoursiere, Y.,
      Raynaud, J.P., Gareau, J., Fazekas, A.T.A., Monfette, G.,
      Girard, J.G., Emond, J., and Houle, J.G. (1983): Prostate,
      4:579-594.
20. Labrie, F., Dupont, A., Belanger, A., Lefebvre, F.A., Cusan,
      L., Monfette, G., Laberge, J.G., Emond, J.P., Raynaud, J.P.,
      Husson, J.M., and Fazekas, A.T.A. (1983): J. Steroid
      Biochem., 19:999-1007.
21. Mason-Garcia, M., Vigh, S., Comaru-Schally, A.M., Redding,
      T.W., Somogyvari-Vigh, A., Horvath, J., and Schally, A.V.
      (1985): Proc. Natl. Acad. Sci. U.S.A., 82:1547.
22. Mathe, G., VoVan, M.L., Duchier, J., Misset, J.L., Morin, P.,
      Keiling, R., Schwarzenberg, L., Kerbat, P., Achille, E.,
      Tronc, J.C., Machover, D., Fendler, J.P., Pappo, E., Metz,
      R., Prevot, G., Comaru-Schally, A.M., and Schally, A.V.
      (1984): Med. Oncol. Tumor Pharmacother., 1:119-122.
23. Menon, M., and Walsh, P.C. (1980): In: Prostatic Cancer,
      edited by G.P. Murphy, pp. 175-199. PSG Publishing Co.,
      Inc., Littleton, MA.
24. Mukamel, E., Nissenkorn, E., and Servadio, C. (1980): Urology,
      16:257-260.
25. Murphy, G.P., Beckley, S., Brady, M.F., Chu, T.M., deKernion,
      J.B., Dhabuwala, C., Gaeta, J.F., Gibbons, R.P., Loening,
      S.A., McKiel, C.F., McLeod, D.G., Pontes, J.E., Prout, G.R.,
      Scardino, P.T., Schlegel, J.U., Schmidt, J.D., Scott, W.W.,
      Slack, N.H., and Soloway, M.S. (1983): Cancer,
      51:1264-1272.
26. Neumann, F., and Schenck, B. (1976): J. Reprod. Fertil.
      (Suppl.), 24: 129-145.
27. Parmar, H., Lightman, S.L., Allen, L., Phillips, R.H.,
      Edwards, L., and Schally, A.V. (1985): Lancet,
      ii:1201-1205.
28. Raynaud, J.P., Bonne, C., Moguilewsky, M., Lefebvre, F.A.,
      Belanger, A., and Labrie, F. (1984): Prostate, 5:299-311.
29. Redding, T.W., Coy, D.H., and Schally, A.V. (1982): Proc.
      Natl. Acad. Sci. U.S.A., 79:1273-1276.
30. Redding, T.W., and Schally, A.V. (1981): Proc. Natl. Acad.
      Sci. U.S.A., 78:6509-6512.
31. Redding, T.W., and Schally, A.V. (1985): Prostate, 6:219-232.

32. Redding, T.W., Schally, A.V., Tice, T.R., and Meyers. W.E. (1984): Proc. Natl. Acad. Sci. U.S.A., 81:5845-5848.
33. Roger, M., Duchier, J., Lahlou, N., Nahoul, K., and Schally, A.V. (1985): Prostate, 7:271.
34. Rost, A., Schmidt-Gollwitzer, M., Hantlemann, W., and Brosig, W. (1981): Prostate, 2:315-322, 1981.
35. Sandow, J., VonRechenberg, W., Jerzabek, G., and Stoll, W. (1978): Fertil. Steril., 30:205-209.
36. Schally, A.V., Comaru-Schally, A.M., and Redding, T.W. (1984) Proc. Soc. Exp. Biol. Med., 175:259-281.
37. Schally, A.V., Coy, D.H., and Arimura, A. (1980): Int. J. Gynaecol. Obstet., 18:318-324, 1980.
38. Schally, A.V., and Redding, T.W. (1985): Proc. Natl. Acad. Sci. U.S.A., 82:2498-2502.
39. Schally, A.V., Redding, T.W., Cai, R.Z., Paz, J.I., Ben-David, M., and Schally, A.M. (1986): In: International Symposium on Hormonal Manipulation of Cancer: Peptides, Growth Factors and New (Anti) Steroidal Agents, edited by J. Klein, (In press). Raven Press, New York.
40. Schally, A.V., Redding, T.W., and Comaru-Schally, A.M. (1983): Prostate, 4:545-552.
41. Schmidt, J.D., Scott, W.W., Gibbons, R., Johnson, D.E., Prout, G.R., Jr., Loening, S., Soloway, M., deKernion, J., Pontes, J.E., Slack, N.H., and Murphy, G.P. (1980): Cancer, 45:1937-1946.
42. Smith, R.B., Walsh, P.C., and Goodwin, W.E. (1973): J. Urol., 110:106-108.
43. Sogani, P.C., Ray, B., and Whitmore, W.F., Jr. (1975): Urology, 6:164-166.
44. Stoliar, B., and Albert, D.J. (1974): J. Urol., 111:803-807.
45. Sundaram, K., Cao, Y.Q., Wang, N.G., Bardin, C.W., Rivier, J., and Vale, W. (1981): Life Sci., 28:83-88.
46. Tolis, G., Ackman, A., Stellos, A., Mehta, A., Labrie, F., Fazekas, A., Comaru-Schally, A.M., and Schally, A.V. (1982): Proc. Natl. Acad. Sci. U.S.A., 79:1658-1662.
47. Walker, K.J., Nicholson, R.I., Turkes, A., Robinson, M., Crispin, Z., and Dris, S. (1983): Lancet, ii:413-415.
48. Walsh, P.C., and Korenman, S.G. (1971): J. Urol., 105:850-851.
49. Warner, B., Worgul, T.J., Drago, J., Demers, L., Dufau, M., Max, D., and Santen, R.J. (1983): J. Clin. Invest., 17:1842-1853.
50. Waxman, J.H., Wass, J.A.H., Hendry, W.F., Whitfield, H.N., Besser, G.M., Malpas, J.S., and Olivier, R.T.D. (1983): Br. Med. J., 286:1309-1312.

Hormonal Manipulation of Cancer: Peptides, Growth Factors, and New (Anti) Steroidal Agents, edited by Jan G. M. Klijn et al. Raven Press, New York © 1987.

STUDIES WITH NAFARELIN AND A LONG ACTING LHRH ANTAGONIST

B.H. Vickery[*], G.I. McRae[*], L.M. Sanders[†], P. Hoffman[ξ] and S.N. Pavlou[§]

Institutes of [*]Biological Sciences, [†]Pharmaceutical Sciences and [ξ]Clinical Medicine, Syntex Research, 3401 Hillview Avenue, Palo Alto, California 94304, USA and [§]Dept. of Medicine, Vanderbilt University, Nashville, Tennessee 37232, USA

The gonadal suppressive effects of LHRH agonists, resulting from a complex mechanism of pituitary receptor desensitization and down regulation and perhaps stimulation of release of non-biologically active gonadotropins, are being increasingly exploited as therapy for a variety of gonadal steroid dependent syndromes (17,27,36). Possibilities for contraception have also been explored (21,25,26). One of the more actively pursued uses is in the induction of a chemical orchiectomy in patients with prostatic cancer (9,10). Two analogs have reached the market place for this indication and a number of others are in various stages of clinical evaluation (27).

In more recent developments, competitive antagonists of LHRH have become available with sufficient potency to warrant clinical evaluation for much the same indications as the LHRH agonists (28). Nafarelin ([D-Nal(2)^6]LHRH; RS-94991) and RS-68439 ([D-Nal(2)^1,D-pCl-Phe^2,D-Trp^3,D-hArg(Et$_2$)^6, D-Ala^{10}]LHRH), are the Syntex LHRH agonist and antagonist, respectively (18,19). They each appear to be the most potent representatives of their class presently under clinical evaluation. This article will describe the endocrine effects of these compounds and, as appropriate, studies in prostatic cancer patients.

STUDIES WITH NAFARELIN

Nafarelin (fig. 1) is an LHRH agonist which in vitro has approximately one half the binding affinity and LH releasing potency of the well described analog [D-Trp^6]LHRH (30). However, in vivo in rats, its potency multiple relative to the same analog increases 4-fold, with a final potency relative to LHRH of about 200 (18). Plasma t$_{1/2}$ in rats is 34 minutes for nafarelin and 7 minutes for LHRH; in addition nafarelin is 80% plasma protein bound whereas LHRH is only 25% bound (7,8). A similar situation holds true in primates including man in that the plasma t½ of 2.5-3.5 hours for nafarelin is 5-7 times that of LHRH.

Figure 1. Structural formula of nafarelin

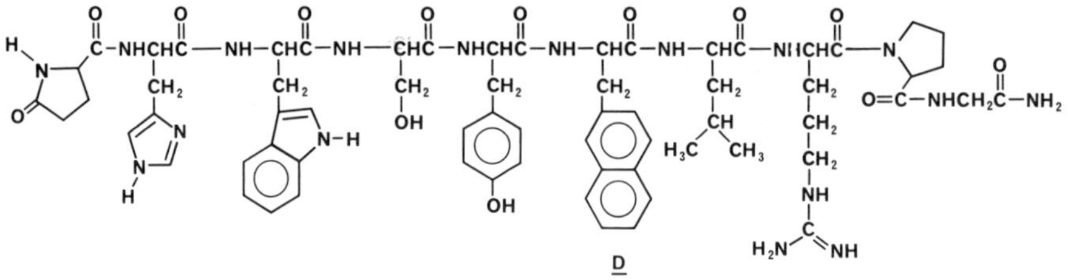

Early animal studies, particularly those conducted in dogs, indicated the ability of once daily injection of nafarelin to suppress testicular function (32,33). However primates, including normal volunteer men, appeared resistant to the effects of daily treatment and complete suppression was not achieved (12,13,35). Similar findings have been made with other analogs (3). Gonadal function is completely suppressed in prostatic cancer patients by such a regimen (14,22), probably reflecting an increased sensitivity of this older, more debilitated population (6,37). In fact, in an ongoing Phase III trial nasal administration of only 300 µg nafarelin twice daily is achieving and maintaining castrate levels of circulating testosterone within 4 weeks of starting treatment (14). The nasal formulation (4) is well tolerated, and there is no sign of acute-on-chronic stimulation of testosterone levels in patients studied 6 months into dosing.

More recently we have been evaluating the effect of continuous administration of nafarelin. Early studies performed with either pelleted material (29) or using implantable minipumps (2,31) had revealed a quantitative, even qualitative, increase in responsivity and suppressibility of the pituitary-gonadal axis when analogs were administered in this way. A prototype formulation incorporating nafarelin in PLGA microspheres at the level of about 1% was suppressive after an initial lag period (23) (figs. 2 and 3). The present formulation incorporates nafarelin at levels of up to 10%. These higher loading levels produce superior release kinetics with no discernable lag phase in release of nafarelin. An additional advantage is that a reduced mass of injected material is required. After injection to rhesus monkeys testicular suppression is rapidly achieved and maintained for 32 days (fig. 4).

Figure 2.   Plasma testosterone and nafarelin levels in rhesus monkeys after a single 3 mg i.m. injection of a prototype 0.8% PLGA formulation.

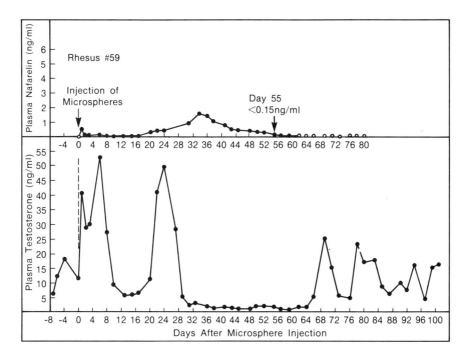

Figure 3.   Plasma testosterone (T) and nafarelin levels in men after a single 4 mg i.m. injection of nafarelin in a prototype 0.8% PLGA formulation.

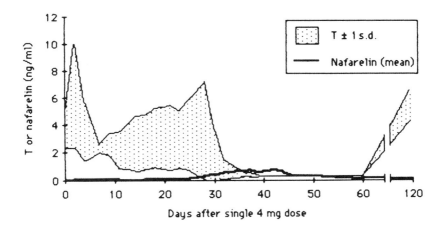

Figure 4.   Plasma levels of nafarelin and testosterone in rhesus
monkeys following a single injection of PLGA microspheres
containing 3 mg of nafarelin at a 4% loading.

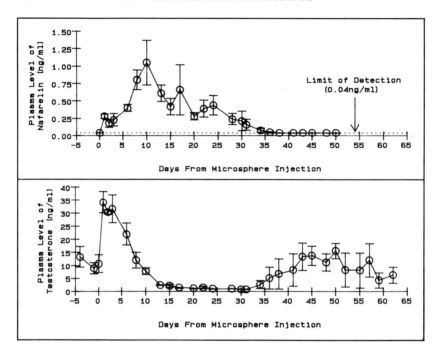

STUDIES WITH RS-68439

RS-68439 (fig. 5) is a competitive antagonist of LHRH which
competes at the level of the pituitary receptors and prevents
stimulation of release (and synthesis) of the gonadotropins.

Figure 5.   Structural formula of RS-68439

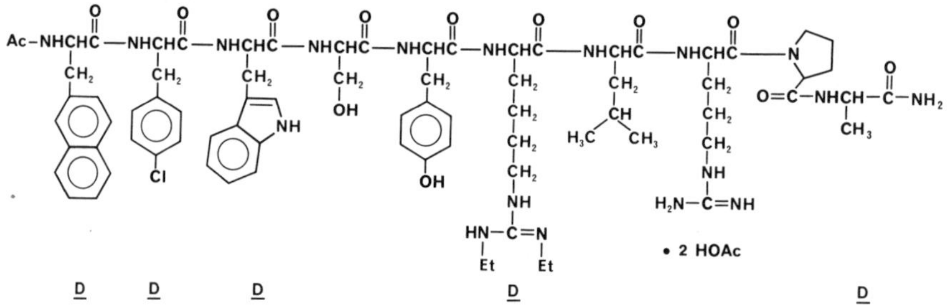

In addition to having high receptor binding affinity it has a long circulatory $t_{1/2}$: 96 minutes in rats and 22 and 48 hours in dogs and men respectively (R. Chan and M.D. Chaplin, personal communication) resulting in an analog of high potency. In rats, RS-68439 is excreted to a large extent intact in the bile indicating that the structural modifications have rendered it metabolically inert, and that the circulatory half life reflects the rate of clearance. The analog is suppressive of pituitary and testicular function in all species so far evaluated (26,28, 34). In contrast to results with the agonists, macaques are readily suppressed on either an acute (1) or chronic basis (5,20). Complete azoospermia can be achieved even in the face of concomitant administration of testosterone (5).

Schmidt et al. (24) first noted anaphylactoid reactions in rats due to dosing with [N-AC-D-Nal(2)[1],D-pF-Phe[2],D-Trp[3], D-Arg[6]]LHRH at levels required for suppression of the pituitary-gonadal axis. It has since become clear that many of the LHRH antagonists, in particular those with [D-Arg[6], L-Arg[8]] substitution share a propensity to degranulate, and release mediators from, mast cells (11,15,16). Although RS-68439 shares this ability when added to rat mast cells in vitro, perhaps because of altered pharmacokinetic characteristics, these effects are only seen at very high doses in vivo.

However before proceeding into clinical testing in man, all subjects were screened for possible histamine sensitivity reaction with a skin test. This test involved intradermal administration of 10 µg of RS-68439. None of the subjects developed more than a mild, 2[+] reaction, and therefore, none was excluded from the study.

First, normal male volunteers were given seven different doses of the LHRH antagonist, from 1 µg to 20 mg. Six men received the first six doses and two men received the 20 mg dose. A decline in circulating levels of LH and testosterone first became apparent at the 100 µg dose. Serum immunoreactive (IR)-FSH fell only by 30%, even with the 20 mg dose. IR-LH decreased by about 50% after all doses. In contrast, the decrease in bioactive LH was dose dependent and reached a nadir of 12% above baseline after the 20 mg dose. Testosterone decline closely reflected the bioactive LH values and fell to less than 10% after the higher doses. The duration of hormonal suppression was also clearly dose related. There was a good correlation between doses and area under the response curve for IR-LH (r=0.86, P<0.001), FSH (r=0.8, P<0.03) and T (r=0.95, P<0.001).

Then, RS-68439 was given as a single subcutaneous injection to 9 normal men at 3 dose levels: 5, 10 and 20 mg. Each volunteer received all 3 doses at least 7 days apart. The nadirs of FSH, LH and testosterone after administration of the antagonist are shown in Table 1.

Table 1. Lowest values of FSH, LH and testosterone observed in
normal male volunteers following various doses of RS-68439
administered subcutaneously.

Dose (mg)	FSH (mIU/ml)	LH (mIU/ml)	Testosterone (ng/ml)
Baseline	6.9 ± 0.5	6.2 ± 0.3	5.1 ± 0.2
5	4.4 ± 1.1	3.3 ± 0.4	1.3 ± 0.3
10	3.6 ± 0.9	2.9 ± 0.3	0.9 ± 0.3
20	4.1 ± 0.9	2.7 ± 0.3	0.6 ± 0.1

FSH levels decreased by 8-10 h and remained suppressed
($p<0.05$) for up to 48 h by 23 ± 2.0%, 44 ± 1.7% and 44 ± 2.1%
after the 5, 10, and 20 mg doses of the antagonist (fig. 6). LH
levels decreased within 2-4 h and remained suppressed ($p<0.05$)
for up to 36 h by 26 ± 3.2%, 41 ± 3.1% and 39 ± 2.4%.
Testosterone decrease was more pronounced than that of FSH or
LH. It remained suppressed ($p<0.05$) by 52 ± 2.6%, 57 ± 2.3% and
76 ± 3.2% for up to 72 h after the 3 doses of the antagonist.
The area under the response curve, describing hormone
concentrations as a function of time during the study,
diminished by 19 ± 6.2%, 39 ± 5.6% and 37 ± 7.1% for FSH, by
13 ± 9.1%, 33 ± 12% and 36 ± 6.6% for LH, and by 43 ± 7.9%, 49 ±
6.7% and 66 ± 4.7% for testosterone with the same doses
respectively. Bioassayable LH and FSH were decreased to a
greater extent than immunoreactive, correlating better with
suppression of T than did the IR-gonadotropins.
Serum levels of the RS-68439 reached a maximum of 40 to
140 ng/ml by 2 hours and levels of 10 to 50 ng/ml were still
present at 48 hours. The apparent half-life of this antagonist
was calculated from these data to be between 44 and 48 hours.
A small degree of erythema developed at the site of injection
but the extent was not dose related and involvement of the
propylene glycol vehicle has not been ruled out. No systemic
side effects were observed.
It was concluded from these studies that a dose of 5 mg
(~70 μg/kg) of RS-68439 was adequate to suppress testicular
function for 24 hours. However, based on the circulating $t_{1/2}$
of RS-68439 in men, computer modelling studies suggested that
circulating levels of RS-68439 from consecutive daily dosing
would increase for 7-9 days before steady state conditions were
achieved. Studies are therefore planned to evaluate the ability
of daily doses of 1-2 mg to achieve and maintain full testicular
suppression.

Figure 6. <u>Effects of single subcutaneous injection of 5, 10 or 20 mg of RS-68439 on circulating levels of RS-68439, LH, FSH and testosterone in men.</u>

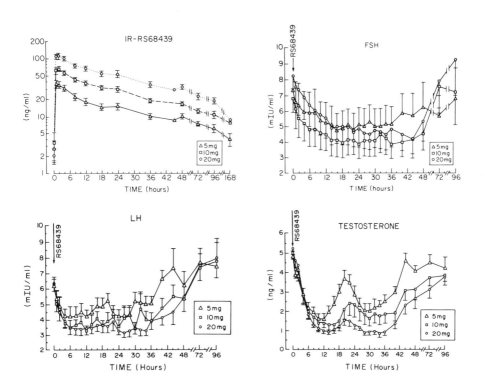

CONCLUSIONS

Nafarelin, as other LHRH agonists, is highly effective in long term suppression of gonadal function. Its high potency and prolonged circulatory half life make it particularly suitable for convenient administration by either twice daily nasal insufflation or low dose controlled release formulation injected once monthly. No doubt nafarelin will become a valuable alternative to orchiectomy and estrogen therapy for treatment of prostate cancer. However, because of their mechanism of action, LHRH agonists cause an initial stimulation of gonadotropin and gonadal steroid output for the first few days of treatment. This "flare" in prostatic cancer patients results in elevated serum alkaline phosphatase and, in a percentage of cases, increased bone pain (38). In extreme cases it may lead to pulmonary collapse, spinal compression or ureteral obstruction.

For these reasons it may be that LHRH antagonists such as RS-68439, even if having a reduced risk: benefit ratio compared to the agonists, will find a niche for treatment of a subpopulation of prostatic cancer patients. This subpopulation would be composed of patients with bilateral hydronephrosis, extensive metastatic disease to the lungs or spine and in whom the cardiovascular risks of estrogen therapy are deemed unacceptable. In these cases, particularly if the patients have a poor prognosis for surgery, the rapidity with which the LHRH antagonists can achieve a medical orchiectomy would make them the therapy of choice.

REFERENCES

1. Adams, L.A., Bremner, W.J., Nestor, J.J. Jr., Vickery, B.H., and Steiner, R.A. (1986): J. Clin. Endocrinol. Metab., 62:58–63.
2. Akhtar, B.F., Marshall, G.R., Wickings, E.J., and Nieschlag, E. (1983): J. Clin. Endocrinol. Metab., 56:534–540.
3. Akhtar, B.F., Wickings, E.J., Zaidi, P., and Nieschlag, E. (1982): Acta Endocrinol., 101:113–118.
4. Anik, S.T., Benjamin, E.J., Masciewicz, R., McRae, G.I., Nerenberg, C., Hwang-Felgner, J., Schneider, J., Worden, A., and Foreman, J. (1986): J. Pharm. Sci., in press.
5. Bremner, W.J., and Steiner, R.A. (1986): Clin. Res., 34:642A.
6. Bremner, W.J., Vitiello, M.V. and Prinz, P.N. (1983): J. Clin. Endocrinol. Metab., 56:1278–1281.
7. Chan, R.L., and Chaplin, M.D. (1985): Biochem. Biophys. Res. Commun., 127:673–679.
8. Chu, N.I., Chan, R.L., Hama, K.M., and Chaplin, M.D. (1985): Drug Metab. Dispos., 13:560–565.
9. Faure, N., Lemay, A., Laroche, B., Robert, G., Plante, R., Thabet, M., Roy, R., Jean, C., Forest, J.-C., and Fazekas, A.T.A. (1985): In: A New Approach to the Treatment of Prostatic Cancer: Buserelin (Suprefact), edited by F. Labrie and U.K. Wenderoth, pp. 17–33, Excerpta Medica, Amsterdam.
10. Garnick, M., and Glode, M., for The Leuprolide Study Group (1984): N. Eng. J. Med., 311:1281–1286.
11. Hahn, D.W., et al. (1986): In: LHRH and Its Analogs: Contraceptive and Therapeutic Applications, Part II, edited by B.H. Vickery and J.J. Nestor Jr., MTP Press, Lancaster, in press.
12. Heber, D., Bhasin, S., Steiner, B., and Swerdloff, R.S. (1984): J. Clin. Endocrinol. Metab., 58:1084–1088.
13. Heber, D., Swerdloff, R.S., and Henzl, M. (1984): In: LHRH and Its Analogs: Contraceptive and Therapeutic Applications, edited by B.H. Vickery, J.J. Nestor, Jr., and E.S.E. Hafez, pp. 257–269, MTP Press, Lancaster.

14. Hoffman, P.G., Henzl, M.R., Chaplin, M.D., and Nerenberg, C.A. (1986): Submitted for publication.

15. Hook, W.A., Karten, M., and Siraganian, R.P. (1985): Fed. Proc., 44:1323. Abstr. #5336

16. Karten, M., et al. (1986): In: LHRH and Its Analogs: Contraceptive and Therapeutic Applications, Part II, edited by B.H. Vickery, and J.J. Nestor Jr., MTP Press, Lancaster, in press.

17. Labrie, F., Belanger, A., and Dupont, A., editors (1985): LHRH and Its Analogs: Basic and Clinical Aspects. Excerpta Medica International Congress Series 656. Elsevier/N. Holland, Amsterdam.

18. Nestor, J.J. Jr., Ho. T.L., Simpson, R.A., Horner, B.L., Jones, G.H., McRae, G.I., and Vickery, B.H. (1982): J. Med. Chem., 25:795-801.

19. Nestor, J.J. Jr., Tahilramani, R., Ho., T.L., McRae, G.I., and Vickery, B.H. (1983): In: Peptides - Structure and Function, Proceedings of the Eighth American Peptide Symposium, edited by V.J. Hruby, and D.H. Rich, pp. 861-864, Pierce Chem. Co., Rockford, Illinois, USA.

20. Nieschlag, E., Akhtar, F.B., Schurmeyer, T., Weinbauer, G. (1984): In: LHRH and Its Analogs: Basic and Clinical Aspects, edited by F. Labrie, A. Belanger, and A. Dupont, pp. 277-286, Elsevier Science Publishers, B.V., Amsterdam.

21. Nillius, S.J. (1984): Clin. Obstet. Gynecol., 11:551-572.

22. Rajfer, J., Swerdloff, R.S., and Heber, D.M. (1984): Fertil. Steril., 42:765-771.

23. Sanders, L.M., McRae, G.I., Vitale, K.M., Vickery, B.H., and Kent, J.S. (1984): In: LHRH and Its Analogues: Basic and Clinical Aspects, edited by F. Labrie, A. Belanger, and A. Dupont, pp. 53-62, Elsevier Science Publishers B.V., Amsterdam.

24. Schmidt, F., Sundaram, K., Thau, R.B., and Bardin, C.W. (1984): Contraception 29:283-289.

25. Vickery, B.H. (1985): In: Male Fertility Regulation, edited by T.J. Lobl, and E.S.E. Hafez, pp. 303-318. MTP Press, Lancaster.

26. Vickery, B.H. (1985): J. Steroid Biochem., 23:779-791.

27. Vickery, B.H. (1986): Endocrine Reviews, 7:115-124.

28. Vickery, B.H. (1986): In: Pharmacology and Clinical Uses of Inhibitors of Hormone Secretion and Action, edited by B.J.A. Furr, and A. Wakeling, Praeger Scientific, Eastbourne, in press.

29. Vickery, B.H., and McRae, G.I. (1984): In: LHRH and Its Analogs: Contraceptive and Therapeutic Applications, edited by B.H. Vickery, J.J. Nestor Jr., and E.S.E. Hafez, pp. 91-106, MTP Press, Lancaster.

30. Vickery, B.H., Anik, S., Chaplin, M., and Henzl, M. (1985): In: Transnasal Systemic Medications, edited by Y.W. Chien, pp. 201- 215, Elsevier Science Publishers B.V., Amsterdam.
31. Vickery, B.H., McRae, G.I., and Tallentire, D. (1983): Fertil. Steril., 39:417.
32. Vickery, B.H., McRae, G.I., Briones, W., Worden, A., Seidenberg, R., Schanbacher, B.D., and Falvo, R. (1984): J. Androl., 5:28-42.
33. Vickery, B.H., McRae, G.I., Briones, W.V., Roberts, B.B., Worden, A.C., Schanbacher, B.D., and Falvo, R.E. (1985): J. Androl., 6:53-60.
34. Vickery, B.H., McRae, G.I., Donahue, D.J., Roberts, B.B., and Worden, A.C. (1985): J. Androl., 6:48P.
35. Vickery, B.H., McRae, G.I., Nestor, J.J. Jr., and Bremner, W. (1983): J. Androl., 4:35.
36. Vickery, B.H., Nestor, J.J. Jr., and Hafez, E.S.E., editors (1984): LHRH and Its Analogs: Contraceptive and Therapeutic Applications. MTP Press, Lancaster.
37. Warner, B.A., Dufau, M.L., and Santen, R.J. (1985): J. Clin. Endocrinol. Metab., 60:263-268.
38. Waxman et al. (1985): Brit. Med. J., 291:1387-1388.

*Hormonal Manipulation of Cancer: Peptides,
Growth Factors, and New (Anti) Steroidal
Agents,* edited by Jan G. M. Klijn et al.
Raven Press, New York © 1987.

THE IMPORTANCE OF COMBINATION THERAPY WITH FLUTAMIDE AND CASTRATION (LHRH AGONIST OR ORCHIECTOMY) IN PREVIOUSLY UNTREATED AS WELL AS PREVIOUSLY TREATED PATIENTS WITH ADVANCED PROSTATE CANCER

F. Labrie, A. Dupont, A. Bélanger, M. Giguère, J.P. Borsanyi,
Y. Lacourcière, J. Emond, G. Monfette and R. Lachance

Departments of Molecular Endocrinology, Medicine, Nuclear Medicine and Urology, Laval University Medical Center, Quebec G1V 4G2,
Canada

SUMMARY

The combination therapy with Flutamide and castration (medical or surgical) has been applied in 136 previously untreated stage D_2 patients with prostate cancers as well as in 204 patients having received previous endocrine therapy. In the first study, we have administered the pure antiandrogen Flutamide in association with orchiectomy (13 patients) or the LHRH agonist [D-Trp[6]]-LHRH ethylamide (123 patients) to previously untreated men with clinical stage D_2 prostate cancer. The mean duration of treatment was 610 days (88 to 1367 days). The response was assessed according to the criteria of the U.S. National Prostatic Cancer Project. A complete response has been observed in 35 patients (26%) while partial and stable responses have been achieved in 52 (38%) and 43 (32%) patients, respectively. A positive objective response has thus been observed in 130 of 136 patients (96%), thus leaving only 4% of progression. When comparing to recent studies, the complete response rate following combination therapy is 5.6 times superior while the rate of progression is 4.1 times lower. The probability of continuing positive response after 2 years of treatment (according to Kaplan and Meier) is 56.2%, while the probability of survival at the same time interval is 82.4%. This survival should be compared to values of 40 to 60% achieved with previous endocrine therapy limited to inhibition of testicular androgen secretion or action.

In the second study, two hundred and four patients having clinical stage D_2 prostate cancer previously treated by orchiectomy, estrogens or LHRH agonists alone received, at the time of relapse, the same combination therapy. Complete, partial and stable objective responses assessed according to the same objective criteria were obtained in 11 (5.4%), 17 (8.3%) and 39 (19.1%) patients, respectively, for a total objective response rate of 32.8%. Progression continued in 137 (67.2%) patients. The present data obtained in a large population of relapsing patients clearly demonstrate that a large number of tumors were left growing under the influence of androgens still present after standard treatment limited to blockade of testicular androgens. By adding the pure antiandrogen Flutamide to block the action of adrenal androgens remaining active after castration, a positive objective response is seen in one third of cases, thus providing those patients with a marked improvement in quality of life and most likely survival. Without this treatment, progression would have continued in all cases. The present data demonstrate that the combined blockade of androgens achieved with Flutamide and castration provides an objective response in approximately 95% of patients, and markedly prolongs the period of remission while the death rate within the first two years is lower than that obtained with previous treatments. In addition, the prolongation of survival is achieved with an excellent quality of life.

Although more efficient when applied as first treatment, the combination therapy with Flutamide remains the best treatment, even for those who relapse after castration or estrogens.

INTRODUCTION

Since the observations of Huggins and his colleagues in 1941 (3), orchiectomy and treatment with estrogens have been the cornerstone of the management of advanced prostate cancer. These two approaches cause improvement for a limited time interval in 60 to 80% of cases, thus leaving 20 to 40% of the patients without improvement of their disease (5, 13, 15). Moreover, progression of the cancer usually occurs within 6 to 24 months in those who initially responded (16) and 50% of the patients are then expected to die within the next 6 months (4, 18). In addition to the questionable improvement in survival, orchiectomy is often psychologically unacceptable while estrogens cause serious and often lethal side effects (2).

LHRH agonists can avoid the psychological limitations of orchiectomy as well as the serious side effects of estrogens (2, 7, 8). However, despite their excellent tolerance and efficacy as inhibitors of testicular androgen secretion (7, 8), one cannot expect results better than those already achieved with castration. Man, in fact, is unique among species in having a high secretion rate of adrenal steroids which are converted into potent androgens in the prostatic tissue itself (for review, see 9). In order to achieve a more complete blockade of androgens, we have associated a pure antiandrogen with castration (chemical with an LHRH agonist or orchiectomy) at the start of treatment of 136 patients with advanced prostate cancer. We have also applied the same combination therapy to 204 patients showing relapse after orchiectomy or treatment with estrogens or LHRH agonists alone.

RESULTS AND DISCUSSION

Previously untreated patients

Starting in March 1982, 136 previously untreated patients with histology-proven prostatic carcinoma and bone metastases identified by bone scan and X-Ray received the combined treatment for more than 3 months as first therapy for an average period of 610 days of treatment and could thus be evaluated objectively (Table I). Pain was originally present in 66% of patients and it subsided completely in more than 90% of cases during the first month of treatment.

TABLE 1   Objective response rate to combination therapy in previously untreated patients (NPCP criteria)

Total evaluated	Days of RX means limits	Objective response			
		Complete	Partial	Stable	Progression
136	610	35	52	43	6
	88-1367	25.7%	38.2%	31.6%	4.4%

The serum levels of PAP were initially elevated in 87% of the patients, the values ranging between 0.2 and 896 ng/ml, the normal being < 2.0 ng/ml. In all cases, the start of treatment was followed by an extremely rapid fall in serum PAP, a decrease to 21% of control being already reached before 10 days of treatment ($p < 0.01$). Serum PAP values returned to normal in all except 8 patients before 6 months of treatment.

As can be seen in Table 1, a positive objective response assessed according to the criteria of the US NPCP (18) has been observed in 96% of the patients. As illustrated in Fig. 1, such a high level of complete objective responses (25.7%) is far superior (5.6 times) to comparable recent studies where the treatment was limited to a blockade of testicular androgens. On average, only 4.6% of patients showed a complete response in these studies (14, 19, 20). It should be mentioned that the 26% complete response rate observed in the present study includes patients recently entered into the study, a situation which does not take into account the chances of complete response which can be achieved at longer time intervals. In fact, for the 50 patients who have reached 2 years of combination treatment, 23 (46%) of them showed a complete objective response as best response.

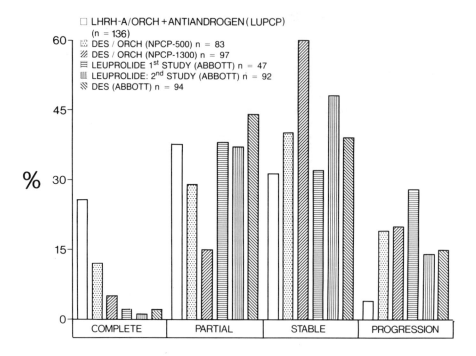

FIG. 1 Comparison of objective responses (complete, partial,
stable and progression) to combination therapy (LHRH
agonist or orchiectomy associated with Flutamide) versus
therapies limited to the blockade of testicular androgens
(orchiectomy, estrogens or LHRH agonist alone) (14, 19,
20).

The other striking finding illustrated on Fig. 1 is that only
4.4% of the patients did not show an objective response at the
start of combination therapy while, on average, 18% of patients
continued to progress at the start of treatment in the other
studies (14, 19, 20). In all these six cases who were classified
as non responders, however, regression of uptake on the bone scan
could be seen in some lesions while disease continued to progress
in one or more areas. In the four patients having pain at start
of treatment, disappearance of pain was observed for a few
months. Such data clearly indicate various levels of androgen
sensitivity of different tumors in the same patient. Thus, while
a positive objective response could be documented in 96% of
cases, a subjective improvement is observed in more than 99% of
patients upon start of the combination therapy, thus indicating
that almost (if not all) tumors are androgen-sensitive at the
start of treatment.

In addition to the improved percentage of positive responses at the start of treatment, another most important aspect of the effect of the combination treatment is the marked increase in the duration of the positive response. While the percentage of patients still in remission at 2 years is 56.2% with the combination therapy, it has already decreased to 0% before reaching 2 years with Leuprolide (14). There is thus a remarkable advantage of the combination therapy, not only on the percentage of initial responses, but even more strikingly, upon the duration of the

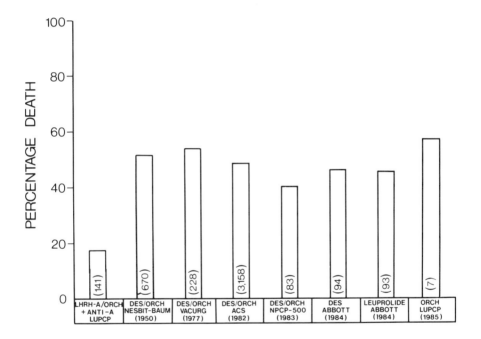

FIG. 2. Comparison of the death rate after 2 years of treatment with the combined androgen blockade (Laval University Prostate Cancer Program (LUPCP) with results obtained with no treatment (15) and the standard hormonal therapies (orchiectomy (ORCH) and/or estrogens) in previously untreated stage D patients: Nesbit and Baum's study (15), study of the Veterans' Administration Cooperative Urology Research Group (VACURG) (5); survey of the American College of Surgeons (ACS) (1982) (13); and study 500 of the USNPCP (1983) (14); Leuprolide alone (1984) (20), and orchiectomy alone (LUPCP) (1985) (10).

positive response. The most medically significant result is
however that observed on survival. In fact, as shown on Fig. 2,
the probability of survival following combination therapy is
82.4% at 2 years as compared to 40 to 60% by previous therapies
(p < 0.01) (5, 13–15, 19, 20).

Previously treated patients

An important question is the relative benefits of the combination therapy administered as first treatment as compared to the
same therapy applied as a second step at the time of disease progression in patients previously orchiectomized or treated with
estrogens or LHRH agonists alone. As illustrated in Fig. 3, the
survival is markedly improved (p < 0.01) in the group of stage D2

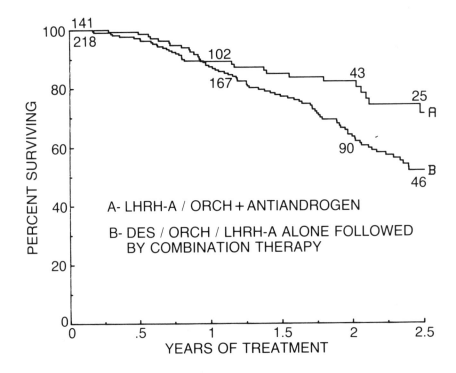

FIG. 3.   Comparison of the death rate in previously untreated
patients having clinical stage D2 prostate cancer who
received the combination therapy as first treatment and
those who had orchiectomy or received estrogens or LHRH
agonists alone before administration of the combination
therapy at the time of progression. Survival was calculated according to Kaplan–Meier from the time of first
treatment in the two groups and is thus comparable.

patients who received the combined treatment with the pure antiandrogen as first treatment as compared to the group of patients
who had orchiectomy or received estrogens or LHRH agonists alone
prior to the administration of Flutamide. In fact, as mentioned
earlier, the survival at 2 years is 82.4% in the group of
patients who received the combination therapy at the start of
treatment as compared to only 63.8% in those who had partial
androgen blockade for various time intervals before receiving the
combination therapy. Up to 2 years of treatment, the death rate
is thus increased by approximately 2-fold by delaying Flutamide
administration (from 17.6 to 46.2%, $p < 0.01$).

Of major interest in Table II is the finding that 32.8% of
previously treated patients showed a positive objective response
to the combined antiandrogen blockade, thus demonstrating the
benefits of adding Flutamide in relapsing patients. Patients
previously castrated received only Flutamide while those treated
with DES or an LHRH agonist alone received [D-Trp^6]LHRH ethylamide in combination with Flutamide. By comparison, 130 of 136 (96%)
of previously untreated patients showed a positive objective
response at start of treatment ($p < 0.01$, Fisher's exact test)
(Table 1).

TABLE 2   Objective response to combination therapy in previously
treated patients

Number of patients	Days of RX limits	Objective response			
		Complete	Partial	Stable	Progression
204	690	11	17	39	137
	64-3237	5.4%	8.3%	19.1%	67.2%

There is ample clinical and biochemical evidence for a role of
adrenal androgens in prostate cancer. Although it seems logical
to remove all androgens as first treatment of androgen-sensitive
diseases such as prostate cancer, the relative benefits of early
versus late blockade of adrenal androgens had to be determined.
The finding of a 96% rate of positive objective response at start
of treatment following combination therapy in previously untreated patients (Table 1) indicates that prostate cancer, even at the
advanced stage of metastases, remains exquisitely sensitive to
androgens when continuously exposed to normal levels of androgens. However, when exposed for some time to the low level of

adrenal androgens, an important proportion of tumors become "autonomous" or, using a more appropriate term, treatment-insensitive, thus loosing their property to respond to the combined antiandrogen blockade. This loss of response to the combination treatment occurs in approximately 66% of patients, thus leaving 33% of responders to the combination therapy applied late at the time of relapse from previous endocrine therapy (orchiectomy, estrogens or LHRH agonists alone).

The recent finding that the antiandrogen Flutamide can prevent the loss of androgen sensitivity (12) in the presence of low androgen levels may partially explain the favorable results observed in the present study in patients who received the combination therapy at start of treatment. In fact, Flutamide not only blocks the stimulatory action of the adrenal androgens which remain present in prostatic cancer tissue following medical or surgical castration but the drug may well block the spontaneous action of the free androgen receptor (17) and thus prevent or delay the development of treatment-resistant tumors (11).

The present data confirm that a large proportion of prostatic cancer tumors are treatment-resistant at the time of relapse following medical or surgical castration. As a consequence, the delay in administering the combination therapy has a major negative impact on the quality of life and survival, the death rate during the first 2 years being approximately 2-fold higher in the group of previously treated patients as compared to those who received the combination therapy as first treatment. It should be mentioned that survival was calculated in the two groups from the time of first treatment, thus permitting comparison of the data obtained.

The common belief that patients in relapse after castration or treatment with estrogens have exclusively "androgen-insensitive" tumors should be abandonned. In fact, it is most likely that androgen-sensitive tumors are present at all stages of prostate cancer in all patients and that optimal androgen blockade should be performed in all cases. Instead of being androgen-insensitive, most of the tumors which continue to grow after castration are most likely to be "androgen-hypersensitive". These tumors are able to grow in the presence of the "low" level of androgens of adrenal origin left after castration. Inhibition of the growth of these tumors requires further androgen blockade. This affirmation is supported by convincing clinical data (see 9 for review) as well as by well-established fundamental observations (1, 6, 11).

Since the combined antiandrogen blockade provides a much higher rate of positive response at the start of treatment (96 vs 60-80%), and provides additional years of excellent quality of life with no side effects other than those related to the blockade of androgens (hot flashes and a decrease or loss of libido), it seems logical to propose that the combination therapy should be given as first treatment with no exception to all patients having advanced prostate cancer and should be continued for life without interruption. For all those who have received previous hormonal therapy, the combination treatment remains the best available therapy and can still permit a positive objective response in a large proportion of patients with a good quality of life and most likely, a prolongation of survival. In order to avoid the development of resistance to treatment, compliance is an essential requirement: the combination therapy with flutamide + LHRH agonist (in non castrated patients) should be taken for life without any interruption. Similarly, the antiandrogen should be started 24 hours before orchiectomy or first administration of the LHRH agonist. As clearly indicated by fundamental (11, 12) and clinical (9) data, any lack of compliance could permit the development of resistance to the antiandrogen treatment. When this resistance has developed, very little, if any, therapeutical alternative can be offered to the patient.

REFERENCES
1. Bartsch, W., Knabbe, M., and Voigt, K.D. (1983): Regulation and compartmentalization of androgens in rat prostate and muscle. J. Steroid Biochem., 19:929–937.
2. Glashan, R.W., and Robinson, M.R.G. (1981): Cardiovascular complications in the treatment of prostatic carcinoma. Br. J. Urol., 53:624–630.
3. Huggins, C., and Hodges, C.V. (1941): Studies of prostatic cancer. I. Effect of castration, estrogen and androgen injections on serum phosphatases in metastatic carcinoma of the prostate. Cancer Res., 1: 293–297.
4. Johnson, D.E., Scott, W.W., Gibbons, R.P., Prout, G.R., Schmidt, J.D., Chu, T.M., Gaeta, J., Sarott, J. and Murphy, G.P. (1977): National randomized study of chemotherapeutic agents in advanced prostatic carcinoma: progress report. Canc. Treat. Rep., 61:317–323.
5. Jordan, W.P., Blackard, C.E. and Byar, D.P. (1977): Reconsideration of orchiectomy in the treatment of advanced prostatic carcinoma. South Med. J., 70:1411–15.
6. King, R.J.B., Cambray, G.J., Jagus–Smith, R., Robinson, J.H. and Smith, J.A. (1977): In Receptors and mechanisms of action of steroid hormones, edited by J.R. Pasqualini, p. 215, Marcel Dekker, New York.
7. Labrie, F., Bélanger, A., Cusan, L., Séguin, C., Pelletier, G., Kelly P.A., Lefebvre F.A., Lemay A. and Raynaud J.P. (1980): Antifertility effects of LHRH agonists in the male. J. Androl., 1:209–228.
8. Labrie F., Dupont A., Bélanger A., Lachance, R., Giguère M. (1985): Long-term treatment with luteinizing hormone-releasing hormone agonists and maintenance of serum testosterone to castration concentrations. Brit. Med. J., 291:369–370.
9. Labrie F., Dupont A., and Bélanger A. (1985). Complete androgen blockade for the treatment of prostate cancer. In: Important Advances in Oncology, edited by V.T. De Vita Jr., S. Hellman and S.A. Rosenberg, pp. 193–217. J.B. Lippincott Company, Philadelphia.

10. Labrie, F., Dupont, A., Bélanger, A., Giguère, M., Lacourcière, Y., Emond, J., Monfette, G. and Bergeron, V. (1985): Combination therapy with flutamide and castration (LHRH agonist or orchiectomy) in advanced prostate cancer: a marked improvement in response and survival. J. Steroid Biochem., 23:833-841.

11. Labrie, F. and Veilleux, R. (1986): A wide range of sensitivities to androgens develops in cloned Shionogi mouse mammary tumor cells. The Prostate, 8:293-300.

12. Luthy I. and Labrie, F. (1986). The development of androgen resistance in mouse mammary tumor cells can be prevented by the antiandrogen Flutamide. The Prostate (in press).

13. Mettlin, C., Natarajan, N. and Murphy, G.P. (1982): Recent patterns of care of prostatic cancer patients in the United States: results from the surveys of the American College of Surgeons Commission on Cancer. Int. Adv. Surg. Oncol., 5: 277-321.

14. Murphy G.P., Beckley S., Brady M.F., Chu M., DeKernion J.B., Dhabuwala C., Gaeta J.F., Gibbons R.P., Loening S., McKiel C.F., McLeod D.G., Pontes J.E., Prout G.R., Scardino P.T., Schlegel J.U., Schmidt J.D., Scott W.W., Slack N.H., and Soloway M. (1983): Treatment of newly diagnosed metastatic prostate cancer patients with chemotherapy agents in combination with hormones versus hormones alone. Cancer, 51:1264-1272.

15. Nesbit, R.M., and Baum, W.C. (1950): Endocrine control of prostatic carcinoma: clinical and statistical survey of 1818 cases. JAMA, 143:1317-20.

16. Resnick, M.I., and Grayhack, J.T. (1975). Treatment of stage IV carcinoma of the prostate. Urol. Clin. North. Amer., 2: 141-161.

17. Simard J. and Labrie F. (1984). Unoccupied androgen receptors are biologically active in rat pituitary gonadotrophs. Proc. 7th Int. Congr. Endocrinology, Excerpta Medica ICS 652, Amsterdam), p. 973.

18. Slack, N.H., Murphy, G.D., and NPCP participants (1984): Criteria for evaluating patient responses to treatment modalities for prostatic cancer. Urol. Clin. North Amer. 11, 337-342.

19. Smith, J.A., Glode, L.M., Wettlaufer, J.N., Stein, B.S., Glass, A.G., Max, D.T., Anbar, D., Jagst, C.L., and Murphy, G.P. (1985): Clinical effects of gonadotropin-releasing hormone analogue in metastatic carcinoma of the prostate. Urology, 20:106-114.

20. The Leuprolide Study Group (1984): Leuprolide versus diethylstilbestrol for metastatic prostate cancer. New Engl. J. Med., 311:1281-1286.

Hormonal Manipulation of Cancer: Peptides, Growth Factors, and New (Anti) Steroidal Agents, edited by Jan G. M. Klijn et al. Raven Press, New York © 1987.

LEUPROLIDE VERSUS DIETHYLSTILBESTROL

FOR METASTATIC PROSTATIC CANCER

Linda J. Swanson, Ph.D., and Marc B. Garnick, M.D.*

Abbott Laboratories, Abbott Park, IL 60064
*Division of Medicine, Dana Farber Cancer Institute
and Department of Medicine, Brigham and Women's Hospital
Harvard Medical School, Boston, MA   02115

INTRODUCTION

For the past 40 years since the observation by Huggins and Hodges that surgical castration or diethylstilbestrol (DES) could bring relief of symptoms from metastatic prostate cancer, these have been the standard therapies for the initial treatment of that disease (7,8). However, during that time the search for less toxic and more acceptable forms of therapy has continued.

The potent analogues of gonadotropin releasing hormone (GnRH) offer an important alternative to DES or orchiectomy. Chronic administration of these analogues, in both animals and man, results in an initial stimulation, followed by inhibition, of the release of follicle stimulating hormone (FSH) and luteinizing hormone (LH) (3,10). The suppression of LH and FSH leads to a decrease in circulating testosterone levels, critical in the treatment of prostate adenocarcinoma (1,2,4,5,6,9,13,14).

METHODS

The efficacy and safety of the superactive analogue of GnRH, leuprolide acetate (Lupron® Injection, TAP Pharmaceuticals), was compared to that of DES in patients with previously untreated, Stage D_2, prostate cancer. The study was conducted in 20 centers in the United States, Canada and Mexico, beginning in October 1981.

Upon entry into the study patients were randomly assigned to receive leuprolide, 1 mg subcutaneously daily or DES, 3 mg orally per day. Ninety-eight patients were randomized to leuprolide as initial treatment and 101 were randomized to

DES. Patients could cross over to the other treatment when
disease progression occurred or because of intolerable side
effects. When disease progression occurred, or if intolerable
side effects were observed on the second treatment, patients
were discontinued from the study and were followed from that
time on to determine survival. Patients were examined every
six weeks during the study, and were evaluated for objective
response every three months. Objective response was determined
using the criteria of the National Prostatic Cancer Project
(12).

Patients were enrolled in the study who fulfilled the
following entrance criteria: Carcinoma of the prostate with
bone metastases, lymph node metastases above the aortic
bifurcation, or metastases to other soft tissues (Stage D_2); two
measurable or evaluable manifestations of prostate cancer (e.g.,
metastases, nodules in the prostate, or elevation of the serum
acid phosphatase level); performance status no higher than 2,
according to the Eastern Cooperative Oncology Group scale
(ambulatory for more than 50 percent of waking hours, unless
incapacitated by bone pain); no previous systemic therapy or
radiotherapy, except for local radiotherapy of nonindicator
lesions; complete recovery from the effects of major surgery;
and informed consent given voluntarily. Patients were excluded
from the study if they had had an orchiectomy. In addition,
they were excluded if they had a history of other cancer or of
life-threatening renal, hepatic, or cardiovascular disease, or
if life expectancy was less than three months because of their
cancer.

There were no significant differences in patient characteristics at study entry between the two initial treatment groups,
with respect to age, performance status, acid phosphatase
levels, tumor burden or cardiovascular history. A "high tumor
burden," seen in 77 and 79 percent, respectively, of leuprolide
and DES patients was defined as any of the following: more than
three lesions on bone scan or the presence of hepatic metastases
or the presence of both lung and osseous lesions. This
represented a relatively high risk group of patients. The
presence of cardiovascular history was defined by an abnormal
ECG, historical evidence suggestive of cardiovascular disease or
the ingestion of cardiovascular medicines seen in 73 and
71 percent, respectively, of leuprolide and DES patients.

RESULTS AND DISCUSSION

Serum testosterone (T) and dihydrotestosterone (DHT) levels
during the study are shown in Figures 1 and 2. After an initial
increase (not shown) T and DHT levels fell to castrate (less
than 50 ng/dl) by Weeks 3 and 4 and remained there throughout

the study. Although testosterone levels appear to be more variable in patients receiving DES 3 mg/day, mean T and DHT levels remain at castrate for both groups.

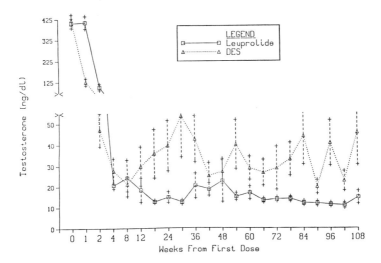

FIGURE 1: Mean (± S.E.M.) serum testosterone levels over 108 weeks of study. N decreased from 89 to 27 in the leuprolide group and from 82 to 24 in the DES group as patients discontinued study. N at any point was never less than 12.

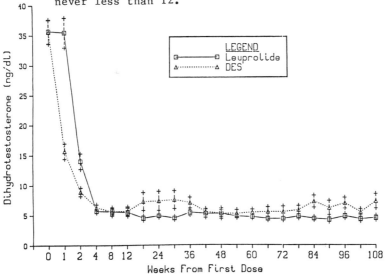

FIGURE 2. Mean (± S.E.M.) serum DHT levels over 108 weeks of study. N varies as described in the legend to Figure 1.

The best objective responses determined during the study for 92 and 94 evaluable patients initially treated with leuprolide or DES, respectively, are shown in Table 1.

TABLE 1. Best Objective Response to Treatment

	Leuprolide N=92 N (%)	DES N=94 N (%)
CR	1 (1)	2 (2)
PR	34 (37)	41 (44)
NC	44 (48)	37 (39)
NO PROGRESSION	79 (86)	80 (85)
PD	10 (11)	2 (2)
SE*	3 (3)	12 (13)

*Patients discontinued secondary to side effects.

Based on NPCP criteria 86% of the patients in the leuprolide group and 85% of the patients initially treated with DES showed "No Progression" of disease (which includes Complete Response, Partial Response and Disease Stabilization).

One of the difficulties in analyzing data generated from crossover designed studies is different patterns of crossover and dropouts. Patients whose initial therapy was DES crossed over or dropped out at a much earlier time in their presentation compared to those patients assigned to leuprolide. Therefore, leuprolide patients were at a much higher risk for a longer period of time of developing progressive disease. Because of this, the most reasonable means of analysis was to evaluate the time to treatment failure. Treatment failure for this analysis was defined as one of the following: the development of progressive disease, death, or the development of adverse side effects.

The time to treatment failure in evaluable, Stage D_2 patients is shown in Figure 3. The time to treatment failure was comparable between the leuprolide population and the DES population.

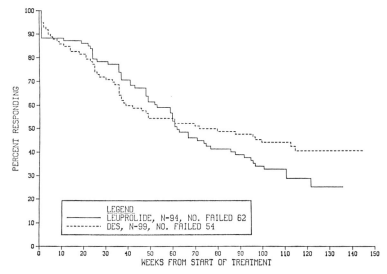

FIGURE 3.   Time to treatment failure, on their initial treatment, in evaluable patients treated with leuprolide
or DES.

Figure 4 exhibits the distributions of time from start of
study to death for evaluable leuprolide and DES patients. There
were no differences observed between the two groups. It is
important to note that when survival is examined, one is not
comparing survival in patients treated only with DES to those of
patients treated only with leuprolide. Rather, one is comparing
the survival of patients treated with leuprolide as first treatment, followed by DES, any other treatment, or no treatment to
the survival of patients treated with DES as primary therapy,
followed by leuprolide, another treatment or no treatment. The
two curves, then, include cohorts of patients who crossed over
to the alternative treatment. The two cohorts do not make
similar contributions to the two survival curves and a bias in
favor of the DES group may be present.

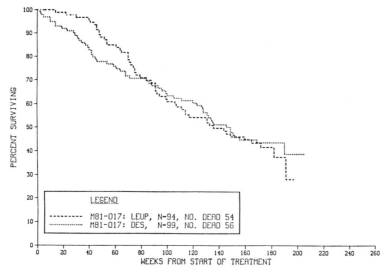

FIGURE 4.   Time from study entry to death in evaluable Stage D_2 patients initially treated with leuprolide or DES.

The importance of the long term complications of DES therapy in older men with prostate cancer is becoming increasingly clear. Although therapy with 1 mg/day DES may be less toxic, it may not be as effective as the standard therapy of 3 mg/day in reducing testosterone to castrate (11).

There were marked differences between the two treatment groups in terms of side effects. Overall 13% of patients on DES discontinued treatment because of intolerable side effects as compared with only 3% in the leuprolide group. Hot flashes were much more common in the leuprolide group. They usually occurred within the first 7 to 10 days of starting therapy and tended to last throughout treatment.

However, other side effects were consistently more numerous in the DES group. There was a higher incidence of gynecomastia and painful breasts. No difference was found between the DES subgroup that had received prophylactic irradiation and the subgroup that had not. Nausea and vomiting were more frequent with DES, as were cardiovascular complications, in terms of peripheral edema. Although the incidence of venous complications, thrombosis, phlebitis or pulmonary embolus showed a tendency towards an increased frequency with DES as compared to leuprolide, their difference did not achieve statistical significance.

In conclusion, leuprolide is a safe and effective palliative
treatment for metastatic prostatic cancer. We feel that
leuprolide offers an important alternative to the use of
estrogens in the initial management of prostatic cancer because
of the marked difference in the side effect profile between
leuprolide and DES.

REFERENCES

1. Ahmed SR, Brooman PJC, Shalet SM, Howell A, Blacklock NJ,
    Rickards D (1983): Treatment of advanced prostatic
    cancer with LHRH analogue ICI 118630: clinical response
    and hormonal mechanisms. Lancet 2:415-9.
2. Allen JM, O'Shea JP, Mashiter K, Williams G, Bloom SR
    (1983): Advanced carcinoma of the prostate: treatment
    with a gonadotropin releasing hormone agonist. Br Med J
    286:1607-9.
3. Belchetz PE, Plant TM, Nakai Y, Keogh EJ, Knobil E (1978):
    Hypophysial responses to continuous and intermittent
    delivery of hypothalamic gonadotropin-releasing hormone.
    Science 202:631-3.
4. Borgmann V, Hardt W, Schmidt-Gollwitzer M, Adenauer H,
    Nagel R (1982): Sustained suppression of testosterone
    production by the luteinizing-hormone releasing-hormone
    agonist buserelin in patients with advanced prostate
    carcinoma: a new therapeutic approach? Lancet
    1:1097-9.
5. Faure N, Lemay A, Laroche B, et al. (1983): Preliminary
    results on the clinical efficacy and safety of androgen
    inhibition by the LHRH agonist alone or combined with an
    antiandrogen in the treatment of prostatic carcinoma.
    Prostate 4:601-24.
6. Garnick MB, Glode LM and the Leuprolide Study Group (1984):
    Leuprolide versus diethylstilbestrol for Metastatic
    Prostate Cancer. New Engl J Med 311:1281-6.
7. Huggins C, Hodges CV (1941): Studies on prostatic cancer.
    I. The effect of castration, of estrogen and of androgen
    injection on serum phosphatases in metastatic carcinoma
    of the prostate. Cancer Res 1:293-7.
8. Huggins C, Stevens RE Jr, Hodges CV (1941): Studies on
    prostatic cancer. II. The effects of castration on
    advanced carcinoma of the prostate gland. Arch Surg
    43:209-23.
9. Koutsilieris M, Tolis G (1983): Gonadotropin-releasing
    hormone agonistic analogues in the treatment of advanced
    prostatic carcinoma. Prostate 4:569-77.

10. Linde R, Doelle GC, Alexander N, Kirchner F, Vale W, Rivier J, Rabin D (1981): Reversible inhibition of testicular steroidogenesis and spermatogenesis by a potent gonadotropin-releasing hormone agonist in normal men: an approach toward the development of a male contraceptive. N Engl J Med 305:663-7.

11. Robinson, MRG, Thomas BS (1971): Effect of hormonal therapy on plasma testosterone levels in prostatic carcinoma. Br Med J 4:391-4.

12. Schmidt JD, Scott WW, Gibbons R, et al. (1980): Chemotherapy programs of the National Prostatic Cancer Project. Cancer 45:1937-46.

13. Walker KJ, Nicholson RI, Turkes AO, et al. (1983): Therapeutic potential of the LHRH agonist, ICI 118630, in the treatment of advanced prostatic carcinoma. Lancet 2:413-5.

14. Waxman JH, Wass JAH, Hendry WF, et al. (1983): Treatment with gonadotrophin releasing hormone analogue in advanced prostatic cancer. Br Med J 286:1309-12.

Hormonal Manipulation of Cancer: Peptides, Growth Factors, and New (Anti) Steroidal Agents, edited by Jan G. M. Klijn et al. Raven Press, New York © 1987.

COMPARATIVE STUDIES WITH LHRH-AGONISTS

H.J.de.Voogt

Department of Urology, Free University Hospital, De Boelelaan 1117, 1007 MB Amsterdam, The Netherlands

The arrival of LHRH-agonists carried high hopes for a new medication of advanced prostatic cancer. A drug was found that lowered serum-Testosteron values to castration levels with minimal side-effects. Would that mean also a better survival or a longer time-to-progression for these patients? Already on theoretical grounds this can hardly be expected. Since Huggins' work we know that androgen-deprivation alleviates the complaints of patients which are caused by urinary obstruction and/or most-ly) bone metastases. The androgen sensitive part of the tumor (cells) is retarded in growth and probably disappears largely (but we do not know whether they disappear completely) and sooner or later androgen-insensitive cells will take over and cause pro-gression (Coffey (1)). Unless a hitherto undetected direct effect of LHRH-a on tumor cells plays a role (as has been sugges-ted for oestrogens), survival and time-to-progression will not change. Results of phase-II-studies with LHRH-a point in that direction. However proof can only be given by randomized, compara-tive studies with large numbers of patients. Garnick (2) was the first to publish such a study which fulfils the criteria and is presen-ted today. There are however a few other, smaller studies, that can be mentioned as well.

To begin with, there is a small, non-randomized pilot study which was performed in Holland, running parallel to the phase-II-study that Schröder (6) presented this morning.13 patients were treated with LHRH-a (Buserelin) combined with CPA 150 mg daily. Interestingly not only was there a rapid decrease in PAP-values during the first 2 weeks, but later, after follow-up of 12 months, the rate of progression in these 13 patients who were age-matched with the group of 58 patients of our phase-II-study, was the same, namely 41% of the 13 patients and 39% in the group of 58.

The other studies are presented in table I and as one can see the numbers of patients are divergent and certainly not all stu-dies can be regarded as phase-III-studies, although they are randomized, except the study of Singer (7) which does not indicate that, but in which the number of patients with buserelin is 45

Table I. Comparative studies of LHRH-a versus androgen deprivation in advanced prostatic cancer.

authors	number of patients	disease-stage	LHRH-a used	Androgen deprivation	remarks
Trachtenberg et al. '86	30	D_2	Buserelin per nasal	orchidectomy and/or RU 23908	randomized prosp.
Parmar et al.'85	79	D_2	D-T2P-6-LHRH	orchidectomy	randomized prosp.
Singer et al.'85	63	D_2	Buserelin per nasal	orchidectomy	?
Koutsilieris and Tollis '84	29	$C_1D_1D_2$	Buserelin per nasal	orchidectomy	randomized prosp.
Garnick et al.'85	199	D_2	Leuprolide s.c.inj.	DES 3 mg	randomized prosp.

Table II. Percentage of overall Response and Progression

	LHRH-a		orchidectomy		DES		time of follow-up
	Resp.	Progr.	Resp.	Progr.	Resp.	Progr.	
Parmar '85	87%	13%	81%	19%			3 month
Singer '85	66%	33%	80%	20%			10-19 months
Koutsilieris '84	93%	7%	100%	0%			6 months
'84	79%	21%	84%	16%			12 months
Garnick '86	86%	14%			85%	15%	12 months

and those with orchidectomy only 18. Also time of follow-up was not the same. The 3 months follow-up of Parmar et al. (4), who gave preliminary results, is too short to give any meaningfull figures. The other 3 studies have follow-up times of 6-12 months respectively. The data as to response (overall) and progression are given in table II. Recently Trachtenberg (9) presented his results in 30 patients after a follow-up of 1 year. There was no difference in progression rate between the 3 groups of patients, in which the treatments were castration and placebo, castration and RU 23908 and Buserelin with RU 23908.

It should be clear that at this moment from these studies a clear-cut evidence of time-to-progression cannot be given as follow-up is not yet long enough and Kaplan-Meier curves could not be calculated from these data. However the first impression is certainly, that differences between LHRH-agonists and androgen deprivation by orchidectomy or DES did not exist. In fact Garnick's study which is the best evaluated with the longest follow-up time, did not see any difference at all.

Also as to laboratory parameters: T-levels in all studies came down to castration level in due time (2 weeks after start treatment) and remained down throughout the duration of the studies. PAP-levels and subjective parameters equally showed the kind of expected response rates, and finally in none of the studies other side-effects than hot flushes and loss of libido were noted with LHRH-therapy, while the patients on DES showed the expected C.V.-side effects.

So at the moment, and once again it has to be stressed that it is still too early to give any definitive answers, there are no signs that treatment with LHRH-agonists is better than the traditional androgen-deprivation such as orchidectomy, estrogens, or anti-androgens.

The EORTC Urologic Group (5) has in the meantime accumulated data on several randomized studies with these drugs . With the exception of Medroxy progresteron acetate all drugs showed the same rates of time-to-progression or survival. Only MPA showed a statistically significant higher progression in M_1 prostatic cancer.

Also in a study, comparing orchidectomy with orchidectomy + CPA and with DES no difference in time-to-progression and survival was observed.

When we ask ourselves the question: which hormonal therapy is the best at this moment, the answer is not determined by the rate of response or progression nor by the survival time. The answer is determined by:
- amount and seriousness of side-effects
- expense of treatment (cost-effectiveness)
- psychological effect

We than see that DES is still the cheapest drug, but with a "price" of C.V.-side-effects.

Orchidectomy is the simplest method, but with the "price" of psychological after-effects.

Anti-androgens like CPA are good for C.V.-risk patients but expensive. Pure anti-androgens such as Flutamide or Anandron should only be given after orchidectomy or together with other androgen deprivating drugs.LHRH-agonists have the clear advantage of no serious side-effects, but the price is still considerable. There is however no psychological effect to be feared, because treatment is reversible, as can be shown by our study of testes examined after progression at 3 and 15 months. No difference in histology was observed and vital Leydig cells were still present. T-production was resumed when the drug was stopped at the time of progression

The answer is that probably only the quality of life at this moment determines which therapy will be preferred by patients when we inform them honestly and extensively.

The EORTC has started 2 phase III-studies to compare LHRH-agonists, daily intranasally or depot injections monthly, with and without anti-androgens against orchidectomy alone.

Simular studies are underway in the USA. Not before these studies are finalized and fully analysed, will we know exactly which choice is the best.

However returning to my statement at the beginning: there is no theoretical basis to expect a real difference as far as response, time-to-progression and survival are concerned. The quality of life might improve, but prostatic cancer and its treatment have not changed since Huggins' experiments.

REFERENCES

1. Coffey, D.S. (1984):The Role of tumor cell Heterogeneity in controling Prostate Cancer. In: Proceedings Lustrum N.V.v.Urol. ed. by H.J. de Voogt

2. Garnick, M.B. (1985): Leuprolide versus DES for previously untreated Stage D_2 Prostate Cancer. "Urology". Suppl. vol. 27:21-28.

3. Koutsilieris, M. and Tolis, G. (1985): Long term follow-up of Patients with Advanced Prostatic Carcinoma treated with either Buserelin (Hoe 766) or orchiectomy: Classification of variables associated with disease outcome. The Prostate, 7: 31-39.

4. Parmar, H., Lightman, S.L., Allen, L., Philips, R.H., Edwards, L., Schally, A.V. (1985): Randomised controlled study of orchidectomy V.S. long-acting D-TRP-6-LHRH microsapsules in advanced prostatic carcinoma. Lancet, 8466: 1201-1205.

5. Pavone Macaluso, M. de Voogt, H.J., Viggiano, G., Baratolo, E., Lardennois, B., de Paauw, M., Sylvester, R. and members of the EORTC Urological Group (1986): Comparison of DES, CPA and MPA in the treatment of advanced prostatic cancer. J.Urol. In press.

6. Schröder, F.H., Debruyne, F.J.M., de Voogt, H.J., Klijn, J.G., and de Jong, F.H.(1986): Metastatic Cancer of the Prostate managed by Buserelin in Acetate versus Buserelin Acetate

plus Cyproterone Acetate. J.Urol.135:4, pt 2, 392 (abstract).

7. Singer, J.H., Block, N.K. and Politano, V.A. (1985): A Comparison of metastatic prostate carcinoma treated with GNRH or orchiectomy. J.Urol. 133: 4, pt 2, 154 A (Abstract).

8. Smith, P.H., Pavone Macaluso, M., Viggiano, C, de Voogt, H.J., Lardennois, P., Robinson, M.R.G., Richards, B., Glashan, R.W., de Paauw, M., Sylvester, R. and tne EORTC Urological Group (1984). EORTC protocols in Prostatic Cancer.
In: Controlled clinical trials in Urologic Oncology, edited by L.Denis, G.P.Murphy, G.R.Pronk and F.Schröder, pp.107-117. Raven Press, New York.

9. Trachtenberg, J., Zadra, J. (1985): Is total androgen ablation superior to testicular androgen ablation in the treatment of metastatic prostatic cancer. J.Urol. 133: 4, pt 2, 374A (abstract).

10. Zadra, J, Bruce, A.W., Trachtenberg, J. (1986): Total androgen ablation therapy in the treatment of advanced prostatic cancer. J.Urol. 135: 4, pt 2, 388 (abstract).

Hormonal Manipulation of Cancer: Peptides, Growth Factors, and New (Anti) Steroidal Agents, edited by Jan G. M. Klijn et al. Raven Press, New York © 1987.

LH-RH AGONIST : BREAST AND PROSTATE CANCER

G. Mathé[1] MD, R. Keiling[2] MD, G. Prévot[3] MD,
ML Vo Van[1] MD, J. Gastiaburu[1] MD, JM Vannetzel[1] MD,
R. Despax[1] MD, C. Jasmin[1] MD, F. Lévi[1] MD,
M. Musset[1] MD, D. Machover[1] MD,
P. Ribaud[1] MD and JL Misset[1] MD.

[1] SMST & ICIG, Hôpital Paul-Brousse
12-16, avenue Paul-Vaillant Couturier
94804 Villejuif - France.

[2] Hôpital Civil, 1 place de l'Hôpital
67004 Strasbourg - France.

[3] Centre Hospitalier de Mulhouse, Boîte postale 1070
68051 Mulhouse Cédex - France.

Prostatic carcinoma, even in its usual disseminated form, has been shown by Huggins and Hodges to be sensitive to castration (1). Luteinizing-Hormone Releasing-Hormone (LH-RH), an hypothalamic polypeptide, controls the release of Luteinizing-Hormone (LH) from pituitary. Chronic administration of the synthetic LH-RH analog, D Trp6 LH-RH and other agonists were shown to cause desensitization of the pituitary receptors and inhibits LH release from pituitary (2). Testosterone secretion from testis is inhibited to castrate levels as well as women sex steroids concentrations. Thus, these analogs were showed to reduce gonadotropin secretion without involving administration of steroid hormones. D Trp6 LH-RH reduces gonadotropin and sex steroid plasma concentrations and also Prolactin secretion and prolactin receptor content (3). There is enough theoretical and clinical data to suggest a direct antitumoral effect at the level of peripheral cells although the mechanism of action is not fully explained (4). D Trp6 LH-RH was demonstrated to inhibit the growth of various hormone-dependent tumors in rats, including the Dunning R3327H prostate adenocarcinoma (5).

We started two oriented phase II trial of D Trp6 LH-RH (in lyophilised form) one in advanced prostatic carcinoma and the second in advanced breast carcinoma. Inclusion's criteria in the first study were the following : patients with biopsy proven prostatic adenocarcinoma and evaluable disease. Every patient had a close monitoring of LH and testosterone levels. Each of them were evaluable since they have completed 3 months of therapy. D Trp6 LH-RH was injected subcutaneously (s.c.) once a day at the dose of 500 mcg for the first seven days and then at the dose of 100 mcg for three months. The therapy was continued in responders.

We registered 90 patients in the trial. Five could not be evaluated as in three cases the follow-up was not satisfactory and in two cases, the protocol was the object of violation. Among the 85 evaluable patients, four died very early from the disease and 81 followed the protocol without violation during the three months required for the completion of this phase II study of short term efficacy and early tolerance. The average of age was 69 years, the youngest patient being 52 and the oldest 88. Eight subjects were at stage B, nine at stage C and 64 at stage D. 24 patients were previously untreated, 40 had previous hormonal therapy, 11 previous surgery and 6 previous radiotherapy. The patients were followed according to the clinical, radiologic and laboratory criteria of prostatic carcinoma and according to NPCP criteria.

RESULTS

Administration of D Trp6 LH-RH induced in the overall study a marked suppression of plasma LH and testosterone levels. The decrease in LH was significant after 30 days and testosterone levels were reduced to castrate level following 15 days of treatment. The suppression of LH and testosterone levels continued during the period of treatment. The first condition to show an improvement and relief symptoms was prostatism, especially urinary outflow, and obstruction. The intensity of prostatism was markedly reduced or disappeared in 36 out of 63 patients with prostatism before treatment. The decrease in pain, mainly in bones, was also rapid, starting during the second week of therapy. Significant improvement or disappearance of pain was observed on 39 out of 53 patients who had pain before treatment. The prostatic size evaluated by transabdominal ultrasonography was normalized in 9 out of 34 patients in which the echographic image was initially abnormal (Complete response rate = 26,4%) and was reduced by 50% or more in 6 patients (Partial response rate = 17,6%).

Thus the overall rate of complete and partial response was 44%. There were also 29,4% of regression smaller than 50% in volume but which still considerably improved the quality of patient's life.

The bone scan showed a marked improvement in 14,5% of the cases and an overall response rate including the regression smaller than 50% in 18,5% of patients. We also observed a complete regression of a lung metastasis. The evolution of prostatic size evaluated by rectal clinical examination and by the prostatic transabdominal ultrasonography showed a good correlation.

The prostatic acid phosphatase level decreased to normal in 50% of patients and reduced by more 50% of the initial value in 11% of patients, which makes a total of 61% but there was no significant correlation between prostate volume and phosphatase level regressions. According to NPCP criteria, we observed a complete and partial response rate of 44% on the overall patients, previously treated and untreated.

Impotence was the common side effect of the treatment, as it is in all other hormonal therapies of prostatic cancer. Hot flushes were observed.

We are conducting a second trial in prostatic cancer with the sustained release formulation of D Trp6 LH-RH, an intramuscular injection delivering a daily dose of 100 mcg during 28 days. The modality and schedule of administration was a daily s.c. injection of 500 mcg of D Trp6 LH-RH supplied in lyophilized form during seven days as a loading dose followed by an intramuscular injection of D Trp6 LH-RH supplied in sustained release formulation every 28 days. The evaluation was made at 3 months of therapy. The treatment was continued in responders. Inclusion's criteria were the same as the first trial. We included so far 39 patients. Three could not be evaluated as in one case the follow-up was not satisfactory and in two cases, the protocol was the object of violation. Among the 36 evaluable patients, 6 discontinued the therapy before three months for progression or early death.

The youngest patient was 58 years old and the oldest 83. Two patients were at stage B, two at stage C and 32 at stage D. Five subjects were previously untreated, 31 had previous chemotherapy and/or hormonal therapy and/or radiotherapy and/or surgery.

Administration of D Trp6 LH-RH induced a marked decrease of plasma LH and testosterone levels. Testosterone levels were induced to castrate level in all patients. We observed an improvement on 11 out of 16 patients who had bone pain, on 15 out of 24 patients who had urinary symptoms.

The prostatic size evaluated by transabdominal ultrasonography was normalized or reduced by 50% or more in 3 out of 12 patients who had initially an abnormal ultrasonography and was reduced by less than 50% in 5 out of the 12 patients.

The bone scan showed a marked improvement in 3 out of 18 patients at 3 months.

Prostatic acid phosphatase level regressed to normal in 2 out of 8 patients, reduced by more 50% of initial level in 2 patients and less to 50% of initial level in 2 patients.

No side effect that could be attributed to the treatment were observed except hot flushes which was an expected consequence of the hormonal treatment.

D Trp6 LH-RH induced objective response, early action on subjective symptoms, bone pain and urinary symptoms effective hormonal suppression is achieved without the side effects of oestrogens, and the sustained release formulation of D Trp6 LH-RH while more convenient than the lyophilised form requiring daily injections, seems to yield comparable response rates.

In the advanced breast carcinoma group the inclusion criteria were the following: patients with histologically proven advanced breast carcinoma regardless of the previous menopausal status of hormonal marker status or of previous therapy. As in the prostatic carcinoma group every patient had a dose monitoring of LH and estrogens levels. We tried when possible to get samples of neoplastic tissues for estrogens receptors determination.

23 patients (pts) with advanced breast carcinoma were treated with an LH-RH analogue   D Trp6 LH-RH (Debiopharm, Lausanne) with a starting dose of 500mcg s.c. for 7 days, followed by either daily s.c. injection of 100mcg (12 pts) or one monthly i.m. injection (11 pts) of its sustained release formulation. Eight pts had local therapy and 15 pts were previously treated with hormonal and/or chemical therapy. Age ranged from 35 to 85 years. Decrease levels of LH were efficiently obtained with both schedules. Eight pts were premenopausal (PM) and 15 postmenopausal (PMP). 5/8 PM pts were ER+, 3 of which were responders (2CR+1PR). ER were unknown in the remaining three pts, none of which responded; 3/15 PMP pts were also responders. 2 of these pts were ER+ (1CR+1PR).

We conclude that sustained release formulation (SRF) D Trp6 LH-RH is as efficient as the immediate formulation one (IF) to obtain LH decrease levels. SRF D Trp6 LH-RH was better tolerated locally. Both D Trp6 LH-RH showed antitumor activity in advanced breast cancer heavily pre treated. These data suggest that D Trp6 LH-RH is preferentially active in ER+ pts, and also that it may have a direct antitumoral action, independant of that of the hypothalamic-hypophysial gonadal axis.

REFERENCES

1. Belchetz, P.E., Plant, T.M., Nakai, Y., Keogh, E.J., Knobil, E. (1978): Science 202:631-3.

2. Cundarm, K., Cao, Y.Q., Wang, N.G., Bardin, C.W., Rivier, J., Vale, W. (1981): Life Sci 154:83-88.

3. Eidne, A.E., et al (1985): Science 229:989-981.

4. Hierowski, M.T., Altamirano, P., Redding, T.W., Schally, A.V. (1983): 154:92-96.

5. Huggins, C., Hodges, C.V. (1941): Cancer Res 1:293.

Hormonal Manipulation of Cancer: Peptides, Growth Factors, and New (Anti) Steroidal Agents, edited by Jan G. M. Klijn et al. Raven Press, New York © 1987.

LHRH AGONIST TREATMENT OF BREAST CANCER:

A PHASE II STUDY IN THE U.S.A.

Harold A. Harvey, Allan Lipton, *Devorah T. Max

Department of Medicine, The Milton S. Hershey Medical Center, The Pennsylvania State University, P.O. Box 850, Hershey, PA   17033; *Abbott Laboratories, Chicago, IL   60064

INTRODUCTION

The pioneering work of Schally et al. and Guilemin and co-workers in elucidating the physiology and synthesis of gonadotrophin releasing hormone (GnRH, LHRH) led in the early 1970's to the development of several analogs of the human hormone (12). These various analogs were soon shown to exhibit potent agonist properties of the native GnRH and were introduced into clinical trials ranging from contraception to cancer (1). Clinical experience with these analogs revealed that chronic parenteral injection of the peptides in animals or patients led, paradoxically, to inhibition of the production of LH & FSH. This mechanism of action has now been clearly defined and has become the basis of most therapeutic applications of these compounds (11). The observation that chronic administration of potent LHRH agonists to rodents bearing chemically induced hormone dependent mammary carcinoma caused tumor regression, provided a basis for initiating clinical studies in women with metastatic breast cancer (2,4,8). Our initial studies demonstrated the safety and feasibility of administering leuprolide (D-Leu^6-Pro^{9}LHRH ethylamide (NEt) on a daily basis to women with advanced advanced metastatic breast cancer (3). The studies of Klijn et al. using another LHRH analog (buserelin) also demonstrated the validity and therapeutic benefit of this approach (5). This paper reports the results of a Phase II trial of leuprolide in premenopausal women with metastatic breast cancer.

MATERIALS AND METHODS

This multi-center trial was begun in May 1979 and enrolled 26 premenopausal patients with metastatic breast cancer. One patient was declared to be ineligible after receiving one dose of leuprolide when it was discovered that she had pre-existing thrombocytopenia. All patients entered the study with locally advanced or progressive metastatic breast cancer with measurable disease and all had given informed consent. Patients were treated with leuprolide initially at a dose of 1 mg. s.c. daily. However, each investigator had the option of increasing the dose to 5 or 10 mg daily at any time during the study based on the patient's clinical condition: Treatment was continued until there was evidence of progressive disease. Criteria of response to therapy were as follows: Objective remission was classified as a decrease of 50% or greater in the sum of the products of the two largest perpendicular diameters in all measurable lesions, partial recalcification of osteolytic lesions for at least 3 months, or both. Stabilization of osteoblastic lesions with regression of other lesions was also considered an objective response. Stable disease was defined as a decrease of less than 50% or an increase of less than 25% in metastatic lesions with marked symptomatic improvement for at least 3 months. Progression required an increase of 25% or greater over original measurement or appearance of new metastatic lesions.

TABLE 1. Characteristics of 25 Premenopausal Women Treated with Leuprolide

Median Age:	43 years (range 23 to-52 years)
ECOG Performance Status:	0-3 (capable of at least limited self-care)
Race:	12 Caucasians, 12 Mestizas (all living in Mexico) and 1 Black
Estrogen Receptors (ER):	14 ER(+), 10 ER(-), 1 ER unknown
Sites of Metastasis:	Soft tissue in 12, bone in 3, viscera in 3 and two or more sites in 7
Prior Treatment:	None in 23, tamoxifen in 2

Serial hormonal assays performed in all patients included radioimmunoassay of LH, FSH, prolactin, estrone, estrone sulfate, estradiol, androstenedione and cortisol in serum. A central reference laboratory performed the hormonal assays using standard techniques. Estrogen receptor assays were performed at the laboratory of choice of the individual investigator. Menstrual histories were carefully recorded. Monitoring for toxicity included history and physical examination, hematologic and biochemical surveys, urinalysis and periodic slit lamp eye

examinations. The characteristics of patients entered on study
are summarized in Table I. Of particular note is the fact that
14 of the 25 evaluable patients had ER positive (>10 fmmol/mg.
cytosol protein) tumors and 10 had ER negative tumors.

RESULTS

Of the 25 evaluable patients, (11 (44% - 95% confident
confidence intervals 22-65) experienced a partial response. The
median duration of benefit in this group was 39 weeks (mean, 49
weeks: range, 12 to 141 weeks). Five patients (20%) had a
stabilization of disease with a median duration of benefit of 19
weeks (mean, 33 weeks; range, 16 to 93 weeks). Thus, the overall
response rate with leuprolide - CR + PR + stable - was 64%. Nine
patients (36%) had progression of the disease. Six of these
patients had rapid disease progression within two to nine weeks
of initiating leuprolide treatment. Twenty patients had an
increase in dosage of leuprolide during the study from 1 to 5 or
1 to 10 mg daily. In only two of these patients did an increased
dosage lead to an improvement in objective response.

Table 2 shows the response rate for different individual sites
of involvement in the 25 evaluable patients. Responses were
primarily seen in soft-tissue and bony sites of involvement.

TABLE 2. Response by Individual Site of Involvement.

	Response			
Type of Tissue Involved	PR	Stable	Progression	Total
Soft-Tissue only	7	3	2	12
Visceral only	0	1	2	3
Bone only	3	0	0	3
Multiple sites of involvement	1	1	5	7
Total	11	5	9	25

Hormonal Effects

Of the 25 evaluable patients, 11 had no menstrual cycles while
receiving leuprolide and nine patients had only one menstrual
cycle. The remaining five patients had two menstrual cycles
within the first ten weeks of treatment. All of the 19 patients
who received leuprolide for more than ten weeks had cessation of
their menses by week 11, and ammenorrhea persisted as long as
they remained on therapy.

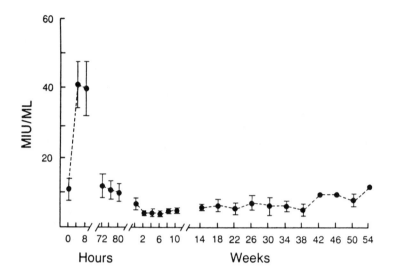

FIG. 1.   Serum FSH levels in premenopausal patients with
metastatic breast cancer treated chronically with
leuprolide.   Numbers in parenthesis indicate sample
size.   Mean value ±SEM is shown.

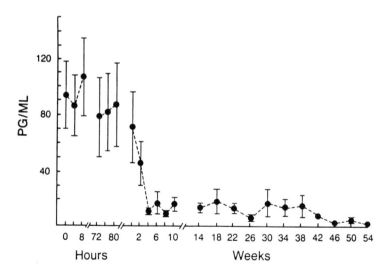

FIG. 2.   Serum estradiol levels during chronic treatment with
leuprolide.

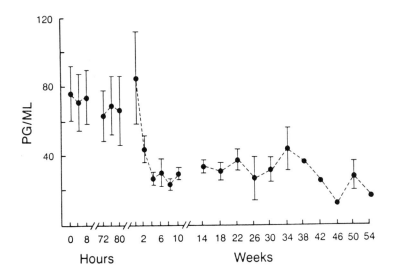

FIG. 3.   Serum estrone levels during chronic treatment with leuprolide.'

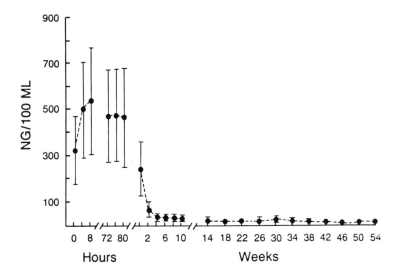

FIG. 4.   Serum progesterone levels during chronic treatment with leuprolide.

Hormonal measurements in the entire patient population revealed that after an initial rise,both FSH (Figure 1) and LH levels became suppressed after 1 week of therapy and remained so throughout the treatment period.   Serum estradiol (Figure 2) was suppressed into the postmenopausal range after 4 weeks of therapy and remained so for as long as leuprolide was administered. Similarly, serum estrone (Figure 3) and estrone sulfate were profoundly suppressed during treatment with this LHRH analog. Progesterone levels were likewise suppressed, (Figure 4) whereas no consistent changes were observed in the serum levels of androstendione, prolactin, or cortisol.

Toxicity

Toxicity in this group of patients was generally mild or nonexistent.   There were no changes in hematologic or biochemical parameters that could be attributed to leuprolide.   The reported side effects are summarized in Table 3.   Two patients experienced an initial increase in bone pain which could be attributed to a flare phenomenon resulting from the transient early increase in serum FSH produced by leuprolide.

TABLE 3.   Side Effects from Leuprolide

	Mild	Severity Moderate	Severe
Hot flushes	2	3	
Nausea/Vomiting	3	1	1
Headache	1	3	
Dizziness	2	1	
Taste in mouth	1	1	
Increased bone pain	0	1	1
Diarrhea	1	1	
Local reaction	1	1	
Nervous/Irritable	0	1	
Hives	0	1	
Vaginal bleeding	1	0	
Polyuria and Polydipsia	0	0	1

Clinical outcome was also assessed with regard to the estrogen-receptor result.   Objective responses were noted in both estrogen-receptor-positive (6/11) and estrogen-receptor-negative patients (4/10).

DISCUSSION

The overall objective response rate of 44% observed in this

trial is remarkably similar to the response rates reported by Klijn, et. al. and Walker, et. al. using different LHRH analogs in a similar group of premenopausal women with metastatic breast cancer (6,13). The hormonal changes noted, clearly indicate that leuprolide in this group of patients produces an effective chemical castration. These findings are different from those observed when premenopausal women are treated with tamoxifen (7). The clinical responses seen in 4 of 10 ER negative tumors, raises the interesting possibility that the LHRH analog might be acting through some mechanism independent of ovarian suppression of estrogen production. More likely however, these receptors may represent false negative values since in this study it was not possible to standardize assays and also specimens were frequently shipped via long distances prior to assay for receptor. Our previous trial of leuprolide in a total of 42 postmenopausal women with metastatic breast cancer produced a less than 10% objective response rate suggesting the absence of any significant extra gonadal mechanism of action of the analog in breast cancer therapy (3). Nevertheless, several recent reports make a case for a direct anti-tumor effect of LHRH analogs in humans and this possible mechanism of action needs to be pursued in further clinical trials (10).

Chronic parenteral administration of leuprolide is able to induce a medical castration in premenopausal patients with breast cancer as assessed by hormonal measurements and the cessation of menses. In addition, this compound has an antitumor effect which is comparable to that observed with surgical ovariectomy.

This and other pilot trials with the LHRH super agonist analogs in women with breast cancer provide a basis for future investigations. Controlled trials of LHRH agonists vs. surgical oophorectomy are initially required. Later, these compounds could be studied as adjuvant endocrine treatment or as components of regimens of hormonal synchronization and chemotherapy. A final potential clinical use of LHRH analogs in the treatment of breast cancer may be in association with antiestrogen therapy. The rationale for this combined approach would be to obtain a complete blockade of estrogen action. The administration of antiestrogens could, in fact, potentiate the antitumor effect of these compounds by blocking the action of the residual postmenopausal levels of estrogens observed during chronic therapy with LHRH analogs. Furthermore, co-administration of antiestrogens may prevent the flare phenomenon observed in some patients and may shorten the time required for tumor regression to occur, since it takes several weeks for the LHRH analogs to

suppress ovarian steroidogenesis. Such a treatment
strategy is currently being applied with encouraging preliminary
results in the management of advanced prostate cancer where
therapy with LHRH analogs is combined with antiandrogens (9).

Finally, the imminent availabilty of long acting preparations
of LHRH agonists will greatly facilitate the planned clinical
studies and enhance patient acceptability of treatment with this
exciting new class of compounds.

ACKNOWLEDGEMENTS

The authors wish to acknowledge the participation of several
physicians in the conduct of this study: P. Band, R. Diaz-
Perches, A. Glass, J. De La Garza, L. Glode, H. Lerner, Y. Van
Loon, D. Plotkin, A. Segaloff, G. Tollis, C. Vogel. The authors
also wish to acknowledge the assistance Mrs. Judith Weigel in
preparation of this manuscript. Leuprolide was kindly provided
by TAP Pharmaceuticals, N. Chicago, Illinois.

REFERENCES

1. Corbin, A., (1981): Yale J. Biol. Med., 55:27.

2. DeSombre, E.R., Johnson, E.S., White, W.F., (1976): Cancer
    Res., 36:3830-3833.

3. Harvey, H.A., Lipton, A., Santen, R.J., et al, (1981): Proc.
    Am. Soc. Clin. Oncol., 22:444.

4. Johnson, E.S., Seely, J.H., White, W.F., et al, (1976):
    Science, 194:329-330.

5. Klijn, J.G.M., de Jong, F.H., (1982): Lancet, 2:1213-1216.

6. Klijn, J.G.M., de Jong, F.H., Blankenstein, M.A., et al,
    (1984): Breast Cancer Res. Treat., 4:209-220.

7. Manni, A., Pearson, O.H., (1980): Cancer Treat. Rep.,
    64:779.

8. Nicholson, R.I., Finney, E.J., Maynard, P.V., (1976): J.
    Endocrinol., 79:51-52.

9. Labrie, F., Dupont, A., Belanger, A., and Members of the
    Laval University Prostate Cancer Program, (1984):
    Proceedings of the seventh International Congress of
    Endocrinology, 98.

10. Miller, W.R., Scott, W.N., Morris, R., Fraser, H.M., Sharpe, R.M., (1985): Nature, 313:231-233.

11. Rabin, D., McNeil, L.W., (1980): J. Clin. Endocrinol. Metab., 51:873-876.

12. Schally, A.V., Arimura, A., Kastin, A.J., Matsuo, H., Baba, Y., Redding, T.W., Nair, R.M.G., Debeljuk, L., White, W.F., (1971): Science, 173:1036.

13. Walker, K.J., Nicholson, R.I., Turkes, A., et al, (1984): J. Steroid Biochem., 20:1409.

Hormonal Manipulation of Cancer: Peptides, Growth Factors, and New (Anti) Steroidal Agents, edited by Jan G. M. Klijn et al. Raven Press, New York © 1987.

THE BRITISH EXPERIENCE WITH THE LH-RH AGONIST ZOLADEX

(ICI 118630) IN THE TREATMENT OF BREAST CANCER

R.I. Nicholson, K.J. Walker, A. Turkes, J. Dyas, K.E. Gotting, P.N. Plowman*, M. Williams[†], C.W. Elston[††] and R.W. Blamey[†]

Tenovus Institute for Cancer Research, University of Wales College of Medicine, Heath Park, Cardiff

*Department of Radiology, St. Bartholomew's Hospital, London

[†]Department of Surgery, City Hospital, Nottingham

[††]Department of Pathology, City Hospital, Nottingham

INTRODUCTION

The first report of the biological characteristics of Zoladex (ICI 118630, D-Ser(Bu^t)^6 Azgly^{10} -luteinizing hormone-releasing hormone (LH-RH)) was published in 1978 when Dutta and his colleagues (4) showed that the drug, in addition to inducing ovulation in androgen-sterilised constant-oestrus rats after intravenous injection of doses as low as 5ng/rat, also inhibited human chorionic gonadotrophin-stimulated uterine growth when given at higher doses (0.5-5µg/rat/day). These observations were quickly followed by a series of publications reinforcing the antifertility effects of high concentrations of Zoladex in male and female rats and demonstrating its ability to reduce circulating levels of gonadal steroids and cause atrophy of the accessory sex organs (6,12,18). Indeed, when administered at pharmacological dose levels Zoladex blocked follicular maturation, inhibited ovarian aromatase activity, reduced plasma oestradiol and decreased the size of oestrogen target tissues (24), including oestrogen receptor positive dimethylbenzanthracene (DMBA)-induced mammary tumours (15,18), in female rats and decreased circulating levels of testosterone and caused atrophy of the testes, prostate and seminal vesicles in male rats (6). Many of these effects were recognised as being similar to those induced by castration and form the basis for the use of Zoladex in cancer therapy (17).

Endocrinological and clinical actions of Zoladex in premenopausal women. The studies were carried out in the Breast Cancer Surgical Unit (Head, RWB) at the City Hospital in

Nottingham with endocrinological assays being performed at the Tenovus Institute. Patients with histologically diagnosed breast cancer were entered into the study if they were menstruating regularly and if their initial plasma FSH concentration fell below 50 IU/L. In all instances Zoladex was given as the first-line systemic therapy. Two modes of administration of the LH-RH agonist were examined: daily subcutaneous injections of the drug (0.5 or 1mg/day) in citrate buffer and a sustained-release formulation of Zoladex (3.6mg/28 days, see ref. 25). Since the latter formulation of Zoladex possesses the advantages of ease of administration and assured patient compliance and since the effects of the daily injections have been described in detail elsewhere (16,19,20), only the endocrine results obtained using the sustained-release formulation will be presented in detail in this communication. The clinical data, however, is drawn from both formulations of the drug.

Figure 1 shows the effects of Zoladex on circulating concentrations of LH and FSH in 24 patients who started therapy during the follicular phase of the menstrual cycle (days 1 to 10). Within 1 day of the subcutaneous implantation of the sustained-release formulation of the LH-RH agonist, substantial increases in the circulating concentrations of the gonadotrophins were recorded. The levels of LH and FSH, however, decreased on continued administration (7-14 days) and remained low during the 28 day duration of the first depot. Administration of subsequent depots evoked no measurable release of the pituitary gonadotrophins and their levels remained low at 6 months (n=11) and 1 year (n=5). One patient has remained on the sustained-release formulation of Zoladex for 2 years and still shows suppressed gonadotrophin levels (not illustrated). Although small rises in circulating concentrations of progesterone and oestradiol were often associated with the early increased serum levels of LH and FSH, they remained within the normal premenopausal range (19,20). On continued treatment the group mean levels of progesterone and oestradiol fell and reached the castrate or postmenopausal range by 14 and 21 days respectively. These values were maintained at 6 and 12 months. Oophorectomy performed immediately after Zoladex therapy did not produce any further fall in circulating levels of progesterone or oestradiol. Some individual variability of response to Zoladex was observed for oestradiol and 3 patients exhibited recurrent, although suppressed, peaks of this steroid throughout a maximum of 6 months active therapy (25). Interestingly, one of these patients showed objective signs of response (sclerosis in lytic bone metastases) during the first three months of therapy despite recurrent oestradiol peaks. This remission was not maintained for six months and no response was subsequently found to oophorectomy. Measurement of serum concentrations of Zoladex in these partially refractory patients showed the presence of the drug both during the first and second months of treatment (25). Comparison of these data with patients showing a greater suppression of oestradiol production did not reveal any striking

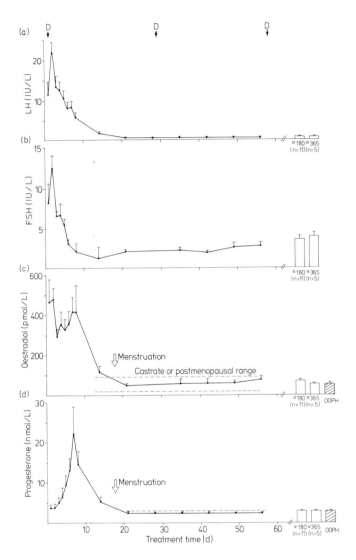

FIG. 1. <u>Influence of the sustained-release formulation of Zoladex on serum hormone levels in 24 premenopausal women with advanced breast cancer.</u> Treatment was initiated during the follicular phase of the menstrual cycle. Blood samples were withdrawn on the days indicated. The results are represented as mean values ± s.e.m. The time of administration of the depots is recorded by the letter D. Oophorectomy after Zoladex therapy was performed in a subgroup of patients (n=6). The circulating concentrations of oestradiol and progesterone in these women (two weeks after the operation) are shown in the hatched area.

difference   in   circulating   concentrations   of   Zoladex.   The
endocrine data presented for the sustained-release formulation of
Zoladex   are   largely   similar   to   those   obtained   with   daily
injections of the drug (cf refs 19,20).

The   side effects relating to treatment with the LH-RH agonist
were   minimal   and   included   cessation   of   menstruation   in
association with suppressed oestradiol, hot flushes (20 patients)
and   occasional   nausea.   All suppressed patients had ceased to
have   normal   menstrual periods by two months after initiation of
therapy,   although   7   patients   experienced   spotting   after   the
second month of Zoladex.   No tumour flare was recorded.

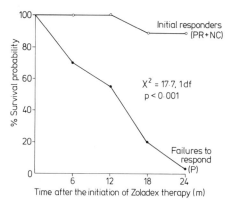

FIG.   2.   <u>Survival of patients after Zoladex therapy</u>.
The survival of patients after the initiation of Zoladex
was   recorded   and analysed by Life Table Analysis.   The
data   is   divided   according   to   the   initial   patient
response to Zoladex.

To   date   45   premenopausal   patients   have been evaluated for
their   clinical   response   to   Zoladex and are reported in detail
elsewhere   (28).   Briefly, tumour remissions lasting a minimum of
6   months   and   externally assessed on the basis of UICC criteria
(9)   have been observed in 14 patients (31%).   Three women showed
no evidence of disease progression (static disease) over 6 months
of   therapy   and   in   28   patients   disease   progressed   despite
treatment.   Responding   patients   were   characterised as having
longer disease-free intervals than those women who failed Zoladex
therapy   (26.7   ±   12.5 and 14.5 ± 12.6 months respectively) and
contained   a   lower   proportion   of poorly differentiated cancers
(22%   and   65% respectively; tumours were graded on the Bloom and
Richardson   scale   (2)   by   C.W.E.).   Comparison of the survival
curves   for   these patients shows a significant advantage for the
patients   who   responded to Zoladex therapy versus those women in
which   the   disease   progressed   (Fig.   2).   Ten   out of the 14
patients   showing   a response presented with bone metastases with
additional   intra-abdominal   involvement   in two of the cases.   A
further   patient   responding   to   Zoladex   received   treatment   for

inoperable locally recurrent axillary nodes and three responding patients presented with stage III disease. The oestrogen receptor (ER) status of the tumour, as determined by a [³H]-oestradiol ligand binding assay (14), was available in 38/45 assessible patients. Responses to Zoladex were observed in 11/20 (55%) patients with ER positive disease, 0/18 in women with ER negative disease and 3/7 (40%) in patients of unknown receptor status. These data parallel the results obtained in a series of breast cancer patients who underwent surgical oophorectomy in the same clinic, where 8/19 patients with ER positive breast cancer and 0/13 patients with ER negative disease showed a worthwhile remission. Application of an ER-immunocytochemical assay (10) to frozen sections of a small number (n=10) of the ER positive tumours revealed considerable heterogeneity of receptor expression within the tumour cell population (Nicholson, manuscript in preparation). Tumours from patients responding to Zoladex therapy, however, contained a higher proportion of strongly oestrogen receptor positive cells than did tumours from women who failed Zoladex therapy. It is noteworthy, however, that all of the oestrogen receptor positive tumours examined contained cells which did not express detectable concentrations of oestrogen receptor proteins.

Oophorectomy after disease progression was performed on 24/45 patients. Of 22 women who failed to respond to Zoladex 18 subsequently failed to respond to oophorectomy. Thirteen (72%) had ER negative disease. The 4 patients in this group who benefitted from the surgical procedure all possessed ER positive tumours and consisted of one woman whose serum oestradiol had not been fully suppressed to castrate levels after 6 months of treatment with the LH-RH agonist and 3 patients who progressed from Zoladex therapy to oophorectomy after short and possibly insufficient treatment periods of 2, 2 and 3 months. No response to oophorectomy was observed in two women who had previously responded to Zoladex. The endocrine actions of Zoladex were similar in responding and non-responding patients (Fig. 3).

The data are largely consistent with Zoladex and oophorectomy acting on the same subgroup of patients, that is those with ER positive hormone sensitive disease and do not provide any major evidence for differing modes of antitumour activity between the two treatments. Moreover, the relative quiescent state within the gonads of long-term LH-RH agonist treated patients most likely relates to the ability of these compounds to down-regulate pituitary LH-RH receptors and hence desensitise the pituitary gland to the releasing properties of the drugs. This process eventually results in a fall in circulating levels of LH and FSH and a withdrawal of their support for gonadal steroidogenic activity. The data does not produce any evidence for an early deleterious effect of the drug on tumour growth.

Menopausal status and response to oophorectomy. The functional activity of the ovaries has an obvious and profound influence on the clinical response of breast cancer patients to oophorectomy. Several studies have now reported that the

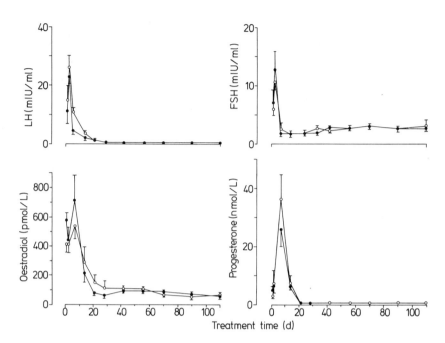

FIG. 3.   Endocrine   effects   of Zoladex: Influence of
response to therapy.   Mean hormone levels in initial
responders   to   Zoladex   (O—O); Levels in failures to
respond (●—●).

likelihood of a patient obtaining a worthwhile improvement in
their disease after oophorectomy decreases progressively with
increasing time from cessation of menstruation. Very little
benefit may be expected beyond the 5 year mark. These clinical
observations correlate with the transition of the perimenopausal
ovary towards its relatively quiescent state in the
postmenopausal woman. This environment of low gonadal steroid
output may, however, increase the importance of other tumour
growth regulatory pathways and allow the expression of
alternative mechanisms by which tumour remissions may be achieved
by LH-RH agonists.

Endocrinological   and   clinical   actions   of   Zoladex   in
postmenopausal women.   The studies were carried out in the
Department of Radiology (PNP), St. Bartholomew's Hospital, London
with endocrinological assays being performed in the Tenovus
Institute. Patients with asymptomatic breast cancer were entered
into the study if they had ceased to menstruate (>2 years
previously). Two formulations of Zoladex (250μg/day, n=6 and
3.6mg/28 days, n=4) were given as first-line systemic therapy.

Administration of daily subcutaneous injections of Zoladex
resulted in an initial rise in the already high circulating
concentrations of LH and FSH (Table 1). On continued therapy
(7-14 days), however, both formulations of the drug caused

Table 1. Effect of Zoladex on plasma hormone levels in
postmenopausal women

Daily injections (n=6 ± SD)

	LH(IU/L)	FSH(IU/L)	Oestradiol (pmol/L)	Progesterone (nmol/L)
Day 0	17.1 ± 15.3	25.9 ± 22.3	36.0 ± 7.9	0.68 ± 0.30
Day 1	42 ± 15.6	63.9 ± 19.0	34.5 ± 9.4	0.70 ± 0.30
Day 7	6.5 ± 5.3	12.1 ± 10.6	26.6 ± 10.8	0.44 ± 0.26
Day 21	2.9 ± 1.6	10.4 ± 5.9	31.0 ± 6.1	0.53 ± 0.30
Day 28	3.7 ± 3.0	9.2 ± 5.7	31.8 ± 11.3	0.55 ± 0.30

Sustained-release formulation (n=4 ± SD)

	LH(IU/L)	FSH(IU/L)	Oestradiol (pmol/L)	Progesterone (nmol/L)
Day 0	19.0 ± 7.5	28.6 ± 7.3	50 ± 8.0	< 2
Day 7	17.9 ± 4.0	13.3 ± 1.3	53 ± 1.5	< 2
Day 21	0.7 ± 0.2	4.6 ± 6.4	45 ± 16.6	< 2
Day 28	1.1 ± 1.0	2.8 ± 3.1	107 ± 100.0	< 2

pituitary gland desensitisation and lowered basal levels of the
gonadotrophins.   No alterations were observed in the already low
levels of oestradiol or progesterone.   Similarly, no marked
response to Zoladex was seen at 1 month in the serum
concentrations of oestrone, androstenedione, testosterone,
dehydroepiandrosterone sulphate, cortisol, prolactin and growth
hormone (not illustrated).

     To date 9 patients with asymptomatic breast cancer have been
assessed for their response to Zoladex and are reported elsewhere
(21).   Responses to the LH-RH agonist have been recorded in a 58
year old woman with bone metastases (ER positive primary tumour)
and in a 54 year old woman with pulmonary metastases (ER status
unknown).   An early pituitary gland desensitisation was achieved
in both responding patients. Disease progression or no response
to Zoladex therapy was recorded in the remaining women of which
two subsequently responded to tamoxifen (20mg bd).

     The above data are in agreement with other studies
demonstrating tumour remissions in postmenopausal women with
breast cancer following LH-RH agonist therapy (8,22) and infer
extragonadal actions of this class of compounds. The results
were obtained in women administered Zoladex as a first-line
systemic therapy.   Application of LH-RH agonist treatment to
postmenopausal women following either endocrine or cytotoxic
measures appears to reduce the effectiveness of the treatment
(27).   Unfortunately, to date we have been unable to detect any
changes in plasma hormone concentrations that are likely to
account for the tumour remissions. Indeed, in our studies only

gonadotrophin concentrations were suppressed by Zoladex treatment. Since several reports have failed to correlate plasma gonadotrophin levels with the development of breast cancer (1), response to various endocrine therapies (7,11,23) and rates of relapse of patients with early breast cancer (26) it seems unlikely that the decreases in LH and FSH observed in our study are relevant to the tumour remissions. Moreover, Bates et al (1) have reported a clinical remission in a postmenopausal woman with breast cancer following an incomplete ablation of the pituitary gland in which the plasma gonadotrophin concentrations were only reduced by half and pituitary gland responsiveness to injected LH-RH was evident. Similarly, in virgin female Sprague-Dawley rats Zoladex causes regression of hormone dependent DMBA-induced mammary tumours in the absence of a complete suppression of pituitary gland responsiveness to the drug (18). The data, therefore, imply an action of Zoladex on tumour growth in addition to those normally identified by routine hormone measurements. Thus, while it is possible that a more dynamic sampling procedure might unravel the complexities of LH-RH action on the hormonal environment of tumours, it is also feasible that these drugs may influence the release of other pituitary factors that potentiate the mitogenic actions of oestrogens (3) or have inherent antitumour activity themselves. Certainly, the recent identification of LH-RH binding sites on human breast tumours (5) and the reported inhibitory effects of the LH-RH agonist buserelin on MCF-7 human breast cancer cells grown in culture (13), add weight to the latter proposal. Conversely, studies designed to detect direct inhibitory actions of Zoladex in oestrogen-sensitive tissues and carcinogen-induced mammary tumours of the rat have proved negative (6, 17). Indeed, implantation of the sustained-release formulation of Zoladex directly into this tumour type has produced no evidence for either localised inhibitory actions of LH-RH agonists on tumour morphology (not illustrated) or additional benefit in terms of rate of tumour remission (Fig. 4). Similarly, Zoladex appears unable to prevent the oestradiol supported growth of uteri and MCF-7 human breast cancer cell xenografts in ovariectomised nude mice (Fig. 5).

Conclusions and future prospects

Clearly, LH-RH agonists represent a fascinating addition to the spectrum of drugs used to treat breast cancer. They appear to be active in patients with hormone-sensitive oestrogen receptor positive disease and although in the immediate future it is likely that their main clinical value will centre around their ability to elicit a chemical castration-like response within the ovaries of premenopausal women, their actions in postmenopausal women are of considerable clinical and biological interest. Projecting further ahead, it is noteworthy that studies in animals have shown that LH-RH agonists are effective in the adjuvant setting (6) and in preventing the initiation (17) and

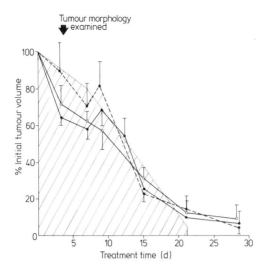

FIG. 4. Influence of intra-tumour administration of Zoladex on the rate of regression of DMBA-induced mammary tumours. Depots (1mg) of the sustained-release formulation of Zoladex were directly implanted into established tumours and the rate of tumour regression, (●—●; n=12) compared with that produced by depots subcutaneously implanted diametrically opposite to the tumours under study O—O; n=14). Also shown are the tumour regressions produced when depots were implanted in another tumour in the same animal (●--●, n=6) and after twice daily injections of 5μg of the drug (▨▨, ref. 18). Results are expressed as mean ± S.D.

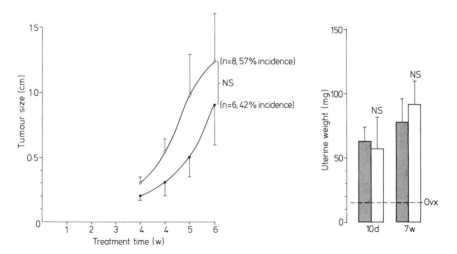

FIG. 5. Effect of Zoladex on the growth of MCF-7 human breast cancer cell xenografts and uterine weights in

ovariectomised nude mice. Mature ovariectomised Balbc nude mice bearing subcutaneously implanted MCF-7 breast cancer cells (3.4×10^6) were administered 5mg depots of oestradiol (steroid released over a 6 month period) in the presence (O—O) or absence (●—●) of 0.5mg depots of the sustained-release formulation of Zoladex (replaced after 21 days). Animals were palpated weekly and tumour growth recorded as changes in the mean diameter ± SD. After 7 weeks the animals were killed, their uteri removed and weighed. The results were compared with those obtained in animals treated for 0 or 10 days. Oestradiol alone,▨; oestradiol plus Zoladex, ☐ .

promotion (6) of carcinogen-induced mammary tumours. This information, taken together with their impending use both in the treatment of benign diseases of the breast and as contraceptive agents, points to LH-RH agonists playing a central and expanding role in the control of the development and growth of breast cancer.

ACKNOWLEDGEMENTS

The authors are grateful to the Tenovus Organisation and to ICI Pharmaceuticals Division for generous financial support, and to Dr. B.J.A. Furr and Dr. A. Todd for the provision of Zoladex.

REFERENCES

1. Bates, T., Ruben, R.D., Bulbrook, R.D. et al (1976): Europ. J. Cancer, 12: 775-782.
2. Bloom, H.J.G. and Richardson, W.W. (1957): Brit. J. Cancer, 11: 359-377.
3. Dembinski, T.C., Leung, C.K.H. and Shiu, R.P.C. (1985): Cancer Res. 45: 3083-3089.
4. Dutta, A.S., Furr, B.J.A., Giles, M.B., Valcaccia, B. and Walpole, A.L. (1978): Biochem. Biophys. Res. Comm. 81: 832-390.
5. Eidne, K.A., Flanagan, C.A. and Millar, R.P. (1985): Science, 229: 989-991
6. Furr, B.J.A. and Nicholson, R.I. (1982): J. Reprod. Fert., 64: 529-539
7. Golder, M.P., Phillips, M.E.A., Fahmy, D.R. et al (1976): Europ. J. Cancer, 12, 719-723.
8. Harvey, H.A., Lipton, A., Santen, R.J. et al (1981): Proc. Am. Assoc. Cancer Res./Am. Soc. Clin. Oncol. 22, p444
9. Hayward, J.L., Carbone, P.P., Heuson, J.C., et al. (1977): Cancer, 39: 1289-1293.
10. King, W.J. and Greene, G.L. (1984): Nature, 307: 745-747
11. Manni, A., Trujillo, J.E., Marshall, J.S., Brodkey, J. and Pearson, O.H. (1979): Cancer, 43: 444-450.
12. Maynard, P.V. and Nicholson, R.I. (1979): Brit. J. Cancer, 39: 274-279

13. Miller, W.R., Scott, W.N., Morris, R., Fraser, H.M. and
    Sharpe, R.M. (1985): Nature, 313 (5999): 213-233
14. Nicholson, R.I., Campbell, F.C., Blamey, R.W., Elston, C.W.,
    George, D. and Griffiths, K. (1981): J. Steroid Biochem.
    15: 193-199
15. Nicholson, R.I. and Maynard, P.V. (1979): Brit. J. Cancer,
    39: 268-273
16. Nicholson, R.I. and Walker, K.J. (1985): Chemioterapia, 4:
    249-251
17. Nicholson, R.I., Walker, K.J., Harper, M., Phillips, A.D.
    and Furr, B.J.A. (1983): In: Reviews on Endocrine-Related
    Cancer, edited by R.I. Nicholson and K. Griffiths, Suppl.
    13. pp 55-62. ICI Publications, U.K.
18. Nicholson, R.I., Walker, K.J. and Maynard, P.V. (1980):
    In: Breast Cancer, experimental and clinical aspects,
    edited by H.T. Mouridsen and T. Palshof, pp 295-297.
    Pergamon Press, Oxford.
19. Nicholson, R.I., Walker, K.J., Turkes, A., Dyas, J., Plowman,
    P.N., Williams, M. and Blamey, R.W. (1985): J. Steroid
    Biochem., 23: 843-847.
20. Nicholson, R.I., Walker, K.J., Turkes, A., Turkes, A.O.,
    Dyas, J., Blamey, R.W., Campbell, F.C., Robinson, M.R.C.
    and K. Griffiths (1984): J. Steroid. Biochem. 20: 129-135.
21. Plowman, P.N., Walker, K.J. and Nicholson, R.I. (In Press).
    Europ. J. Cancer and Clin. Oncol. Abst. III-18.
22. Schally, A.V., Redding, T.W. and Comaru-Schally, A.M. (1984):
    Cancer Treat. Rep. 68: No1.
23. Tanaka, M., Abe, K., Ohnami, S. et al. (1978): Jap. J. Clin.
    Oncol. 8: 141-145.
24. Walker, K.J. (1983). PhD Thesis, University of Wales.
25. Walker, K.J., Turkes, A., Williams, M., Blamey, R.W.
    Nicholson, R.I. (In Press). J. Endocrinol.
26. Wang, D.Y., Goodwin, P.R., Bulbrook, R.D. and Hayward, J.L.
    (1976). Europ. J. Cancer, 12: 305-311.
27. Waxman, J.H., Harland, S.J., Coombes, R.C. et al. (1985):
    Cancer Chemother. Pharmacol. 15: 171-173.
28. Williams, M., Walker, K.J., Turkes, A., Blamey, R.W. and
    Nicholson, R.I. (In Press): Brit. J. Cancer.

Hormonal Manipulation of Cancer: Peptides, Growth Factors, and New (Anti) Steroidal Agents, edited by Jan G. M. Klijn et al. Raven Press, New York © 1987.

LONG-TERM LHRH-AGONIST (BUSERELIN) TREATMENT IN METASTATIC PREMENOPAUSAL BREAST CANCER

J.G.M. Klijn and F.H. de Jong

Depts. of Endocrinology and Internal Medicine
The Dr Daniel den Hoed Cancer Center, Groene Hilledijk 301,
P.O.Box 5201, Rotterdam, and Erasmus University, Rotterdam, The
Netherlands

INTRODUCTION

Different steroid and peptide hormones, growth factors and other trophic substances are involved in the growth regulation of breast cancer cells (17). Especially oestrogens play an important role. Since the observation of tumour growth remission after surgical castration by Beatson (1896) various treatment modalities have been developed, which suppress gonadal, adrenal or peripheral oestrogen production or antagonize the stimulatory effects of oestrogens at the level of the tumour cells. Apart from castration by surgical and radiotherapeutical means it appeared possible to suppress pituitary-gonadal function by different kinds of medical treatment. During the last 5 years, it became apparent that LHRH analogues are of interest for suppression of pituitary gonadotrophin secretion and for reaching "medical castration", especially because of the absence of side effects (25). The effectiveness of this type of treatment has been established in patients with prostate cancer by a large number of investigators (see previous chapters and review, 25) as well as by our group (13,14,26) and the number of studies in breast cancer patients has been increasing since our first report in 1982 (9). Since that time we have treated 32 premenopausal patients with metastatic breast cancer with at present a minimal follow-up of 1.5 years. Part of the endocrine and clinical results have been published before in detail (9-12,15, 16). In this report we present our updated results and a review on this subject in the literature.

PATIENTS, TREATMENT AND METHODS

Thirty-two premenopausal patients with metastatic breast cancer gave consent for treatment with the potent LHRH-agonist Buserelin (Hoe 766) as a single agent or in combination with other agents like tamoxifen or megestrol acetate. The characteristics of this group of patients with respect to age, disease-free interval, oestradiol receptor status and follow-up are indicated in Table 1. All patients were unselected with the exception of the patients in group IB (see treatment scheme),

TABLE 1.

PATIENTS

- 32 premenopausal patients with metastatic breast cancer

- mean age: 40 yr (range 30 - 53 yr)

- disease-free interval: $\bar{x}$ = 2.5 yr (range 0.5 - 5.0 yr)

- oestradiol receptor: 18 x pos., 2 x neg., 12 x unknown

- mean follow-up: 3.5 yr (range 1.5 - 4.5 yr)

who were selected on the basis of having an oestradiol receptor positive tumour.

During the first week all subgroups of patients were treated parenterally (Table 2) with a daily dose of 3 mg Buserelin as described before (11). Subsequently 12 patients (group IA) were treated chronically with 3 x 400 µg Buserelin intranasally (i.n.) and 11 patients (group IB) with 2 x 1 mg Buserelin subcutaneously (s.c.), decreasing this daily dose after 2 months with 2 x 0.1 mg for every next month and switching to intranasal administration in the presence of continuous medical castration after one year of treatment. Ultimately the patients in this subgroup IB have been treated with doses between 2 x 1000 µg s.c. and 3 x 400 ug i.n. ($\sim$ 25 µg s.c.) per day (Table 2). Five women (group IIA) were treated daily with 3 x 400 ug

TABLE 2.

PATIENTS AND TREATMENT SCHEME

May 1986

Group	n	first week	long-term treatment
IA	12	3 mg Hoe 766 i.v.	3 x 400 µg i.n.
		or s.c.	
IB	11	3 mg Hoe 766 i.v.	2000 ---▶ 100 µg s.c. --▶ i.n.
IIA	5	3 mg Hoe 766 i.v.	3 x 400 µg i.n. + 2 x 20 mg TAM[*]
IIB	4	3 mg Hoe 766 i.v.	3 x 400 µg i.n. + 4 x 45 mg MA[*]

Total	32	patients

[*] TAM = tamoxifen

[*] MA = megestrol acetate

Buserelin i.n. in combination with 2 x 20 mg tamoxifen from the start of treatment, while in 9 out of the 12 patients of group IA tamoxifen was added later because of tumour progression or recurrent peaks of plasma oestradiol. Four patients (group IIB) were treated with 3 x 400 µg Buserelin i.n. in combination with 4 x 45 mg megestrol acetate s.c.

Blood sampling, measurement of plasma luteinising hormone (LH), follicle stimulating hormone (FSH), oestradiol (E2), progesterone (Prog), prolactin (PRL) and oestradiol receptor (ER) were done as described previously (4,8). Measurement of tumour response were performed according to the UICC criteria. Significances of differences between mean values at various time points within treatment groups were assessed by Student's paired t-test.

RESULTS

Endocrine effects

Gonadotrophins

Results have been described in detail before (11,12,15). During chronic subcutaneous treatment the suppression of gonadotrophin secretion was more pronounced than during intranasal administration. No pre-ovulatory peaks were observed with the exception of data in a few patients treated with Buserelin plus tamoxifen (group IIA), while subnormal immunoassayable gonadotrophin levels occurred rarely.

Sex steroids

Anovulation as indicated by persisting low plasma progesterone levels occurred in all patients of group IA, IB and IIB; however, subnormal peaks of progesterone were observed in 7 out of 14 patients treated with Buserelin i.n. in combination with tamoxifen (10,11).

During chronic subcutaneous treatment plasma E2 concentrations showed a striking fall to castration levels within 3 weeks with a mean concentration of 19 pmol/l (5 pg/ml) during 1-4 months after start of treatment (Fig.1). During subcutaneous treatment mean plasma E2 was much more suppressed than during intranasal treatment, during which a great variation in plasma E2 concentrations was observed as expressed by a large SEM. During intranasal treatment some patients (40%) reached medical castration values, others showed recurrent peaks of E2.

During gradual decrement of the daily subcutaneous dose, mean plasma E2 slowly increased after 5-12 months of treatment using Buserelin dosages of 0.6 - 1.4 mg per day. Plasma E2 levels reached the same range as observed in patients with medical castration during intranasal therapy (Fig.1) i.e. between 20 and 60 pmol/l. One patient (Fig.2) showed a clear escape of pituitary-gonadal suppression after 32-40 weeks of treatment s.c. while after 20 weeks plasma E2 levels were already

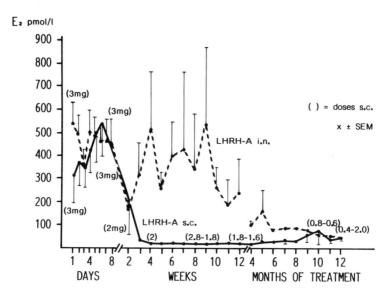

FIG. 1. Mean plasma E_2 concentrations during chronic single treatment with Buserelin intranasally (i.n.) and subcutaneously (s.c.) in 23 patients.

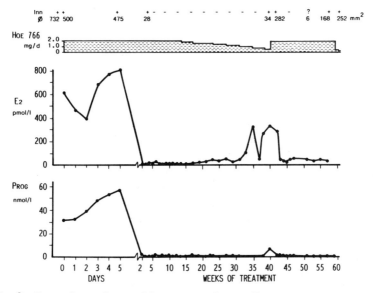

FIG. 2. Dose dependent effects on plasma E_2 and prog levels and lymph node metastasis (lnn) of subcutaneous treatment with Hoe 766 in the same patient.

slightly increased using dosages of 1.4 - 0.6 mg per day. Ultimately a small peak of progesterone occurred. After increment of the dose to 2 x 1 mg s.c. per day a medical castration was reached again. This patient showed a complete remission of her cervical lymph node metastases within 5 weeks after start of treatment, but a recurrence of these lymph node metastases occurred after 9 months, about 7 weeks after the time that plasma E2 increased above levels of 100 pmol/l. When medical castration was reached for the second time after dose increment a complete tumour remission occurred again indicating that the tumour was still hormone dependent. However, after one year of treatment hormone independency occurred with tumour progression in the presence of castration levels of plasma E2. On the other hand, in another patient it appeared possible to decrease the daily dose from 2000 µg s.c. to 1200 µg i.n. (∿25 µg s.c.) in the course of 1 year. In this patient continuous medical castration and nearly complete tumour regression for more than 2 years were observed.

Prolactin
Detailed data were reported in a previous report (15). The main observations were that basal and stimulated (TRH) plasma PRL levels increased during the first day and after one week of treatment respectively. Thereafter there appeared no significant difference with pretreatment values. During parenteral therapy the mean night peak of PRL, however, decreased significantly from 27.2 ± 4.6 to 15.9 ± 3 µg/l (p < 0.05).

Antitumour effects
The effects on tumour growth are summarized in Table 3. In the whole group 14 patients (44%) showed an objective remission with a mean duration of response of more than 19 months. Three patients are still under treatment. In addition 6 patients (19%) showed stable disease. An objective response during single Buserelin treatment was found in 9 out of 23 patients (39%) and in 5 out of 11 (45%) patients selected on the basis of an ER-positive tumour treated subcutaneously. Until now the longest duration of response is more than 53 months. At present, this patient has been treated with an LHRH analogue for the longest period reported. In total, 8 out of 18 patients with an ER-positive tumour responded objectively (44%).

Survival
The overall survival of the whole group of 32 patients is shown in Fig.3. Median survival is 3 years. Eight patients (25%) died within 1.5 years after start of treatment. Thirteen (54%) out of 24 patients, all of them with a follow-up of at least 3 years survived longer than 3 years. The 9 patients with combination treatment showed a somewhat better survival curve than the other patients, but the number is too small for definite conclusions. In general, these results are as good or

better than those reported in the literature.

TABLE 3.

ANTITUMOR EFFECTS IN 32 PATIENTS

May 1986

Group	Treatment	CR + PR	No Change	Failure	n
IA	Hoe 766 i.n.	4 x ($\bar{x}$ = 21$^+$m)	4 x (3-5m)	4x	12
IB	Hoe 766 s.c.	5 x ($\bar{x}$ = 14$^+$m)	1 x (5m)	5x(2x mixed)	11
IIA	Hoe 766 + TAM	3 x ($\bar{x}$ = 15$^+$m)	0 x	2x	5
IIB	Hoe 766 + MA	2 x (22,41$^+$m)	1 x (14m)	1x	4
Total		14 x (44%)	6 x (19%)	12x	32

- Objective response rate during single Hoe 766 treatment (IA+B) = 9/23 (39%)

- Objective response rate in patients with ER + tumors: 45%

- Longest duration of response: 53$^+$ months

Side effects

No side effects occurred with the exception of those caused by the intended hypogonadism, i.e. hot flushes, decreased libido and in a few patients mental depression. Hot flushes were experienced 3-4 weeks after start of treatment at the time of medical castration. The frequency of the flushes varied between 3-30 times per day. During the years of treatment the intensity decreased. Some patients (about 15%) showed short-term (10-60 minutes) urticarial skin irritation at the injection site without pain or itching.

DISCUSSION AND CONCLUSIONS

In our study the objective response rate in premenopausal metastatic breast cancer is 39% during single LHRH agonist treatment. Recently, in 4 other studies (5-7,18,19,23) with a shorter follow-up and with application of 4 different LHRH agonists comparable response rates (between 31 and 47%, Table 4) have been reported. In total, an objective response was found in 44 (38%) out of 116 patients. The overall response rate in patients with ER-positive tumours appeared 53% (30/57). So, chronic LHRH-agonist treatment seems as effective as other common kinds of endocrine treatment in premenopausal breast cancer in the absence of serious side effects, but randomised

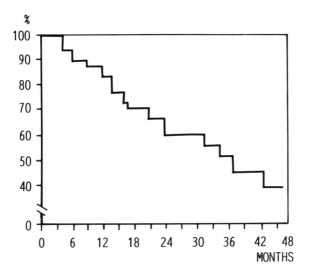

FIG. 3.   Survival of 32 premenopausal patients with metastatic breast cancer treated with Buserelin (9 in combination with TAM or MA).

studies have still to be performed. On the basis of our experience and that of others (21,22), an escape of suppression of pituitary-ovarian function or non-complete medical castration may occur in some women treated with daily dosages of an LHRH agonist lower than 1 mg subcutaneously, especially after initiation of therapy during either the mid-cycle or luteal phase according to Nicholson et al. (21,22). Therefore we advise a daily dose of at least 1 mg s.c. to reach safely medical castration in all patients as also observed by Harvey and Manni et al. (5,6,18).

Although the main mechanism of action of LHRH agonist treatment is medical castration, direct antitumour effects at the level of tumour cells cannot be excluded. We reported before (1,2,15) and in this book (Foekens et al.) on direct antitumour effects of Buserelin using oestrogen stimulated breast cancer cell growth (MCF-7) in vitro in the presence of E2 concentrations as found in castrated or postmenopausal patients. Prolactin stimulated growth of breast cancer cells appeared inhibited too as found by Wiznitzer and Benz (28) using a prolactin responsive cell line (T-47-D). Direct effects were also observed by Miller et al. (20, this book) but not on all cell lines investigated. The suggestion of direct effects of the LHRH agonists in vitro is supported by the in vivo observation that LHRH agonist treatment can cause objective remission in postmenopausal metastatic breast cancer (5,6,19,24, Table 5) and by the presence of (low affinity) binding sites for LHRH agonists

TABLE 4.

RESULTS OF LHRH–AGONIST TREATMENT IN PREMENOPAUSAL METASTATIC BREAST CANCER (Updated 1986)

Author	LHRH-agonist	n	CR + PR
1) Klijn et al.	Buserelin	23	9 (39%)
2) Nicholson et al.	Zoladex	45	14 (31%)
3) Harvey et al.	Leuprolide	25	11 (44%)
4) Mathé et al.	D-Trp-6-LHRH	8*	3 (38%)
5) Höffken et al.	Buserelin	15	7 (47%)
In total		116	44 (38%)

* pretreated

Overall response rate of ER-positive tumors: 30/57 (53%)

TABLE 5.

RESULTS OF LHRH–AGONIST TREATMENT IN POSTMENOPAUSAL METASTATIC BREAST CANCER (Updated 1986)

Author	LHRH-agonist	n	CR + PR
1) Harvey et al.	Leuprolide	41*	4 (10%)
2) Mathe et al.	D-Trp-6-LHRH	15*	3 (20%)
3) Plowman	Zoladex	10	2 (20%)
4) Waxman	Buserelin	18	0 (0%)
In total		84	9 (11%)

* pretreated

in breast cancer cells (3,20). However, the in vivo results could not be reproduced by all authors (27), and the relatively low overall response rate (11%) indicates that this kind of treatment will be of less value in postmenopausal patients. Maybe in some patients with bad drug compliance slow release preparations injected once per 1-3 months may be useful in the future.

In conclusion

1. In premenopausal metastatic breast cancer chronic LHRH-agonist treatment appears as effective as other common kinds of endocrine treatment in the absence of serious side effects.
2. Although intranasal administration appeared to be a pleasant and sufficiently effective way of treatment in some patients, high subcutaneous dosages of LHRH-agonists (at least 1.0 - 1.5 mg per day) are needed for reaching optimal and rapid suppression of the pituitary-gonadal function within 3 weeks in all patients.
3. The reported responses in some postmenopausal patients may indicate direct antitumour effects in vivo at the level of the tumour cells as was observed in vitro.
4. Sustained release preparations of LHRH agonist may be of great advantage if indeed medical castration can be reached in all patients.

REFERENCES

1. Blankenstein, M.A., Henkelman, M.S., and Klijn, J.G.M. (1983): J. Steroid Biochem.,19, Suppl.: 95 S.
2. Blankenstein, M.A., Henkelman, M.S., and Klijn, J.G.M. (1985): Eur.J.Cancer Clin.Oncol., 21:1493-1499.
3. Eidne, K.A., Flanagan, C.A., and Miller, R.P. (1985): Science, 229:989-992.
4. EORTC Breast Cancer Cooperative Group (1980): Eur.J.Cancer, 16:1513-1516.
5. Harvey, H.A., Lipton, A., and Max, D.T. (1984). In: LHRH and its analogues, contraceptive and clinical application, edited by B.H. Vickery, J.J. Nestor and E.S.E. Hafex, pp 329-338, MTP, Lancaster.
6. Harvey, H.A., Lipton, A., and Max, D. (1986): Eur.J.Cancer Clin.Oncol., 22:724.
7. Höffken, K., Miller, B., Fischer, P., Becher, R., Kurschel, E., Scheulen, M.E., Miller, A.A., Callies, R., and Schmidt, C.G. (1986): Eur.J.Cancer Clin.Oncol., 22:746.
8. Klijn, J.G.M., Lamberts, S.W.J., de Jong, F.H., Docter, R., van Dongen, K.J., and Birkenhäger, J.C. (1980): Clin. Endocrinol., 12:341-355.
9. Klijn, J.G.M., and de Jong, F.H. (1982): Lancet, i:1213-1216.

10. Klijn, J.G.M. (1984): Med.Oncol. & Tumor Pharmacother., 1:123-128.
11. Klijn, J.G.M., de Jong, F.H., Blankenstein, M.A., Docter, R., Alexieva-Figusch, J., Blonk-van der Wijst, J., and Lamberts, S.W.J. (1984): Breast Cancer Res.Treatm., 4:209-220.
12. Klijn, J.G.M., and de Jong, F.H. (1984): In: LHRH and its Analogues, basic and clinical aspects, edited by F. Labrie, A. Belanger and A. Dupont, pp 425-437, Excerpta Medica, Amsterdam.
13. Klijn, J.G.M., de Jong, F.H., Lamberts, S.W.J., and Blankenstein, M.A. (1984): Eur.J.Cancer Clin.Oncol., 20:483-493.
14. Klijn, J.G.M., de Voogt, H.J., Schröder, F.H., and de Jong, F.H. (1985): Lancet, ii:493.
15. Klijn, J.G.M., de Jong, F.H., Lamberts, S.W.J., and Blankenstein, M.A. (1985): J.Steroid Biochem., 23:867-873.
16. Klijn, J.G.M. (1986): In: Proceedings of the Symposium on Endocrine Related Tumours (May 1985, Noordwijkerhout), edited by E. Engelsman, in press, The Update Group Limited, London.
17. Lippman, M.E. (1985): Clin.Res., 33:375-382.
18. Manni, A., Santen, R., Harvey, H., Lipton, A., and Max, D. (1986): Endocr.Rev., 7:89-94.
19. Mathé, G., Keiling, R., Vovan, M.L., Gastiaburu, J., Prévot, G., Vannetzel, J.M., Despax, R., Jasmin, C., Lévi, F., Musset, M., Muchover, D., and Misset, J.L. (1986): Eur.J.Cancer Clin.Oncol., 22:723.
20. Miller, W.R., Scott, W.N, Morris, R., Fraser, H.M., and Sharpe, R.M. (1985): Nature, 313:231-233.
21. Nicholson, R.I., Walker, K.J., Turkes, A., Turkes, A.O., Dyas, J., Blamey, R.W., Campbell, F.C., Robinson, M.R.G., and Griffiths, K. (1984): J.Steroid Biochem., 20:129-135.
22. Nicholson, R.I., Walker, K.J., Turkes, A., Dyas, J., Plowman, P.N., Williams, M., and Blamey, R.W. (1985): J.Steroid Biochem., 23:843-849.
23. Nicholson, R.I. (1986): Eur.J.Cancer Clin.Oncol., 22:724.
24. Plowman, P.N., Nicholson, R.I., and Walker, K.J. (1986): Eur.J.Cancer Clin.Oncol., 22:746.
25. Schally, A.V., Redding, T.W., and Comaru-Schally, A.M. (1984): Cancer Treatm.Rep., 68:281-289.
26. Schröder, F.H., Lock, T.M.T.W., Chadha, D.R., Debruyne, F.M.J., de Jong, F.H., Klijn, J.G.M., Matroos, A.W., and de Voogt, H.J. (1986): J.Urol., in press.
27. Waxman, J.H., Harland, S.J., Coombes, R.C., Wrigley, P.F.M., Malpas, J.S., Powles, T., and Lister, T.A. (1985): Cancer Chemother.Pharmacol., 15:171-173.
28. Wiznitzer, I., and Benz, C. (1984): Proc.Ann.Am.Assoc. Cancer Res., 25:208.

Hormonal Manipulation of Cancer: Peptides, Growth Factors, and New (Anti) Steroidal Agents, edited by Jan G. M. Klijn et al. Raven Press, New York © 1987.

LHRH AGONIST TREATMENT IN OVARIAN CANCER

S. Kullander, A. Rausing and A.V. Schally

University of Lund, Depts. of Gyn.Obst. and Pathology, Malmö General Hospital, Malmö, Sweden, and Dept. of Medicine, Tulane University, Medical Center, New Orleans, Lo., U.S.A.

Experimental animal observations as well as human epidemiological and receptor studies suggest that many ovarian tumours are endocrine-related. Especially high gonadodotrophin levels have been suggested to be of possible significance. The protective effects in women of pregnancies and the use of oral contraceptives against ovarian cancer may be associated with low gonadotrophin levels (4). In the experimental model, excess gonadotrophin secretion in many animals is related to the development of ovarian tumours (1). The therapeutic possibilities of antagonizing hormones may lead to new approaches toward the control of neoplastic ovarian growth. An inhibitory effect through the suppression of pituitary FSH and LH secretion by administration of GnRH superagonist has been suggested (2,3) but treatment reports still are scarce. Therefore, this has now been further tested both in an animal rat model and in a pilot-study as second-line therapy in women with advanced ovarian cancer.

16 4-week old female homozygotic rats of the R-strain were castrated and one ovary at the same time autografted under the splenic capsule. One year after the operation when such animals have developed ovarian hormone-producing tumours in the grafts (1) one group (n = 9) started to receive daily subcutaneous injections of 25 ug of GnRH superagonist, D-Trp-6-LH-RH while the control group (n = 7) received sham injections. The tumour growth was monitored for around a year by direct measurements of the geometric diameters of the tumours at repeated laparotomies every second month starting 2 weeks after commencement of the injections. Small biopsies for histologic and electronmicroscopic examinations were taken at the same time and routinely treated.

In the controls the tumours grew continuously and histologically they showed the typical picture earlier well-known and described (1) with mitoses in the tumour cells in all sections examined. After 2 months, suppression of the tumour growth was found in the GnRH superagonist treated rats compared with that in the controls and from then on these tumours remained practically static showing around 15 mm mean geometric diameter after a year compared with 30 mm in the controls.

Tumours from treated animals showed during the treatment year an increasing disturbance histologically in the relation between tumour cells and stroma cells with increasing stroma. The picture somewhat looked like a liver cirrhosis. From the second month the tumour cells began to arrange in alveolar groups surrounded by fibrous tissues and electronmicroscopically irregular electron-dense bodies missing in the control tumours were seen within the tumour cells. These were presumably lysosomes and degenerative processes. After a year large hyalinized areas and pyenotic tumour cells with brownish pigment were found. Electronmicroscopically degenerative processes in the cells with large irregular vacuoles were seen. However, also small intermingling bands and groups of still fully vital tumour cells were always found.

In conclusion it can be said that GnRH superagonist is effective in inhibiting experimental ovarian tumour growth in rats but also that some cell clones survive and escape the consequences of suppression of pituitary gonadotrophin secretion and any direct local superagonist suppression. This is in accordance with the findings earlier of the effects of surgical hypophysectomy on ovarian tumours of the same age in the same experimental model (1). Presumably autonomy is gained by some cell-lines due to progression and selection pressure and those hormone-independant cell clones survive.

The activity of the agonist was also evaluated in 10 patients with advanced ovarian carcinomas. 6 of these tumours were histologically serous cysto-carcinomas and the patient age varied between 40 and 82 years. All patients had received cytotoxic chemo-therapy combined with heavy doses of gestagens (MPA) but due to failure this regime had been abandoned and for one month before starting the agonist. The patients were given 100 ug/day subcutaneously initially for 7 days and subsequently monthly injections of a slow-release preparation of D-Trp-6 LHRH microcapsules designed to release 100 ug/day.

The basal levels of gonadotropins were suppressed by the treatment but were initially rather low, probably a residual effect of the preceeding high MPA doses.

Two patients, in a final stage of the cancer when starting the treatment, died within a month. Of the remaining 8 patients, 2 showed objective tumour regression, disappearing of ascites and lower Ca 125 and a survival of 1-2 years. The disease remained objectively stable in 3 other patients with a survival for 8-24 months. Slow continuous progress was observed in another 2 patients who survived 3 and 6 months, respectively. In conclusion the agonist treatment in half of the 10 patients - earlier under cytotoxic-gestagen regime - induced objective response or objective stabilization of the disease. The survival time, 1-2 years, was then free of chemical side-effects but included recovery of appetite and bone-marrow activity.

Summarizing the results of experimental and clinical trials on the effects of LHRH agonists in ovarian cancer it may be said that this endocrine therapy which has no apparent toxicity appears to hold some promise. The data support the contention that the use of hypothalamic analogs might supplement or in some cases replace conventional procedures for the treatment of advanced ovarian tumours. Attention should be given clinically to combined use of LHRH analogs with chemotherapy and/or gestagens. Coming prospective randomized studies on analogs as first-line therapy should evelute also the importance of the tumour histology and its receptor content as well as the patients' hormonal status.

REFERENCES

1. Kullander, S. Thesis. Lund, 1956

2. Mortel, R., Satyawaroop, P.G., Schally, A.V., Hamilton, T. and Ozols, R. Personal communication, 1986.

3. Parmar, H., Nicoll, J., Stockdale, A., Cassoni, A., Philips, R.H., Lightman, S.L. and Schally, A.V. Cancer Treatment Reports 69, 1341, 1985.

4. Stadel, D.V. Am J Obstet Gynecol 123, 772, 1975.

Hormonal Manipulation of Cancer: Peptides, Growth Factors, and New (Anti) Steroidal Agents, edited by Jan G. M. Klijn et al. Raven Press, New York © 1987.

DIRECT INHIBITION OF HUMAN BREAST CANCER CELL GROWTH BY AN

LHRH AGONIST

W R Miller*, W N Scott*, H M Fraser[+] and R M Sharpe[+]

*University Department of Clinical Surgery, Royal Infirmary, Edinburgh EH3 9YW, [+]MRC Unit of Reproductive Biology, Chalmers Street, Edinburgh EH3 9EW

INTRODUCTION

About one-third of human breast cancers appear to require hormones for their continued growth. Hormone deprivation or anti-hormone therapy results in regression of these tumours. In premenopausal women with advanced breast cancer, treatment usually has taken the form of surgical or radiological castration. Recently, however, such women have also been successfully treated with agonist analogues of LHRH(12,18,14). As this treatment reduces circulating oestrogen to castrate levels(17,11), it seems likely that beneficial effects are achieved by suppressing the pituitary-ovarian axis(21,19). Major clinical studies have, therefore, been performed in pre-menopausal women, but responses to LHRH agonist can occur in postmenopausal patients who are without measurable ovarian function(9). Since administration of LHRH agonists does not significantly change levels of circulating oestrogen in post-menopausal women(18), an alternative mechanism of action must be responsible for these effects. As it is now clear that LHRH analogues are capable of major actions on extra-pituitary tissues(10,13,27,26), it is possible that LHRH and its analogues might have direct effects on breast tumours. To explore this possibility, we have (a) studied the effects of LHRH on the growth of established lines of breast cancer cells maintained in culture and (b) looked for the presence of specific binding sites for LHRH in the same cell lines.

EFFECTS OF LHRH AND ITS ANALOGUES ON BREAST CANCER CELLS IN CULTURE

MCF-7 human breast cancer cells were obtained from the Michigan Cancer Foundation and were used between their 183rd and 192nd passage. T-47D and MDA-MB-231 breast cancer cells and

HBL-100 "normal" human breast cells were obtained from the
American Tissue Type Collection.   All cells were grown at 37°C
in Dulbecco's minimal essential medium containing 10% heat-
inactivated foetal calf serum, under a humidified atmosphere of
5% CO_2:95% air.   Further experimental detail has already been
published(15).

Studies with MCF-7 cells

Because of disparate results from different laboratories
regarding the hormone sensitivity in culture of MCF-7 cells, it
is essential to characterize the particular cultures which are
under investigation.   In the present studies, growth of the cell
line in culture was sensitive to oestrogen being stimulated by
concentrations of oestradiol as low as 10^{-10}M and inhibited by
the anti-oestrogen, tamoxifen(16).   The cells had a human
karyotype and were tumourogenic when innoculated into immuno-
suppressed mice; the resulting xenografts were oestrogen
dependent (appearing only in animals supplemented with oestrogen)
and had a histology consistent with breast carcinoma, including
evidence of vascular invasion.

Effects of the LHRH agonist, Buserelin, on the growth of these
MCF-7 cells in shown in Figure 1.   All concentrations of the
agonist other than 10^{-11}M caused significant (p < 0.001)
inhibition of growth in comparison with control cells.   These
inhibitory effects were dose-related and concentrations of
buserelin in excess of 10^{-9}M produced a net decrease in cell
numbers after four days of culture.   Levels in excess of 10^{-7}M
agonist resulted in a progressive decrease in cell numbers over
the whole test period.   Inhibitory effects were highly
reproducible and could be detected microscopically as early as
day 2 of culture.   Although cell numbers decreased even after
short exposure to LHRH agonist, the remaining cells appeared
viable and, after an initial delay, showed increased growth if
cultured in media without LHRH agonist (Figure 2).   Similar
inhibitory effects have been described by Blankenstein et al(3)
although the LHRH agonist was less potent in their system.

The specificity of these inhibitory effects was studied by
performing similar studies with native LHRH, the 3-10 fragment of
LHRH and the LHRH antagonist, (N-Ac-D-Nal(2)1, D-pCL-Phe2, D-Trp3,
D-hArg(Et2)6, D-Ala10)LHRH.   Native LHRH was also capable of
inhibiting cell growth although much higher concentrations were
required than with the LHRH agonist (Figure 3).   The 3-10
fragment of LHRH did not significantly affect the growth of the
MCF-7 cell line.   The major inhibitory effects of LHRH agonist
on cell growth were completely blocked by addition of the LHRH
antagonist, the combination of the two peptides having no greater
effect than the antagonist alone (Figure 4); the latter only
caused minor but nevertheless significant suppression of cell
growth.

Interestingly, inhibitory effects of LHRH agonist could not be

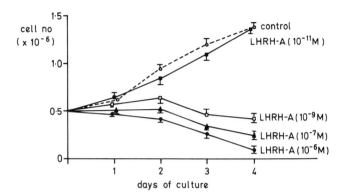

FIG. 1.   Inhibition of breast cancer cells by the LHRH agonist
(LHRH-A), buserelin. Each point is the mean of
triplicate cultures and vertical lines the standard
deviation of the mean.

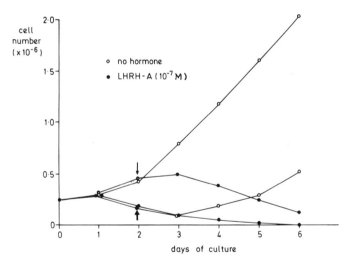

FIG. 2.   Recovery of MCF-7 breast cancer cells after treatment
with LHRH agonist.   At day 2 media from certain
control cultures were changed to include LHRH agonist
and certain cultures with LHRH agonists were switched
to media containing no hormones.

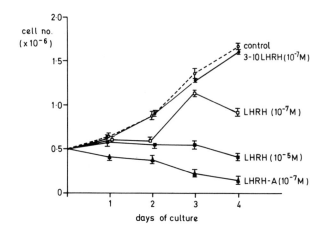

FIG. 3.   The comparative effects of native LHRH, the 3–10
            fragment of LHRH and LHRH agonist (LHRH–A) on the
            growth of MCF-7 breast cancer cells in culture.

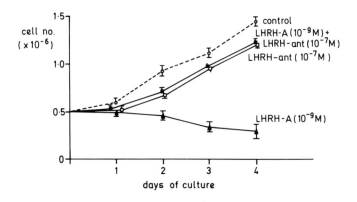

FIG. 4.   The effects of LHRH agonist (LHRH–A) or LHRH antagonist
            (LHRH–ant) alone and in combination on the growth of
            MCF-7 breast cancer cells in culture.

demonstrated if insulin was included in the culture medium
(Figure 5).   Thus the combination of insulin (10ug/ml) and a
concentration of LHRH agonist (10^{-6}M) which alone has a marked
action on cell growth had no greater effect than insulin alone,
cell numbers being slightly less than in the absence of insulin.
Insulin was also able to abolish sensitivity to oestrogen (data
not shown).

The effects of oestrogen and LHRH agonist alone and in
combination are shown in Figure 6.   Oestradiol at a
concentration of 10^{-10}M slightly stimulated cell growth and was
able to reverse in part the inhibitory effects of LHRH agonist.
Nevertheless cell numbers in cultures containing both LHRH and
oestradiol were significantly suppressed as compared with control
and oestrogen-supplemented systems.

Studies with other cell lines

To determine whether inhibitory effects may be observed in
other breast cancer cells, similar studies have been performed
with the T-47D and MDA-MB-231 lines.   These cell lines have a
different sensitivity to oestrogen when compared with MCF-7 cells,
the growth of MDA-MB-231 cells being resistant to both oestradiol
and tamoxifen and that of T-47D cells having only limited
sensitivity to these agents.   The effects of LHRH agonist on the
growth of MDA-MB-231 and T-47D cells are shown in Figure 7.
Concentrations of agonist which were inhibitory in MCF-7 cells
were totally ineffective against MDA-MB-231 and produced minimal
effects in the T-47D (although some inhibition was evident after
4 days of culture).   Major inhibitory effects of LHRH agonist
have, however, been reported against prolactin-stimulated growth
of T-47D cells(28).   Nevertheless, it is clear that the
inhibitory action of LHRH is not a non-specific effect on the
growth of cells in general.   This observation is supported by the
inability of LHRH agonist at any concentration to produce
measurable effects on the growth of the HBL-100 "normal" human
breast cell line (data not shown).

LHRH-BINDING SITES ON BREAST TUMOUR CELLS

The demonstration that the inhibitory effect of the LHRH
agonist on growth of MCF-7 cells in-vitro was blocked completely
by addition of an LHRH antagonist implies that the described
effects are mediated via stereo-specific recognition sites i.e.
receptors.   To test this, MCF-7 cells grown to confluence were
harvested by mechanical agitation and repeated aspirations into a
Pasteur pipette and these cells then incubated with 125I-LHRH
agonist in-vitro.   Initial binding studies were performed at
21°C using a 10 min incubation period(15) but the results
described below were obtained by incubating cells on ice for 90
mins followed by rapid separation of bound and free hormone by
centrifugation at 4°C for 5 min at 1000g.   Comparable results
were obtained using either of these incubation procedures.

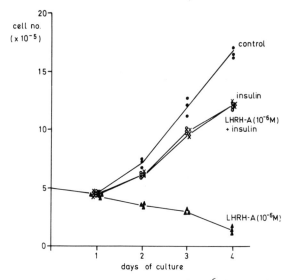

FIG. 5.   The effects of LHRH agonist (10^{-6}M) and insulin (10μg/ml) alone and in combination on MCF-7 breast cancer cells in culture

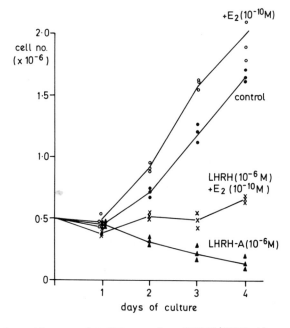

FIG. 6.   The effects of LHRH agonist (LHRH/LHRH-A) or oestradiol (E_2) alone and in combination on MCF-7 breast cancer cells in culture

As judged by the displacement of labelled LHRH agonist by unlabelled LHRH agonist, the MCF-7 cells contained binding sites with a low affinity (Kd ~ 4 x 10^{-5}M) for the LHRH agonist (Figure 8). However, these binding sites showed a high degree of specificity in that only peptides which were LHRH-like competed for binding with 125I-LHRH agonists. Thus, two LHPH antagonists competed for binding with higher affinity (Kd ~ 10^{-6}M) than did the LHRH agonist whilst native LHRH competed very poorly (Kd > 5 x 10^{-4}). Surprisingly, 3-10 LHPH, which is completely devoid of any biological activity in-vitro, displaced binding of 125I-LHRH agonist nearly as effectively as did the unlabelled agonist itself. Of the other peptides tested, at concentrations up to 1mM, only bradykinin caused any displacement of binding and this was considered to be due to alteration of the pH of the incubation medium. Binding sites with similar affinity and specificity were also found in MCF-7 cells grown in the presence of insulin and in T-47D and MDA-MB-231 cells.

Recently LHRH-receptors have been identified in a high percentage of ductal breast carcinomas(8), although these were shown to have a relatively high affinity (Kd ~ 10^{-8}M) for an LHRH agonist, a finding which contrasts with the present findings in culture breast tumour cells.

DISCUSSION

Evidence has been presented that LHRH and its analogues have the potential for direct actions upon breast cancer cells, this being based on the ability of these compounds to inhibit the growth of certain breast cancer cells in monolayer and the presence of specific binding sites for LHRH agonists in breast cancer cells and tumours.

The inhibitory effects of LHRH agonists on growth of the MCF-7 cells appear to be mediated by a specific recognition mechanism in that (a) similar effects could be elicited by native LHRH although much higher concentrations were required; (b) the biologically inactive 3-10 fragment of LHRH was ineffective; and (c) inhibition could be abolished by the simultaneous presence of and LHRH antagonist.

The mechanism by which the effects are achieved is still a matter of conjecture although it is possible that they reflect an anti-steroidal process as has been reported for LHRH agonists in other tissues(19,25). Some circumstantial support for an anti-oestrogenic action can be derived from these studies in that (a) inhibition by LHRH agonist could be partially overcome by oestrogen, (b) inclusion of insulin in the culture system abolished sensitivity to both oestrogen and LHRH agonist and (c) in the limited number of cell lines studied there was a parallelism between sensitivity to LHRH agonist and both responsiveness to oestrogen and levels of oestrogen receptors. Interplay between polypeptides and steroids is not unusual in growth regulation of the breast. Prolactin and oestrogen are

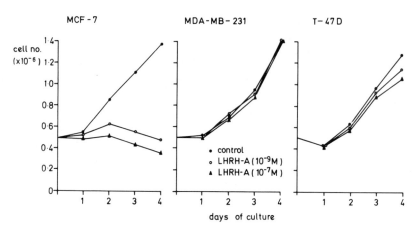

FIG. 7. The effects of LHRH agonist (LHRH-A), buserelin on human breast cancer cells in culture.

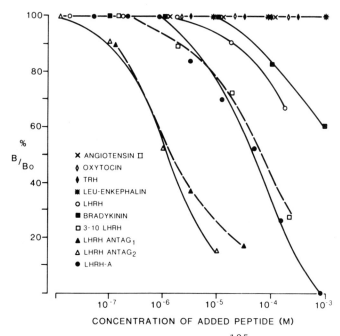

FIG. 8. Displacement of the binding of ^{125}I-labelled LHRH agonist to isolated MCF-7 cells by increasing concentrations of unlabelled LHRH agonist (LHRH-A), two LHRH antagonists (ANTAG$_1$ and ANTAG$_2$), LHRH and 3-10LHRH as well as several other peptides.

synergistic during the development of normal breast and recently it has been proposed that the mitotic effects of oestrogen on breast cancer cell may be mediated by secretion of autocrine growth factors some of which have epidermal growth factor- and somatomedin-like properties(7). It is possible that the inhibitory effects of LHRH described may result from antagonism of endogenous growth-promoting peptides.

The inhibitory action of LHRH agonists is specific, little effects being observed in cultures of other breast cancer cell lines and a "normal" breast cell line. It may be pertinent, however, that whilst we could detect only minimal effects in the T-47D cell line, major inhibitory effects of an LHRH agonist have been described on prolactin-stimulated growth of T-47D cells(28). This perhaps suggests that LHRH exerts its inhibition only when growth of the cancer cells is stimulated, the nature of the stimulus being specific for different cell lines, i.e. oestrogen for MCF-7 cells and prolactin to T-47D cells.

The presence of specific binding sites for LHRH agonists as described in this study in breast cancer cell lines and by Eidne et al(8) in primary breast cancers would support the notion that LHRH-like molecules are capable of exerting direct effects on human breast tumours. It is tempting to assume that the inhibitory effects on the growth of the MCF-7 cells are mediated through these binding sites. However, it should be noted that similar binding sites were detected in cell lines such as the MDA-MB-231 which were not observed to be sensitive to LHRH agonist. The binding sites were also of very low affinity so that biological effects of the agonist on growth of the MCF-7 cells in-vitro was obtained with doses (10^{-9}M) far lower than the apparent affinity (Kd) of the receptor (4×10^{-5}M). It is possible that the MCF-7 cells contain two classes of LHRH-receptors, one of high affinity but low capacity and the other of low affinity and high capacity, with the former mediating the biological effects on growth. Unfortunately, because of the low numbers of LHRH-receptors present and other technical limitations it is not feasible to test directly this possibility.

LHRH-receptors with relatively low affinity have also been reported in other human extra-pituitary tissues such as the placenta(6) and corpus luteum(20,4). Moreover, in the placenta, these receptors have been shown to mediate biological effects of LHRH-like peptides(2), and the gene for LHRH has been isolated from the human placenta(22). Therefore, it appears that several human extra-pituitary tissues contain LHRH-receptors which have a considerably lower affinity for LHRH agonists than do the respective extra-pituitary LHRH-receptors in the rat testis(24) and ovary(5). This may indicate that the human extra-pituitary LHRH-receptors are designed to detect a locally-produced LHRH-like peptide, the structure of which is different from native hypothalamic LHRH. In this respect it is of interest that LHRH has been reported in human breast milk (1) and LHRH-like activity has been located immunohistochemically in certain ductal carcinomas of the breast(23).

Direct inhibitory effects on tumour cells, if reflected in vivo would have important implications in the treatment of breast cancer.   First of all, there would be no reason to restrict the use of LHRH agonists to premenopausal patients.   Indeed the responses reported in postmenopausal women with advanced breast cancer may have resulted from direct anti-tumour effects of LHRH agonist.   Furthermore, effects against oestrogen independent tumours cannot be excluded.

The regimes of LHRH agonist which are now being conventionally employed have been designed for use as a form of medical ovariectomy.   It has to be appreciated that the doses of LHRH agonist necessary to suppress the pituitary-ovarian axis may not be the same as those to inhibit directly breast tumour growth. Methods of administration will have to be developed so that optimal amounts of agonist can reach metastatic deposits of tumour systemically and be maintained in the local environment of the cancer cells.   Infusion or implantation techniques will probably be required.

If the anti-tumour effects of LHRH agonist are to be fully exploited in clinical practice, future research should be directed towards elucidating the mechanism by which LHRH agonists inhibit tumour growth and to determining the optimal regime for administration of the agent.

REFERENCES

1.   Amarant T, Fridkin M and Koch Y (1982):   Luteinizing hormone-releasing hormone and thyrotropin-releasing hormone in human and bovine milk: Europ J Biochem 127:647

2.   Belisle S, Guevin J-F, Bellabarba D and Lelous J-G (1984): Luteinizing hormone-releasing hormone binds to enriched human placental membranes and stimulates in vitro the synthesis of bioactive human chorionic gonadotropin: J Clin Endocrinol Metab 59:119

3.   Blankenstein M A, Henkelman M S and Klijn J G M (1985): Direct inhibitory effect of a luteinizing hormone-releasing hormone agonist on MCF-7 human breast cancer cells: Eur J Cancer Clin Oncol 21:1493

4.   Bramley T A, Menzies G S and Baird D T (1986):   Specific binding of LHRH and an agonist to human corpus luteum homogenates: Characterization, properties and luteal phase levels: J Clin Endocrinol Metab 61-834

5.   Clayton R N, Harwood J P and Catt K J (1979):   Gonadotropin-releasing hormone analogue binds to luteal cells and inhibits progesterone production: Nature 282:90

6.   Currie A J, Fraser H M and Sharpe R M (1981): Human placental receptors for luteinizing hormone releasing hormone: Biochem Biophys Res Commun: 99:332

7. Dickson R B, Huff K K, Spencer E M and Lippman M E (1986): Induction of epidermal growth factor-related polypeptides by 17 beta-estradiol in MCF-7 human breast cancer cells: Endocrinology 118:138

8. Eidne K A, Flanagan C A and Miller R P (1985): Gonadotropin-releasing hormone binding sites in human breast carcinoma: Science 229:989

9. Harvey H A, Lipton A and Max D T (1984): LHRH analogs for human mammary carcinoma in: "LHRH and its Analogs, Contraceptive and Clinical Application" B H Vickery, J J Nestor and E S E Hafez, eds, MTP Lancaster, p 329

10. Khodr G and Siler-Khodr T M (1978): The effect of luteinizing hormone-releasing factor on human chorionic gonadotrophin secretion: Fert Steril 30:301

11. Klijn J G M and de Jong F H (1982): Treatment with a luteinizing-hormone-releasing-hormone analogue (buserelin) in premenopausal patients with metastatic breast cancer: Lancet i:1213

12. Klijn J G M and de Jong F H (1984): Long-term treatment with the LHRH-agonist buserelin (HOE 766) for metastatic breast cancer in single and combined drug regimens, in: "LHRH and its analogues", F Labrie, A Belanger and A Dupont, eds, Elsevier Science, Amsterdam, New York, p 425

13. Lambers S W J, Timmers J M, Oosterom R, Verleun J, Rommerts F G and de Jong F H (1982): Testosterone secretion by cultured arrhenoblastome cells: Suppresion by a luteinizing hormone-releasing hormone agonist: J Clin Endocrinol Metab 54:450

14. Manni A, Santen R, Harvey H, Lipton A and Max D (1986): Treatment of breast cancer with gonadotropin-releasing hormone: Endocrine Rev 7:89

15. Miller W R, Scott W N, Morris R, Fraser H M and Sharpe R M (1985): Growth of human breast cancer cells inhibited by a luteinizing hormone-releasing agonist: Cancer Res 36:3610

16. Miller W R, Scott W N, Morris R, Fraser H M and Sharpe R M (1986): Direct effects of LHRH and agonists on human breast cancer cells in: Proceedings of 13th Annual Meeting of International Foundation for Biochemical Endocrinology, Edinburgh 1985, eds K W Kerns, G Fink, A J Harmer, Plenum Press, New York

17. Nicholson R I and Maynard P V (1979): Anti-tumour activity of ICI 118630, a new potent luteinizing hormone-releasing hormone agonist: Br J Cancer 39:268

18. Nicholson R I, Walker K J, Turkes A, Dyas J, Plowman P N, Williams M and Blamey R W (1985): Endocrinological and clinical aspects of LHRH action (ICI118630) in hormone dependent breast cancer: J Steroid Biochem 23:843

19. Pedroza E, Vilchez-Martinex J A, Coy D H, Arumura A and
     Schally A V (1980): Reduction of LHRH pituitary and
     estradiol uterine binding sites by a superactive analog
     of luteinizing hormone-releasing hormone: Biochem
     Biophys Res Commun 95:1056

20. Popkin R, Bramley T A, Currie A, Shaw R W, Baird D T and
     Fraser H M (1983): Specific binding of luteinizing
     hormone-releasing hormone to human luteal tissue:
     Biochem Biophys Res Commun 114:750

21. Schally A V, Arimura A and Coy A H (1980): Recent
     approaches to fertility control based on derivatives of
     LHRH: Vit and Horm 38:257

22. Seeburg P H and Adelman J P (1984): Characterization of
     cDNA for precursor of human luteinizing hormone-releasing
     hormone: Nature 311:666

23. Seppala M and Wahlstrom T (1980): Identification of
     luteinizing hormone-releasing factor and alpha subunit of
     glycoprotein hormones in ductal carcinoma of the mammary
     gland: Int J Cancer 26:267

24. Sharpe R M and Fraser H M (1980): Leydig cell receptors for
     luteinizing hormone-releasing hormone and its agonists
     and their modulation by administration or deprivation of
     the releasing hormone: Biochem Biophys Res Commun 45:256

25. Sundaram K, Cao Y-C, Wang N-G, Bardin C W, Rivier J and Vale
     W (1981): Inhibition of the action of sex steroid by
     gonadotropin-releasing hormone (GnRH) agonists: a new
     biological effect: Life Sciences 28:83

26. Tan L and Rousseau P (1983): The chemical identity of the
     immuno-reactive LHRH-like peptide biosynthesized in the
     human placenta: Biochem Biophys Res Commun 109:1061

27. Tureck R W, Mastroianni L, Blasco L and Strauss J R (1982):
     Inhibition of human granulosa cell progesterone secretion
     by a gonadotropin-releasing hormone agonist: J Clin
     Endocrinol Metab 54:1078

28. Wiznitzer I and Benz C (1984): Direct growth inhibiting
     effects of the prolactin antagonists Buserelin and
     Pergolide on human breast cancer: Proc Ann Am Assoc
     Cancer Res 25:208

Hormonal Manipulation of Cancer: Peptides, Growth Factors, and New (Anti) Steroidal Agents, edited by Jan G. M. Klijn et al. Raven Press, New York © 1987.

DIRECT EFFECTS OF LHRH ANALOGS ON BREAST AND PROSTATIC TUMOR CELLS

J.A. Foekens (1), M.S. Henkelman (1), J. Bolt-de Vries (3), H. Portengen (1), J.F. Fukkink (1), M.A. Blankenstein (1), G.J. van Steenbrugge (4), E. Mulder (3) and J.G.M. Klijn (2)

Departments of Biochemistry (1) and Endocrinology (2) of The Dr Daniel den Hoed Cancer Center, P.O.Box 5201, Rotterdam, and Departments of Biochemistry II (Chemical Endocrinology) (3) and Urology (4) of the Erasmus University Rotterdam, The Netherlands

INTRODUCTION

Luteinizing hormone-releasing hormone (LHRH) is a hypothalamic secretory decapeptide which stimulates the secretion of gonadotropins from the pituitary. As a consequence these gonadotropins stimulate the gonads resulting in increased steroidogenesis. By chronic treatment with potent long-acting LHRH-agonists in sufficiently high doses a chemical castration can be reached through suppression of the pituitary-gonadal axis, and the underlying mechanism is believed to be a desensitization of the pituitary to LHRH (27). Chronic treatment with LHRH-agonists has appeared to be effective in premenopausal breast cancer (14-16,19,22,25,28) and in prostatic cancer (4,17,18,28,29). Direct inhibitory effects of LHRH-agonists on gonadal steroidogenesis have also been reported (for review see ref. 5). LHRH-like activity has been detected in human breast milk (1), and LHRH-like receptors have been demonstrated in various extra-pituitary tissues such as human breast carcinoma (7,24) and experimental prostate cancer (10). Therefore, in addition to the endocrine effects of LHRH-agonists in vivo, from which the steroid receptor positive tumors are likely to benefit, direct effects at the tumor cell level may also occur in vivo. Direct anti-tumor effects of the LHRH-agonist Buserelin on breast cancer cells in vitro have recently been reported by us (2,3,19) and by others (24,33). These observations lead to the assumption that LHRH-agonist therapy may have additional direct effects to the indirect effects of chemical castrations and may also be effective in postmenopausal breast cancer patients. In the few clinical studies reported so far for postmenopausal patients, however, conflicting results have been described (9,22,23,26,31). In the average, a response rate of 10% has been observed.

More studies are required to elucidate the mechanism of the direct anti-tumor action of LHRH-agonists, and we have therefore studied the effects of the LHRH-agonist Buserelin on the growth of human breast and prostate cancer cells in culture. Its effects on growth and several biochemical parameters were investigated in particular with steroid concentrations which resemble the plasma values in patients chronically treated with LHRH-agonists.

EFFECTS OF BUSERELIN, ESTRADIOL AND TAMOXIFEN ON MCF-7 HUMAN BREAST CANCER CELLS

Methods
MCF-7 human breast cancer cells were obtained from EG&G Mason Research Institute, Worcester, MA, USA. Cells were maintained in culture in a humidified atmosphere of 5% CO_2 and air at $37^\circ C$ and were passaged weekly in RPMI-1640 medium supplemented with 10% heat-inactivated fetal calf serum, 100 U/ml penicillin, 0.1 mg/ml streptomycin and 10 ng/ml insulin (complete growth medium). For experiments cells were trypsinized and seeded in complete growth medium which was replaced by experimental medium after 1 day. Experimental medium consisted of RPMI-1640 medium supplemented with 10% charcoal-treated male human serum. Charcoal treatment was performed either after inactivation (for 60 min at $56^\circ C$) with 0.05%-0.5% (w/v) dextran-coated charcoal for 20 h at $4^\circ C$ or by two incubations with 0.5% charcoal for 2x45 min at $50^\circ C$ each (Table 2, Figure 3) with an intermediate sulphatase incubation step (13). Unless indicated otherwise, medium was refreshed after 3 and 5 days followed by termination of the experiments at day 7 and subsequent protein- or DNA-assays, as described before (3).

Effects on MCF-7 cell proliferation
In medium containing fetal calf serum Buserelin appeared to have direct inhibitory effects, which could be abolished by LHRH-antagonists, on the growth of MCF-7 breast cancer cells (3,24). The mitogenic stimulation of the cell cultures by estradiol only appeared to be about 10% under the experimental conditions used (3). In the search for culture conditions which would result in a higher growth-stimulating effect of estradiol, it was found that by replacement of fetal calf serum for male human serum and by omitting insulin, the growth-stimulating effect of estradiol was much more pronounced. A dose-response relationship is shown in Figure 1 and it appeared that concentrations of estradiol between 10 and 100 pM already resulted in maximal stimulation of MCF-7 cell proliferation. For evaluation of possible physiological significance of direct anti-tumor effects of LHRH-agonists, further experiments were performed with a concentration of 30 pM estradiol, a concentration which falls within the range of the plasma values (5-50 pM) which are observed in chemically castrated premenopausal breast cancer patients when treated chronically with LHRH-agonists. It was found that Buserelin showed a dose-response

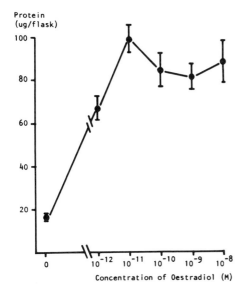

Buserelin concentration	inhibition (%)
8 nM	15 ± 11
72 nM	40 ± 18
270 nM	87 ± 6
760 nM	96 ± 5

Left:
FIGURE 1. Effect of increasing dosages of estradiol on the proliferation of MCF-7 cells. Data represent the mean ± SD of the monolayer protein contents of six incubations.

Right:
TABLE 1. Effect of increasing dosages of Buserelin on the estradiol-stimulated growth of MCF-7 cell cultures. Data represent the mean percent inhibition ± SD of the estradiol (30 pM)-stimulated growth (3.6-fold), as calculated on the basis of monolayer protein contents of six incubations.

relationship with respect to inhibition of the estrogen-induced growth-stimulation (Table 1). Almost complete inhibition was obtained at a concentration above 270 nM Buserelin. In subsequent studies we have observed variable results with respect to growth-stimulation by estradiol (both higher and lower) and subsequent inhibition by Buserelin. Both effects may highly depend on the composition of the different batches of human serum used. One could speculate that certain (autocrine or paracrine) growth factors are present in different amounts in serum batches, or that they are secreted into the medium (20, 21) in different quantities. Due to the experimental conditions used possible differences in interference of these growth factors with the actions of estradiol and/or Buserelin may have occurred. The inconsistency of the effects of Buserelin can also be the result from the frequency of medium refreshment (24).
At a concentration of approximately 500-fold excess of that of estradiol, Tamoxifen was fully able to exert its anti-estro-

genic action (Fig.2). Unexpectedly however, while both Tamoxifen and Buserelin (when added separately) were able to inhibit
the estrogen-induced growth-stimulation, combined addition of
both drugs to the estradiol containing cultures resulted in
less inhibition (Fig.2, right bar).

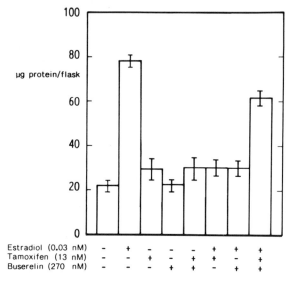

FIGURE 2. Effects of estradiol, Buserelin and Tamoxifen on the
proliferation of MCF-7 cells. Data represent the mean ± SD of
the monolayer protein contents of six incubations.

In subsequent experiments with 3-fold higher concentrations of
estradiol, Tamoxifen and Buserelin, a similar phenomenon was
observed (not shown). Although not completely comparable, these
results are conflicting with those observed by Wiznitzer and
Benz (33) who have used another breast cancer cell line
(T-47D), and found greater than additive growth-inhibition with
Buserelin and Tamoxifen in the presence of prolactin. In a
clinical study tumor regression did occur after administration
of a combination of Buserelin and Tamoxifen to premenopausal
breast cancer patients (15,16). Therefore, further studies are
required to clarify the observed in vitro results.

Effects on secretory proteins
Estradiol affects the synthesis of specific secretory
proteins (32), of which a 52K protein is believed to act as an
autocrine mitogen (30). We have investigated whether the synthesis of specific secretory proteins which are under estrogen
control was altered as a response of Buserelin action. Figure 3
shows that in cultures in the presence of estradiol several
specific secretory proteins are increased or decreased, when

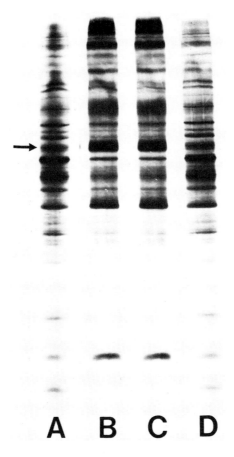

A B C D

FIGURE 3. Effects of estradiol and Buserelin on the synthesis of secretory proteins of MCF-7 cells. Cells were cultured in 24-well dishes in experimental medium in the absence or presence of estradiol (30 pM) and/or Buserelin (0.8 μM).
After incubation for 5 days, cells were labeled for 5 h with 100 μCi ^{35}S-methionine. The labeled proteins of the medium were analyzed by SDS-polyacrylamide gel (11%) electrophoresis and processed for fluorography.

A: control, B: + estradiol, C: + estradiol + Buserelin, D: + Buserelin. Arrow indicates position of 52 K molecular weight protein.

analyzed by SDS-PAGE followed by fluorography. The density of none of these protein bands appeared to be altered as a result of the additional presence of Buserelin in the cultures. Possible effects of Buserelin on posttranslational processes can not yet be excluded.

Another possibility may be that Buserelin affects the synthesis of small peptide growth factors which can serve as autocrine or paracrine regulators of cell proliferation (20,21). Epidermal growth factor (EGF), which secretion by MCF-7 cells is stimulated by estradiol (6,21), could be such a growth factor. We have studied the effects of estradiol and Buserelin, under the conditions of the experiments as described sofar in this report, on the secretion of polypeptides with EGF-like activities. Cells were precultured in medium supplemented with steroid-depleted male human serum with and without the addition of 30 pM estradiol and/or 0.8 µM Buserelin. After culturing for 3 days medium was replaced for serum-free medium containing additionally transferrin, fibronectin and Hepes, as described by Dickson et al (6). Conditioned media of the 24-96 h period was collected and assayed for the presence of EGF-like activities with a radio-receptor assay. In preliminary experiments no significant differences in the amounts of EGF-like activities, in the conditioned media, as a result of Buserelin treatment were found when expressed as ng EGF-like activity per mg DNA (Table 2).

	EGF-like activity (ng/mg DNA)
Control	4.2 ± 1.6
Buserelin	2.5 ± 0.6
Estradiol	5.1 ± 0.9
Estradiol + Buserelin	4.8 ± 1.0

TABLE 2. Effects of estradiol and Buserelin on the secretion of polypeptides with EGF-like activities by MCF-7 cells. Cells were precultured for 3 days in 75 cm^2 flasks in experimental medium in the absence or presence of estradiol (30 pM) and/or Buserelin (0.8 µM). Subsequently, monolayer cells were incubated in the same experimental media without serum but with the additions of transferrin, fibronectin and Hepes (6). Conditioned media were lyophilized and assayed for the presence of EGF-like activity with a radio-receptor assay for EGF using human placental membranes. Data presented are the means ± SD of triplicate cultures and expressed as ng EGF-like activity/mg monolayer DNA.

Moreover, no stimulating effect of estradiol on the secretion of polypeptides with EGF-like activities was observed (Table 2). This is in contrast with observations of Dickson et al (6), who did however use higher concentrations of estradiol (1000 pM vs 30 pM in our experiments) to stimulate the MCF-7 cell cultures. Nevertheless, it is unlikely from the preliminary data (as reported in Table 2) that the inhibition of cell growth caused by Buserelin (Table 1, Fig.2) could be due to effects on the secretion of polypeptides with EGF-like activities.

Effects on steroid receptors
Experiments were performed to study whether the inhibitory effects of Buserelin on the estrogen-stimulated growth of the MCF-7 cell cultures may in some way be related to changes in the amounts of steroid receptors. After culturing of the cells in the absence or presence of estradiol and Buserelin, cytosolic and nuclear estrogen and progesterone receptors were measured. Buserelin (0.8 µM) had no effect on the amount of estrogen receptors (not shown), whereas the estrogen (30 pM)-induced progesterone receptor amounts were reduced (Table 3).

| | progesterone receptor | |
Conditions	cytosol (fmol/mg P)	nucleus (fmol/mg DNA)
Control	1020	2200
Buserelin	1500	2000
Estradiol	4820	2900
Estradiol + Buserelin	1540	830
Estradiol + Tamoxifen	1770	1580
Estradiol + Tamoxifen + Buserelin	2180	3780

TABLE 3. Effects of estradiol (30 pM), Buserelin (0.8 µM) and Tamoxifen (40 nM) on the progesterone receptor content of MCF-7 cells.

In the presence of 40 nM Tamoxifen Buserelin had a less pronounced effect on the estradiol-induced progesterone receptor synthesis. Interference of Buserelin and Tamoxifen on the level of the progesterone receptor synthesis might explain the interference in cell growth inhibition as described in Fig.2. On the

other hand it may not be conceivable to explain the direct
inhibitory action of Buserelin solely by its inhibiting effect
on the estrogen-induced progesterone receptor synthesis, because some anti-estrogens which were able to inhibit breast
cancer cell growth in vitro on the contrary caused an increase
in progesterone receptor synthesis (8). Similar results were
obtained by Tamoxifen at low concentrations (below 0.1 μM),
although the growth inhibitory effects were minor (12).

EFFECTS OF BUSERELIN AND METHYLTRIENOLONE
ON THE GROWTH OF LNCaP HUMAN PROSTATE CANCER CELLS

Methods

The LNCaP-FGC cell line (derived from a lymphe node
carcinoma of the prostate) was a gift of Dr. Horoszewicz
(Buffalo, NY). Cells were maintained in culture in a humidified
atmosphere of 5% CO_2 and air at $37^\circ C$ in RPMI-1640 medium
supplemented with 15% heat-inactivated fetal calf serum (FCS),
10,000 IU penicillin and 10,000 μg streptomycin. Cells were
passaged weekly by trypsinization and for experiments 5×10^5
cells were seeded in T-25 flasks in medium containing 5%
heat-inactivated FCS which had been depleted of steroids by two
incubations with dextran-coated charcoal (0.1% dextran, 1.0%
charcoal). After three days medium was replaced for medium
containing the additions of the components to be studied.
Subsequently every second day the medium was refreshed and
after culturing for 6 days the cells were harvested as
described before (3). For each condition six-fold incubations
were used.

Effects on cell proliferation

The LNCaP human prostate cell line was used as an in vitro
model to study the effect of Buserelin on the growth of prostate cancer cells. The LNCaP cells are androgen responsive in
vitro, produce acid phosphatase, contain androgen receptors and
grow in vitro with a doubling time of 60 h (11). The synthetic
androgen R1881 at concentrations of 10 pM and 100 pM stimulated
the growth of the cell cultures significantly (p < 0.005, Wil-
coxon test) with 20% and 107% respectively. In cultures in the
presence of 100 pM R1881 no inhibiting effect of Buserelin on
the androgen-induced growth was observed (Fig.4). With lower
concentration of R1881 (10 pM), a concentration which is comparable to the free plasma testosterone concentration in
chemically castrated prostate cancer patients, a significant
inhibition of the androgen-stimulated growth (88% inhibition of
the 20% stimulated growth, p < 0.005) was observed (Fig.4).
Also in the absence of added androgen Buserelin inhibited the
growth of the cell cultures (10% inhibition, p < 0.005). This
10%-effect may also have been caused by inhibition of the
androgen-induced growth stimulation, due to traces of androgen

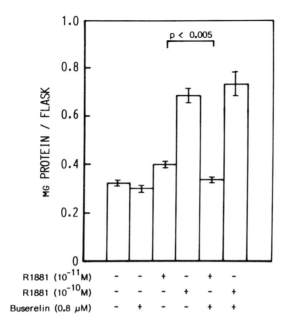

FIGURE 4. Effects of Methyltrienolone (R1881) and Buserelin on the growth of LNCaP human prostate cancer cells. Data represent the mean ± SD of the monolayer protein contents of six incubations.

left behind after charcoal treatment of the serum. Although these preliminary data show that the growth of human prostate cancer cells can be inhibited by the LHRH-agonist Buserelin, no definite conclusions can be drawn yet whether the effect of Buserelin is only on the androgen-stimulated growth or also on the unstimulated growth.

SUMMARY AND CONCLUSIONS

The LHRH-agonist Buserelin has direct inhibitory effects on the growth of breast and prostate (preliminary data) cancer cells in vitro in the presence of low concentrations of steroid hormones. Thus, LHRH-agonists may have the potential to inhibit in vivo the growth of endocrine related tumors directly at the tumor cell level after surgical or medical castration in premenopausal women. Miller et al (24), using different experimental conditions, have shown that concentrations as low as 1 nM Buserelin, which can currently be obtained in plasma of patients, already resulted in a net decrease of MCF-7 cell growth in vitro. The availability of different drug preparations will determine the relative contribution of direct anti-tumor effects, depending on the plasma LHRH-agonist concentration which can be reached.

The mechanism of action which is responsible for the observed growth-inhibiting effects of Buserelin still remains unclear. The effects are probably not a result of altered synthesis of secretory proteins which can be evaluated with SDS-PAGE, and of effects on the secretion of polypeptides with EGF-like activities. Inhibitory effects on the estrogen-induced progesterone receptor synthesis in MCF-7 cells may be one of the events resulting in breast cancer cell growth-inhibition directly at the cellular level. More studies are required to come to the elucidation of the underlying mechanism of action of LHRH analogs, both for breast cancer and prostate cancer cells.

ACKNOWLEDGEMENTS

We thank Hoechst AG, Frankfurt, FRG, and the Medical Department of Hoechst Holland BV for supplies of the LHRH-agonist Buserelin. We thank Mrs M.J. Slotboom and Mrs A. Sugiarsi for administrative help and J. Marselje for preparing the prints.

This study is sponsored in part by the Netherlands Cancer Foundation (KWF) through grant No. RRTI 83-3.

REFERENCES

1. Amarant, T., Fridkin, M., and Koch, Y. (1982): Eur. J. Biochem. 127:647-650.
2. Blankenstein, M.A., Henkelman, M.S., and Klijn, J.G.M. (1983): J. Steroid Biochem. 19, Suppl., 95S.
3. Blankenstein, M.A., Henkelman, M.S., and Klijn, J.G.M. (1985): Eur. J. Cancer Clin. Oncol. 21:1493-1499.
4. Borgmann, V., Hardt, W., Schmidt-Gollwitzer, M., Adenauer, H., and Nagel, R. (1982): Lancet I:1097-1099.
5. Cooke, B.A., and Sullivan, M.H.F. (1985): Molec. Cell Endocrinol. 41:115-122.
6. Dickson, R.B., Huff, K.K., Spencer, E.M., and Lippman, M.E. (1986): Endocrinol. 118:138-142.
7. Eidne, K.A., Flanagan, C.A., and Miller, R.P. (1985): Science 229:989-992.
8. Eckert, R.L., and Katzenellebogen, B.S. (1982): Cancer Res. 42:139-144.
9. Harvey, H.A., Lipton, A., and Max, D.T. (1984). In: LHRH and its analogues, contraceptive and clinical application, edited by B.H. Vickery, J.J. Hestor and E.S.E. Hafex, pp 329-338, MTP, Lancaster.
10. Hierowski, M.T., Altamirano, P., Redding, T.W., and Schally, A.V. (1983): FEBS Lett. 154:92-96.

11. Horoszewicz, J.S., Leong, S.S., Kawinski, E., Karr, J.P., Rosenthal, H., Chu, T.M., Mirand, E.A., and Murphy G.P. (1983): Cancer Res. 43:1809-1818.
12. Horwitz, K.B., Koseki, Y., and McGuire W.L. (1978): Endocrinol. 103:1742-1751.
13. Jakesz, R., Smith, C.A. Aitken, S., Huff, K.K., Schnette, W., Schakney, S., and Lippman, M.E. (1984): Cancer Res. 44:619-625.
14. Klijn, J.G.M., and de Jong, F.H. (1982): Lancet i:1213-1216.
15. Klijn, J.G.M. (1984): J. Med. Oncol. & Tumor Pharmacother. 1:123-128.
16. Klijn, J.G.M., de Jong, F.H., Blankenstein, M.A., Docter, R., Alexieva-Figusch, A., Blonk-van der Wijst, J., and Lamberts, S.W.J. (1984): Breast Cancer Res. Treatm. 4:209-220.
17. Klijn, J.G.M., de Jong, F.H., Lamberts, S.W.J., and Blankenstein, M.A. (1984): Eur. J. Cancer Clin. Oncol. 20:483-493.
18. Klijn, J.G.M. (1985): Lancet ii:493.
19. Klijn, J.G.M., de Jong, F.H., Lamberts, S.W.J., and Blankenstein, M.A. (1985): J. Steroid Biochem. 23:867-873.
20. Lippman, M.E. (1985): Clin. Res. 33:375-382.
21. Lippman, M.E., Dickson, R.B., Bates, S., Knabbe, C., Huff, K., Swain, S., McManaway, M., Bronzert, D., Kasid, A., and Gelmann, E.P. (1986): Breast Cancer Res. Treatm. 7:59-70.
22. Manni, A., Santen, R., Harvey, H., Lipton, A., and Max, D. (1986): Endocrine Rev. 7:89-94.
23. Mathé, G., Keiling, R., VoVan, M.L., Gastiaburu, J., Prévot, G., Vannetzel, J.M., Despax, R., Jasmin, C., Lévi, F., Musset, M., Muchover, D., and Misset, J.L. (1986): Eur. J. Cancer Clin. Oncol. 22:723.
24. Miller, W.R., Scott, W.N., Morris, R., Fraser, H.M., and Sharpe, R.M. (1985): Nature 313:231-233.
25. Nicholson, R.I., Walker, K.J., Turkes, A., Turkes, A.O., Dyas, J., Blamey, R.W., Campbell, F.C., Robinson, M.R.G., and Griffiths, K. (1984): J. Steroid Biochem. 20:129-135.
26. Plowman, P.N., Nicholson, R.I., and Walker, K.J. (1986): Eur. J. Cancer Clin. Oncol. 22:746.
27. Sandow, J. (1983): Clin. Endocrinol. 18:571-592.
28. Schally, A.V., Redding, T.W., and Comaru-Schally, A.M. (1984): Cancer Treatm. Rep. 68:281-289.
29. Tolis, G., Ackman, D., Stellos, A., Menta, A., Labrie, F., Fazekas, A.T.A., Comaru-Schally, A.M., and Schally, A.V. (1982): Proc. Natl. Acad. Sci. USA 79:1658-1662.
30. Vignon, F., Capony, F., Chambon, M., Freiss, G., Garcia, M., and Rochefort, H. (1986): Endocrinol. 118:1537-1544.

31. Waxman, J.H., Harland, S.J., Coombes, R.C., Wrigley, P.F.M., Malpas, J.S., Powles, T., and Lister, T.A. (1985): Cancer Chemother. Pharmacol. 15:171-173.
32. Westley, B., and Rochefort, H. (1980): Cell 20:353-362.
33. Wiznitzer, I., and Benz, C. (1984): Proc. Ann. Am. Assoc. Cancer Res. 25:208.

Hormonal Manipulation of Cancer: Peptides,
Growth Factors, and New (Anti) Steroidal
Agents, edited by Jan G. M. Klijn et al.
Raven Press, New York © 1987.

Mechanisms of Estrogenic and Antiestrogenic
Regulation of Growth of Human Breast Carcinoma

Marc E. Lippman
Robert B. Dickson
Edward P. Gelmann
Cornelius Knabbe
Attan Kasid
Susan Bates
Sandra Swain

Medical Breast Cancer Section, Medicine Branch,
National Cancer Institute, Bldg. 10, Room 12N226
Bethesda, Maryland 20892 USA
Outline

Introduction

Breast cancer growth is strongly regulated in about 1/3 of
clinical cases by therapies which alter concentrations or activities of estrogens (72). Breast cancer occurs in women who have
never had functional ovaries with only 1% of the frequency of
that in women with intact ovaries. Thus estrogens play a critical role, at least initially, in nearly all breast cancers. This
hormonal component of growth control appears to be a remnant of
a normal or differentiated mechanism of epithelial proliferation.
At puberty and throughout menstrual life including pregnancy-
lactation, estrogen exerts mitogenic, anabolic and secretory effects on mammary epithelium. While estrogen is a proximate mitogen for either normal or malignant breast epithelium, the hypo-
thalamus-pituitary axis is indirectly in control of ovarian
estrogen secretion by virtue of GnRH and gonadotropin stimulation
(81). In addition, the pituitary gland (or other organs) may secrete as yet undefined direct or indirect acting mitogens. Such
hypothetical, estrogen induced, endocrine acting mitogens have
been termed estromedins (32,48). The hormonal control of cancer
cell proliferation has recently received an additional potential
regulatory component with the proposal of autocrine or self
stimulating polypeptide growth factors (40).

In this article we will review our studies on the biochemical
and molecular events, induced by estrogen, which are associated

with direct stimulation of proliferation of human breast cancer cell lines in vitro and in vivo. Using clonal lines of cells, usually derived from pleural or ascites fluid of patients, we and subsequently others have succeeded in demonstrating receptors for and direct proliferative responses to physiologic doses of 17β - estradiol $(E_2)(12,69,78,89)$. Several such estrogen responsive lines exist, including MCF-7, T47D, MDA-MB-134 ZR-75-1 and CAMA-1 (33). MCF-7 is the best characterized of these. After summarizing these results we will turn to a consideration of the mechanisms by which such cells respond to estrogens. We will then examine some recent experiments whereby the tumorigenic properties of MCF-7 cells are enhanced by v-ras[H] oncogene transfection, bypassing estrogen controls. Finally, we will provide evidence that growth inhibitors exert their negative effects on cell proliferation, at least in part, by secretion of growth inhibitory substances.

Responses of Human Breast Cancer to Estrogens and Antiestrogens

A systematic search in MCF-7 and other breast cancer cells has led to observations that E_2 induces a large number of enzymes involved in nucleic acid synthesis, including DNA polymerase, thymidine and uridine kinases, thymidylate synthetase, carbamyl phosphate synthetase, aspartate transcarbamylase dihydroorotase, and dihydrofolate reductase (1,2). Physiologic concentrations of E_2 stimulate DNA synthesis by both scavenger and de novo biosynthetic pathways. In two instances recently reported, estrogen regulates thymidine kinase and dihydrofolate reductase at the mRNA level (20,58). Regulation of thymidine kinase mRNA occurs, at least in part, at the transcriptional level (58). Estrogens appear to modulate many enzyme activities involved in growth. Whether, growth is induced by generalized induction of numerous genes or by pleiotropic or cascade mechanisms is not known. The existence of "second message" regulatory systems in this process is possible and much of the data to be reviewed here is supportive of such a pathway. We have also recently observed that E_2 stimulates time the turnover of phosphatidyl inositol in MCF-7 cells (36). In a variety of other model systems, this metabolic effect is quite rapid and tightly coupled to growth control by proteases and hormones, particularly the polypeptide growth factors (17,75). In breast cancer cells, phosphatidyl inositol induction is slower. Estrogen induction of growth factors (to be described below) could explain the delayed time course of the phospholipid effects. Thus, phosphatidyl inositol turnover, with its associated stimulation of protein kinase C and Ca++ fluxes could be a fundamental metabolic mediator of mitogenic effects of E_2.

Others have identified the progesterone receptor (44) as an additional protein induced by estrogen. However, progesterone is apparently not directly growth modulatory of human breast cancer. The presence of the progesterone receptor does, however, appear tightly coupled to functional growth regulation by estrogen. Thus progesterone receptor content of human breast tumors is used (along with the estrogen receptor) as a marker for estrogen and antiestrogen responsiveness of tumors in clinical therapy (72).

In addition to regulation of these essential growth control-ling enzymes and the progesterone receptor, estrogens (and anti-estrogenic compounds) alter the cellular or secreted activity of several other proteins whose function in growth control remains less well characterized. These include plasminogen activator and other collagenolytic enzymes (15), several relatively abundant secreted proteins, including a 24KDa protein described by McGuire and colleagues (18), 52 and 160 KDa glycoproteins described by Rochefort and colleagues (101), a 39 KDa glycoprotein complex (10), a 7KDa protein initially identified by Chambon and col-leagues by detection of an estrogen induced mRNA species (termed pS2) (51), and the cytoplasmic enzyme LDH (14). Plasminogen activator (along with other proteases) is thought to contribute to tumor progression and growth by allowing the tumor to digest and traverse encapsulating basement membrane (68). While this is likely, it is conceivable that proteases may serve additional roles such as facilitating release of mitogenic growth factors like IGF-I (somatomedin C) from carrier proteins, or to process inactive precursor growth factors and proteases to active species (59). Interestingly, one of the major secreted proteins, the 52 KDa glycoprotein, is also reported to have biologic activity in purified form -- it is mitogenic for MCF-7 cells when tested in vitro (97). These investigators have recently discovered that purified 52 has proteolytic activity and thus its mitogenic ef-fects may be linked to cel surface proteolysis. The activities of the 160, 39, 24, and 7KDa proteins are unknown at present. It is of note that at least the 160, 52, and 7KDa secreted proteins may apparently be disassociated from estrogen and antiestrogen modulation of MCF-7 cells growth using two MCF-7 clonal variants aberrant in their growth control by these agents (8,9,21). These three protein species are decreased by antiestrogen to the same extent in MCF-7 and LY2, a stable antiestrogen resistant variant of MCF-7. This suggests that a significant reduction in secre-tion of these proteins has no impact on growth in the case of LY2. In I-13, an MCF-7 clonal variant which is growth arrested by physiologic concentrations of E_2, the same three proteins are induced to the same extent as in MCF-7.

Finally, we have recently demonstrated that estrogen induces another function in MCF-7 cells, the cell surface "receptor" or binding protein for laminin. The laminin receptor is thought to mediate attachment of cells to basement membrane laminin (68) and contribute to cellular invasiveness out of the tumor confines to colonize new areas of the host. E_2 treatment of MCF-7 cells in-creases I^{125}-laminin binding, cell attachment to artificial laminin-coated membranes, and migration of the same cells across an artificial membrane toward a diffusable source of laminin (3).

In summary, while estrogens may exert a considerable number of influences in vivo which may indirectly alter breast cancer progression, direct effects of estrogens on isolated breast cancer cells in vitro are also well established. These effects include growth regulation itself as well as modulation of enzymes and other activities thought to mediate mitogenic and metastatic events. Later we will consider estrogenic influences on a class of secreted proteins which although relatively minor in abundance are very active biologically—the polypeptide growth factors. These factors, along with some of the above-mentioned major secreted proteins, are likely candidates as "second messengers" in the actions of estrogen on breast cancer. Milk, the normal secretory product of untransformed mammary epithelium, is an abundantly rich source of growth factor activities (13, 104). These factors in milk are important in neonatal development and nutrition or have additional actions on the mammary gland. Since, breast cancer cells produce and respond to these growth factors, it seems possible that growth factor secretion either by itself or in the presence of some as yet undefined transforming event may play a critical factor in neoplastic progression.

The triphenylethylene antiestrogen prototype known as tamoxifen has become a mainstay in breast cancer as well as in advanced disease and is used effectively either by itself or when used in combination with cytotoxic chemotherapy. In contrast to cytotoxic agents, antiestrogens appear to be cytostatic rather than cytocidal and have a remarkably low incidence of significant side effects. Many investigators have noted the close correlation between the clinical response to antiestrogens and the presence of the estrogen receptor (and its induced product—the progesterone receptor). Since antiestrogens and their active metabolites have a high affinity for the same receptor, the most likely explanation of antiestrogen action appears to be simple antagonism of the growth promoting effects of estrogen (54,71). However, alternate views involving other microsomal binding sites for antiestrogen have been presented (99).

Antiestrogen treatment of estrogen dependent breast cancer leads to cell cycle blockade (early G_1) of most of the cells in vitro and to arrest in tumor growth in vivo (54,76,77,93). It had been initially observed that MCF-7 cells responded in vitro to both estrogens and antiestrogens under normal cell culture conditions (69). While these experiments could be interpreted to suggest that antiestrogens could act (to arrest growth) independently of an occupied estrogen-receptor complex, recent work by Katzenellenbogen and coworkers has clearly shown that high concentrations of phenol red present in the culture medium of the cells in these studies was a highly significant estrogenic stimulus (7). Removal of phenol red, whose structure resembles that of certain nonsteroidal estrogens, abrogated antiestrogen action on MCF-7 cells and dramatically enhanced the responsiveness of the cells to estrogen induction of cell growth and progesterone

receptor. There remains little compelling evidence at present
that antiestrogens act in any fashion other than by direct antagonism of the initiation of signals generated by an agonist occupied receptor. These studies provide irrefutable evidence for
the direct estrogen responsivity of human breast cancer cells.

The principle limitation with respect to the clinical utility
of antiestrogens is the gradual resistance which develops in tumors treated with these agents. While in some cases, antiestrogen
resistant tumors lack the estrogen receptor, it is not likely
that loss of the estrogen receptors explains even a majority of
the instances of in vivo loss of antiestrogen sensitivity during
treatment. It is of interest that a model system for acquired
resistance, a stable clone of MCF-7 cells stepwise selected in
vitro for antiestrogen resistance, still contains high levels of
the estrogen receptor (9). These data suggest that positive and
negative growth control elements lie distal to the estrogen receptor; data for this contention follows.

A well established system in the study of polypeptide growth
factor action has been the growth of rodent fibroblasts in vitro.
Studies were initially carried out in cell monolayers on plastic
surfaces. Smith, Scher and Todaro, among others, identified
"restriction points" in the cell cycle of "normal" (but immortalized) fibroblasts. Various growth factors abrogated these restriction points, allowing the cell cycle to progress (88).
Platelet derived growth factor (PDGF), a "competence" growth factor, allowed cells to pass a restriction point in early G_1, epidermal growth factor (EGF or the related transforming growth fac
tor $\propto$, TGF $\propto$) acted later, while insulin-like growth factor-I
(IGF-I or somatomedin C) acted still later in G_1 (43). EGF and
IGF-I are "progression growth factors. Malignant transformation
was proposed to result from ectopic production of growth factors,
abolishing both competence and progression restriction points in
a cell's own cycle. One consequence of this appears to be the
serum independent growth of some cancer cells (23,79,90).

An "anchorage independent" growth assay was also developed
using agar or agarose suspensions of cells. It had been observed
that the ability of cells to grow in colonies under anchorage independent conditions was correlated with their tumorigenicity or
state of malignant "transformation" (35). Research from a number
of laboratories over the past few years has identified at least
four growth factor activities which together can reversibly induce the transformed phenotype in murine fibroblasts. These
studies have identified PDGF, EGF (or TGF $\propto$), IGF-I (or IGF-II),
a different somatomedin activity) and an additional growth factor, transforming growth factor β (TGF β) (4,73,88). These growth
factors are considered likely to be involved in cancer growth
control for this reason. However, it should be emphasized that
the murine fibroblast model system may not apply to cancers of
other tissues or species of origin.

The principle restriction points for epithelial cell growth are unknown. A major departure from the fibroblast model, however, is the fact that TGF is a growth inhibitor for many types of primary and malignant epithelial cells (80,96). Therefore, it is likely that while some of the same growth factors may facilitate traverse of the cell cycle in fibroblasts and epithelial cells, control of anchorage independant growth may involve another another less well defined growth factor(s). A candidate for such a growth factor is provided by the work of Halper and Moses (42). Basic pituitary FGF can subserve such a function in cloning of an adrenal carcinoma cell line (SW13), and epithelial cancers produce a related activity which remains relatively uncharacterized at present. A variety of other growth factors have been described. However, description of these is well beyond the scope of the current article - several reviews are now available (40,43,90). Not withstanding the unknown features of cell cycle control in breast cancer, we have begun the analysis of its secreted growth factors with study of representative members of all of the above mentioned activity classes: PDGF, TGFα, IGF-I, TGFβ, and an epithelial transformation factor. We have placed special emphasis on the regulatory effects of the proximate mitogen, estradiol on the activities of these growth factors.

We and others have shown growth regulation of MCF-7 cells in monolayer culture by a variety of lipid soluble trophic hormones other than estradiol. These include glucocorticoids, iodothyronines, androgens and retinoids. MCF-7 cells have receptors but very little growth response to progesterone and vitamin D. Additional studies have demonstrated receptors for and responses to the polypeptides, insulin, EGF, and IGF-I. Receptors, but little cellular response has been demonstrated for other hormones, such as prolactin and calcitonin (70). The multiplicity of growth stimulating hormones for breast cancer cell culture systems in vitro has several interpretations. Obviously, multiple hormones may influence breast cancer growth. Alternatively, serum borne indirect hormonally mediated effects of E_2 (estromedins) may play important contributory roles in vivo (49). Finally, growth factors with a similar spectrum of activities could be elaborated by the breast cancer cells themselves. E_2 is an absolute tumor growth requirement for two human cell lines, MCF-7 and T47D, and a growth stimulator for a third cell line, ZR-75-1, in vivo in the nude (athymic) mouse model system (15, 29,77). McGrath and his colleagues have further defined this system by showing that E_2 need not enter the systemic circulation in nude mice to promote sufficient MCF-7 tumorigenesis; elevation of local E_2 concentration near the tumor was efficient (47). This suggests that if estrogen acts by inducing changes in the host which permit tumor growth, the production and action of such factors is probably restricted to the local area of the tumor. The mammary stroma is however likely to provide an as yet unidentified contributory factor(s) in vivo for full mitogenicity of estrogen (74). Other human breast cancer cell lines, such as Hs578T and MDA-MB-231, lack estrogen receptors and form rapidly growing, estrogen independent tumors in the nude mouse (29,33,41). These 5 human cell lines (MCF-7, ZR-75-1, T47D, Hs578T, MDA-MB-231) have been studied in detail by our laboratory in an attempt to better understand growth regulation of breast cancer in vivo and in vitro.

We have directed our attention to the possible involvement of secreted growth factors in growth control of breast cancer by an observation made with MCF-7 cells plated at various densities. We found that initial growth rate was proportional to number of cells plated (50). While multiple interpretations of these data are possible, they are consistent with the production of auto-stimulatory growth factors by the MCF-7 cells. In preliminary experiments we found that conditioned medium (CME_2) harvested from MCF-7 cells treated with E_2 was capable of stimulating thymidine incorporation and proliferation of other MCF-7 cells. The residual E_2 was removed from CME_2 prior to analyses. This kind of result had also been obtained by Vignon and Rochefort and their colleagues (98) who had noticed that MCF-7 cells grew faster with less frequent medium exchanges as compared to cells in which medium was changed every other day. They had also noted that CME_2 was directly capable of stimulating other MCF-7 cells.

We therefore began the fractionation and purification of CM from MCF-7 and other breast cancer cell lines to identify the growth factors present. These cell lines secrete stimulatory activity for MCF-7 and 3T3 fibroblast monolayer cultures as well as "transforming growth activity" (TGF) for anchorage independent growth of NRK and AKR-2B fibroblasts in soft agar culture (29,30, 62,83). In initial studies using acid Biogel P60 and P150 chromatography we identified a 30 KDa apparent molecular weight peak of transforming activity for NRK fibroblasts. This peak also coincided with a peak of MCF-7 stimulating activity and the principle species of EGF receptor competing activity (29,30). This peak of activity was also identified by an antibody specific for TGF species but not corss reacting with EGF. Thus, this activity may be related to TGFα, but it appears to be larger than the cloned and sequenced 6 KDa species from transformed fibroblasts (24). The 30 KDa TGFα -like species is induced by E_2 treatment of MCF-7, T47D, and ZR-75-1 cells ranging from 2-8 fold depending on cell type and culture conditions. Current experiments are focused on regulation, purification and characterization of this activity. The expected 4.8 Kb TGFα mRNA species has been detected by Derynck and coworkers in MCF-7 and some other human breast cancer cell lines (24,26). It is of interest that some, but not all, estrogen independent breast cancer cells secrete high levels of the TGFα -like activity (29).

Both EGF and TGFα can act via the EGF receptor on both diploid and immortalized cell lines. Many groups of investigators have detected the EGF receptor in human and rodent mammary tumor biopsies and malignant cell lines (22,34). The receptor observed appears to be very similar to or identifcal with the cloned and sequenced human EGF receptor. The apparent molecular size is 170 kDa and the kinase domain is unaltered as determined by S1 ribonuclease analysis (22). At the present time little work has addressed the state of phosphorylation or the tyrosine kinase activity of the receptor. Chronic activation of the EGF/TGF autocrine loop may be achieved by mutation of the EGF receptor (the v-erb-B oncogene) and discussed later.

Using radioimmunoassay, we and others have noted that a second potential autostimulatory mitogen, IGF-I is also secreted by all human breast cancer cells examined to date (6,45). This species, partially purified from MCF-7 cells comigrates with authentic serum-derived IGF-I after acid ethanol extraction. IGF-I mRNA species were also detected with northern blot analysis using a DNA probe to authentic IGF-I (52). One of these, a 300 bp mRNA corresponded to the smallest of 3 RNA transcripts observed in poly A selected RNA from human liver in the same study. We initially observed no E_2 induction of secreted IGF-I in standard culture conditions employing phenol red-containing medium although antiestrogens inhibited IGF-1 secretion. Subsequent studies, utilizing the more substantially estrogen depleted phenol red-free medium, have observed a 2-3-fold IGF-I induction with E_2 treatment (46). IGF-I secretion is inhibited by the growth-inhibitory antiestrogens (in phenol red containing medium) and glucocorticoids. Current work is focussed on the mechanism of IGF-I induction and its possible biological role(s). Interestingly, two highly malignant estrogen receptor negative breast cancer cell lines (MDA-MB-231 and Hs-578T) secrete high levels of IGF-I and have low responsiveness to exogenous IGF-I (45).

IGF-I mitogenesis is mediated by its receptor, a close homologue of the insulin receptor. The receptor in a variety of cell types consists of a 450 kDa complex (2α chains of 130 kDa and 2β chains of 85 kDa)(40). The receptor has not been purified, cloned or sequenced at the present time, but it is thought to possess protein kinase activity (40). Its mechanism of action is largely unknown but is thought to stimulate growth by some as yet undefined post transcriptional mechanism (16). IGF-I receptors of the expected size have been reported on several human breast cancer cell lines. The qualities of IGF-I secreted into the medium are more than sufficient to saturate the IGF-I receptors found on all of the breast cancer cell lines we have thus far studied. We conclude that IGF-I is a hormonally regulated autocrine growth stimulator. This is further substantiated by nude mouse data to be described later.

In addition to IGF-I and the TGF α species previously mentioned, all breast cancer cell lines which we have examined to date secrete a PDGF-related activity detected by anchorage dependent growth stimulation of 3T3 fibroblasts in the presence of platelet poor plasma (11,82). Immunoprecipitation of metabolic labeled MDA-MB-231 breast cancer cell extracts and medium detected the expected 28 KDa and 14 KDa species. Several of the breast cancer cell lines while secreting radioreceptor reactive and immunoreactive PDGF fail to have detectable mRNA transcripts detectable with a human c-sis probe. This will only recognize the chain of PDGF. Normal PDGF is a heterodimer of a and b chains. We are thus exploring the possibilities that these breast cancers may secrete homodimers of a chains. Current research is addressing what its focussed on determining if the PDGF-like species is regulated and what its function might be. Human breast cancer cells are not known to be growth regulated by PDGF. Rather, its role might be paracrine in nature. Interestingly, the highly tumorigenic MDA-MB-231 cell line produces the most PDGF of the cell lines examined so far (11).

PDGF acts through its 185 kDa tyrosine kinase receptor on a variety of mesenchymal cell types (40). The receptor has recently been purified, cloned, and sequenced (102). It has not yet been reported in human mammary carcinoma cell lines.

A Novel Anchorage Independent Epithelial Growth Factor

The hormonal controls on the cell cycle for epithelial cells are only poorly understood. While it is known that EGF and IGF-I are commonly mitogenic and TGFβ commonly growth inhibitory for epithelial cells, the corresponding restriction points in the cell cycle where these growth factors might act is largely unknown. In addition, the controls for anchorage independent growth are also mysterious. Halper and Moses (42) have established a model system with human SW-13 adrenal carcinoma cells in soft agar culture. These cells clone poorly unless basic fibroblast growth factor (FGF) or conditioned medium from certain epithelial cancers is applied. No other growth factors are known to be active. This activity has been only partially characterized from kidney but appears to be 40-42KDa in size.

We have begun to purify a related activity from human breast cancer cells (94). The most tumorigenic lines MDA-MB-231 and Hs578T produce high levels of the activity, while estrogen receptor containing lines produce much lower levels. The activity from MDA-MB-231 cells is very acidic in its isoelectric point, and approximately 60KDa in size by gel filtration and gel electrophoresis. It has been purified to near homogeneity by an acid-ethanol extraction, isoelectric focussing, and HPLC sizing. Current work is directed toward complete purification and characterization of this activity and examination of its regulation (94). This activity has some similarities to a growth factor described by Kidwell (13,104) but preliminary data suggest that they are distinct.

In summary, we have observed that estrogen regulation of MCF-7

cells is associated with inductions of TGF   and IGF-I and re-
pression of TGF β. It is possible that estrogen-antiestrogen regulation of MCF-7 cells is at least partly mediated by coordinant
effects on growth stimulatory and growth inhibitory growth factor
"second messengers." Future studies with blocking antibodies
against growth factors and these receptors should help evaluate
this this hypothesis. Two other growth factors are also secreted
by MCF-7 cells, PDGF and a partially characterized epithelial
transforming factor. These two activities (sometimes in association with high levels of TGF α, TGF β, and IGF-I) are produced
in very large amounts by estrogen receptor negative, highly tumorigenic lines. Estrogen independent cancers are associated
with inceased output of a large number of growth factor activities. The critical growth factors in this type of cancer will
undoubtably require extensive future study. In the next section
we will further evaluate growth factor secretion as it relates
to malignant status in a nude model system for tumor progression.

We wanted to determine if CM proteins were capable of acting
humorally in vivo in the nude mouse to stimulate MCF-7 tumorigenesis (31). For this purpose we developed a serum free culture
system which has supported cell growth for all five above mentioned cell lines for up to one week. The medium consists of
Richter's IMEM + 2 mg/L transferrin + 2 mg/L fibronectin. MCF-7
cells $\pm$ E_2 pretreatment (10^{-9}M, 4 days) were used to condition
serum free medium, collected over a subsequent 2 day period (CM
and CME_2). Media were dialyzed extensively against 1 M acetic
acid, lyophilized, reconstituted in phosphate buffered saline
and precipitated protein removed. This extraction also removed
99.98% of the residual E_2. Reconstituted CM and CME_2 were infused into athymic female oophorectomized mice via Alzet minipumps. The equivalent of 10 ml of CM or CME_2 per day for 4 weeks
were infused from a mid-dorsal, subcutaneous location. MCF-7
injected ($2-5 \times 10^6$ cells/injection) at 4 different mammary fat pad
locations in each mouse. Small tumors (up to 0.5 cm diameter)
appeared at MCF-7 sites within 2 weeks. Tumors in CME_2 infused
animals appeared with 2-3-fold greater frequency than in CM infused animals; animals innoculated with only MCF-7 cells and sham
pump implantations did not have tumors. CM and CME_2 supported
tumors reached maximum size in 2-3 weeks of treatment, usually
declining in size thereafter, whereas, E_2-pellet implanted animals have continuously growing tumors for at least 4 weeks and
they do not regress. CM and CME_2 induced tumors were verified
as adenocarcinoma by histologic analysis. While the CME_2 supported tumor growth, uterine weight was unaffected. In addition,
CME_2 activity was decreased by treatment with trypsin, a reducing
reducing reagent, or heating to 56°C for 1 hour. Therefore the
tumor growth promoting substance(s) in CME_2 was unlike E_2, and
likely to be similar to a polypeptide growth factor(s). These
data suggest that cultured human breast cancer cells under estrogenic stimulation release a tumor-promoting factor(s) which can
act in vivo after release into the general circulation of the

athymic mouse. We do not know why these tumors induce by CM regress. There appear to be 3 potential explanations. First, during the process of growth factor purification concentration one or more essential activities are lost. Second, it should be recalled that these growth factor activities infused via mini-pump are acting via an endocrine route. Thus any of the large number of pharmacologic explanations may explain our failure to induce sustained tumor growth. Third, it remains reasonable that estrogens do exert systemic effects which their induced growth factors do not. Thus estrogen effects on the immune system, etc. are possible.

As an independent line of investigation to evaluate the possibility of autoregulatory growth factors, we have also utilized the MCF-7 cells grown as xenografts in the nude mouse to study the activity of individual growth factors. As previously above, conditioned medium extracts from E_2-treated MCF-7 cells stimulate limited growth of MCF-7 tumor in the absence of E_2 itself. As a test of the hypothesis that E_2-induced growth factors may mediate this effect, we have directly infused human EGF (1 ug/day), human IGF-I (0.6 ug/day) into female oophorectomized nude mice injected at 4 mammary fat pad locations ($2-5x10^6$ cells/injection site) with MCF-7 cells. These concentrations corresponded to those observed in the conditioned medium extracts utilized in the previous studies. As before, growth factors were infused with Alzet minipumps, and the experiment was carried out for 2 weeks. Both growth factors induced tumors, but EGF induced more than twice the tumor incidence as IGF-I. EGF supported development of tumors to 0.5 cm in diameter. As expected, E_2-pellet implanted control animals had a high incidence of continously growing tumors to 0.8 cm over the time of the experiment (31). Thus, based on these experiments with authentic growth factors, it is likely that breast cancer produced and closely related IGF-I and TGF$\propto$ like species have some autostimulatory actions on tumor growth <u>in vivo</u>. In addition, the TGF $\propto$ species induced by E_2 may be relevant in E_2 stimulated tumor growth. Greater availability of TGF$\propto$, TGF β, PDGF, and epithelial transforming activity in the future should facilitate the testing of these activities in this <u>in vivo</u> reconstitution system.

In other studies (66) investigating mouse mammary carcinogenesis, Oka and coworkers have recently demonstrated a likely role of EGF in both mammary tumor onset and subsequent growth support. Using a mouse strain highly susceptible to spontaneous mammary tumors, removal of the submandibular glands (sialoadenectomy) dramatically reduced the incidence of tumor formation and/or the rate of growth of the breast tumors allowed to form. The submandibular gland is a major source of EGF in mammals and reinfusion of EGF into such sialoadenectomized mice returned tumor incidence and growth rate of tumors to their normally high level. TGF$\propto$ - and EGF - like activities thus may have endocrine functions in tumor support. As the data with MCF-7 cells shows, one mechanism of tumor progression might involve local production (estrogen regulated) of TGF α by the tumor. Clearly, TGFα - or EGF-like growth factors are likely to be important regulators of mammary tumor progression by a variety of possible mechanisms. A large body of literature already exists demonstrating that EGF has both tumor promotional and immunosuppressive activities (92).

Interestingly, at least some of the growth factor products of breast cancer appear related to growth factors in milk (13,86, 104). One example is TGFα. The function of such factors may be related to offspring growth rather than parental mammary growth, since TGFα (and EGF) can promote eyelid opening in mice. Though growth factors such as IGF-I and TGFα may be capable of auto-crine stimulation of tumor cells, they and other growth factors may also subserve paracrine functions on surrounding non neoplastic tissue. PDGF promotes fibroblast growth and chemotaxis and its secretion may contribute to the marked stromal proliferation characteristically surrounding breast carcinoma (55). In addition, TGFα and TGFβ stimulate bone resorption and hypercalcemia, also characteristic of breast cancer (95). Other effects of paracrine growth factors might be immunomodulatory in nature. Finally, but potentially the most important paracrine function secreted by cancer is angiogensis factor(s). Though many activities may contribute, both growth factors and proteolytic degra-dation products of basement membranes are likely candidates (39, 84,100). The principle components secreted by breast cancer leading to vascular infiltration of the tumor have not yet been identified. However, Vallee and coworkers have recently isolated sequenced, and cloned an angiogenic protein secreted by human colon carcinoma cells (67).

Recent studies carried out in rodent systems have implicated specific genetic alterations leading to malignant transformation and tumor progression. In the murine model, mouse mammary tumor virus (MMTV) inserts itself into the genome at specific sites and generally induces expression of at least 2 cellular genes (28). In the carcinogen treated rat model system, activation of the oncogene knows as harvey ras (c-ras[H]) occurs by point mutation (103). At the present time, no such unifying statements can be made about human breast cancer. Rather, diverse observations of oncogene activation suggest a plethora of mechanisms at work in malignant progression. In one human breast cancer cell line, Hs578T, as activated c-ras[H] oncogene has been observed, as pre-dicted based on the rat model system. However this potential mechanism appears far from universal (65). Second, a whole series of cellular protooncogenes are observed to be expressed in diverse studies employing cell lines and tumor specimens (34,87). These oncogenes (all members of the ras family, as well as myc, myb, fms, fos, fes) include those localized in plasma membrane, nucleus, and cytoplasm. Two other oncogenes c-erb B and neu (or c-erb b$_2$) are both closely related to the EGF receptor and have also been detected in breast cancer cell lines and tumor biopsies (34,61). Interestingly, c-erb b (the EGF receptor) is expressed to the greatest extent in estrogen receptor negative cell lines and tumor biopsies (22,38). It may represent a new marker for dedifferentiation or malignancy in breast cancer. Recent studies have suggested that a mechanism for its high level of expression is at the transcriptional level. It is not yet known whether overexpression of the cErb B in cancer directly contributes to the transformed phenotype or indirectly mediates the effects of EGF (or TGFα) produced in an autocrine-type loop. Finally, as previously mentioned, PDGF, partially the product of the c-sis protooncogene, is expressed by a variety of breast cancer cell lines (11,82). Though PDGF itself is not generally growth stimulatory of epithelial cells it may contribute in other ways to the transformed phenotype (such as through paracrine actions). It is possible that additional oncogene activities will be observed in breast cancer using different techniques in the future. One such possibility is that an epithelial cell test system will detect transforming genes which go unrecognized by the well established NIH 3T3 fibroblast test system.

The diversity in observations of activated oncogenes and expressed cellular protooncogenes may suggest that many mechanisms or steps exit in the malignant progression of breast cancer. Alternatively, observations of expression of some of these cellular protooncogenes could reflect malignant status rather than induce it. Clearly, to test hypotheses concerning oncogene activity in breast cancer it is necessary to directly insert the oncogene of interest into a relevant cell test system. This objective may recently have been achieved using normal diploid human mammary epithelium first immortalized with brief benzo[a]pyrene treatment and then transfected with oncogenes (91). Stampfer has observed that treatment of normal mammary epithelial cells in culture with benzo[a]pyrene achieved immortalized but non-tumorigenic lines. These lines appear nearly normal by several criteria. Subsequently, using retroviral vectors, Clarke has inserted various oncogenes into one of these lines to determine the phenotype effects (19). Insertion of v-ras[H], v-mos, and SV40 T antigen rendered the cells capable of growth in high levels of serum, but did not confer tumorigenicity. Transfectants containing SV40 T plus either v-ras or v-mos were strongly tumorigenic in nude mice.

We will next describe experiments to test the activity of the v-ras[H] oncogene in MCF-7 cells and its effects on malignant status and assess what growth factor changes are associated with this changed genotype. This type of test has not yet been carried out for other oncogenes of possible importance in human breast cancer.

In many cases, breast cancer patients present initially as responsive to hormonal (tamoxifen) therapy. Following extended treatment, the breast cancer may become hormone unresponsive.

We wished to develop a model system to study the conversion of a hormone responsive to hormone independent cell line. For this purpose we chose to permanently transfer DNA from the tumor-causing retrovirus Harvey sarcoma virus to MCF-7 cells. The tumor inducing portion of this viral DNA (the oncogene) is called v-ras^H, and is closely related to the most commonly detected activated an activated ras oncogene in some highly malignant human cancers. MCF-7 cells did not initially contain this oncogene, but one estrogen independent cell line, Hs578T, does (65). We transferred the v-ras^H oncogene to MCF-7 cells by the calcium phosphate method (57).

MCF-7 cells containing stably integrated v-ras^H genes in their DNA (MCF-7$_{ras}$) had 5-8 times the level of ras mRNA as in control cells, and had detectable phosphorylated p21 (the protein which is the ras gene product). The cellular p21 is not a substrate for phosphorylation. MCF-7$_{ras}$ cells displayed unaltered growth rate under control conditions <u>in vitro</u> but had resistance to growth inhibition by antiestrogens. The transfected cells were tumorigenic in the absence of estrogen in 85% of inoculated female oophorectomized nude mice (57). Interestingly the MCF-7$_{ras}$ cells also exhibited increased rates of turnover of phosphatidyl inositol, analogous to E_2 treatment of MCF-7 cells (36). In addition, these cells also expressed increased levels of the laminin receptor on their surfaces (3).

We next assayed for secreted growth factors by MCF-7 cells. CM prepared from MCF-7$_{ras}$ cultures as compared with control cultures contained 3-4 fold elevated levels of radioreceptor assayable TGF$\propto$ and bioactive TGF $\propto$ as assayed by anchorage-independent growth of NRK fibroblasts. A single peak of TGF$\propto$ -like activity was eluted at an apparent MW of 30 Kd from acid gel chromatography of MCF-7$_{ras}$ CM. Also, secretion of immunoreactive IGF-I and TGFβ were augmented 3-4 fold in MCF$_{ras}$ cells but PDGF secretion was further not elevated. These growth factors may then was be biologically active <u>in vivo</u>. MCF-7$_{ras}$ tumors in the nude mouse were able to induce the development of small tumors derived from MCF-7 cells separately implanted at a distant site in the nude mouse (56). That is, when MCF-7$_{ras}$ cells were innoculated on one side of a nude mouse, and wild type cells on the other, tumors appeared nearly 100% of the time on the MCF-7$_{ras}$ side and about 40% of the time on the wild type side. These do not represent metastases. They do not contain v-ras sequences. When removed from the animal and growth in culture they are still hormone dependent. Thus, the presence of MCF-7$_{ras}$ tumors are able to temper growth of previously hormone dependent cells without permanently altering their phenotype. Ras gene activation could bring about phenotypic and tumorigenic changes in human breast cancer cells, some of which may also be induced by estrogens. However, the cells retained the capacity to bind estrogen and respond to estrogens as shown by E_2 induction of the progesterone receptor. Thus ras gene transfection bypasses estrogen activation of the transformed phenotype and but induces that phenotype via a pathway which appears to be similar but not identical to the E_2 induction pathway. Future studies will more clearly define the similarities and differences between E_2 and v-ras[H] induced malignant progression of MCF-7 cells.

Let us briefly turn to one last hypothesis. That growth inhibition (for example by antiestrogens) not only occurs by a down regulation of growth stimulatory activities but in addition by enhanced production of growth inhibitory substances. Our attention was drawn to this possibility for two reasons. First, work with glucocorticoid regulated systems evidence has been presented that effects occur through induction of gene products capable of inducing cell lysis is sensitive lymphoblasts. Secondly, in preliminary experiments we found that conditioned media derived from antiestrogen treated MCF-7 cells was capable of inducing growth inhibition of estrogen receptor negative, antiestrogen resistant MDA-MB-231 cells. Based on apparent molecular weight of some of this activity, we considered TGFβ as one potential negative regulator.

Breast cancer cells also secrete a TGFβ -related activity (25, 62). A major peak of radioreceptor-competing and AKR-2B fibroblast transforming activity comigrates with authentic platelet derived TGF-β on acid Biogel chromatoraphy. In contrast to its transforming effects on some fibroblasts, authentic TGFβ is growth inhibiting for many breast cancer (and other epithelial derived lines) (62,80,96). All breast cancer cells examined expressed the expected 2.5 Kb mRNA species. Interestingly, TGFβ secretion is inhibited by treatment of MCF-7 cells with growth stimulatory E_2 and insulin. Growth inhibitory antiestrogens and glucocorticoids strongly stimulate its secretion. Intracellular TGFβ did not appear to be modulated. TGFβ from antiestrogen induced MCF-7 cells strongly inhibits the growth of another estrogen receptor negative cell line, MDA-MB-231. This growth inhibitor was reversed in the presence of a polyclonal antibody directed against native TGFβ . Interestingly, in the antiestrogen, but not TGFβ resistant, resistant MCF-7 variant LY2, antiestrogens do not significantly induce TGFβ secretion. Current work is further addressing the mechanism of TGFβ regulation (63).

TGF β acts through a high molecular weight (615 kDa) receptor complex. The receptor subunits have been reported as identical, 330 kDa species. This receptor has not yet been purified, cloned or sequenced, but is not reported to have tyrosine kinase activity (40). High affinity binding sites for TGFβ have been reported on responsive (growth inhibited) human breast cancer cell lines (62). Taken together we believe that these data suggest that growth regulation of some breast cancers (and as a speculation in normal mammary cell(s) may be modulated by secretion of potent growth inhibitors.

Future Prospects

We have presented evidence for involvement of TGFα (EGF-like) IGF-I and TGFβ -related growth factors in E_2 induction of E_2 receptor-containing breast cancer growth. We have also observed elevated levels of these and other growth factors in E_2 receptor negative, highly tumorigenic cell lines. Purified EGF was capable of partially replacing E_2 as tumor growth stimulator in vivo in the nude mouse, and is therefore likely to play a role in vivo as an autostimulatory tumor growth factor. As an independent test of association of growth factor secretion with tumorigenesis, we rendered a cell line E_2 autonomous, and more tumorigenic by DNA mediated transfection of the v-ras^H oncogene. Increased TGFα and IGF-I secretion were observed, confirming their close association with malignant status. Future studies will define the mechanisms of growth factor regulation and attempt to attenuate malignant status by interfering with their action. These studies suggest that future clinical treatment modalities might be designed around inhibition of autocrine or paracrine growth factor action with antibodies or synthetic peptides. Other approaches might involve toxin-antibody targeting to overexpressed cell surface receptors for growth factors.

References

1. Aitken, S.C. and Lippman, M.W. Hormonal regulation of de novo pyrimidine synthesis and utilization in human breast cancer cells in tissue culture. Cancer Res., 43: 4681-4690, 1983.

2. Aitken, S.C., and Lippman, M.E. Effect of estrogens and anti-estrogens on growth-regulatory enzymes in human breast cancer cells in tissue culture. Cancer Res., 45: 1611-1620, 1985.

3. Albini, A., Graf, J.O., Kleinman, H.K., Martin, G.R., Veillette, A., and Lippman, M.E. Estrogen and v-ras^H transfection regulate the interactions of MCF-7 breast carcinoma cells to basement membrane. Proceedings of the East Coast Connective Tissue Meeting, 1986.

4. Assoian, R.K., Grotendorst, G.R., Miller, D.M., and Sporn, M.B. Cellular transformation by coordinated action of three peptide growth factors from human platelets. Nature (London) 309: 804-806, 1984.

5. Bates,S.E., McManaway, M.E., Lippman, M.E., and Dickson, R.B. Characterization of estrogen responsive transforming activity in human breast cancer cell lines. Cancer Res., 46: 1707-1713, 1986.

6. Baxter, R.C., Maitland, J.E., Raisur, R.L., Reddel, R., and Sutherland, R.L. (1983). High molecular weight somatomedin-C (IGF-I) from T47D human mammary carcinoma cells: immuno-

reactivity and bioactivity. In: Insulin-like Growth Factors/ Somatomedins, edited by E.M. Spencer, pp. 615-618 Walter deGruyter Co., Berlin.

7. Berthois, Y., Katzenellenbogen, J.A., and Katzenellenbogen, B.S. Phenol red in tissue culture media is a weak estrogen: implications concerning the study of estrogen-responsive cells in culture. Proc. Nat'l. Acad. Sci. (USA), 83: 2496-2500, 1986.

8. Bronzert, D.A., Triche, T.J., Gleason, P., and Lippman, M.E. Isolation and characterization of an estrogen-inhibited variant derived from the MCF7 breast cancer cell line. Cancer Res., 44: 3942-3951, 1984.

9. Bronzert, D.A., Greene, G.L., and Lippman, M.E. Selection and characterization of breast cancer cell line resistant to the antiestrogen LY 117018. Endocrinology, 117: 1409-1417.

10. Bronzert, D.A., Silverman, S. and Lippman, M.E. Induction of of a secreted protein in human breast cancer cell lines. Proceedings of the 67th Annual Endocrine Society Meeting, Baltimore, MD 1985.

11. Bronzert, D., Davidson, N., Pantazis, P. and Antoniades, H. Synthesis and secretion of PDGF-like growth factor by human breast cancer cell lines. Proceedings of the 68th Annual Meeting of the Endocrine Society, Anaheim, CA, 1986.

12. Brooks, S.C., Locke, E.R., and Soule, H.D. Estsrogen receptor in a human breast cell line (MCF-7) from breast carcinoma. J. Biol. Chem., 248: 6251-6261, 1973.

13. Buno, M., Salomon, D.S., and Kidwell, W.R. Purification of a mammary derived growth factor from human milk and human mammary tumors. J. Biol. Chem. 260: 5745-5752, 1985.

14. Burke, R.E., Harris, S.C., and McGuire, W.C. Lactate dehydrogenase in estrogen responsive human breast cancer cells. Cancer Res., 38: 2773-2780.

15. Butler, W.B., Kirkland, W.L., and Jorgensen, T.L. Induction of plasminogen activator by estrogen in a human breast cancer cell line (MCF-7). Biochem. Biophys. Res. Comm., 90: 1328-1334, 1979.

16. Campisi, J. and Pardee, A.B. Post-transcriptional control of the onset of DNA synthesis by an insulin-like growth factor. Molecular and Cellular Biology, 4: 1807-1814, 1984.

17. Carney, D.H., Scott, D.L., Gordon, E.A., and LaBelle, E.F. Phosphoinositide in Mitogenesis: Neomycin inhibits throm-

bin-stimulated phosphoinositide turnover and initiation of
cell proliferation. Cell, 42: 479-488, 1985.

18. Ciocca, D.R., Adams, D.J., Edwards, D.P., Bjerke, R.J., and
    McGuire, W.L. Distribution of an estrogen induced protein
    with a molecular weight of 24,000 in normal and malignant
    human tissues and cells. Cancer Res., 43: 1204-1210, 1983.

19. Clark, R., Milleg, R., O'Rouke, E., Trahey, M., Stampfer, M.,
    Kreigler, M., and McCormick, F. Transformation of human mam-
    mary epithelial cells with oncogenic retroviruses. Proceed-
    ings of the First Annual Meeting on Oncogenes, Frederick, MD,
    1985.

20. Cowan, K., Levine, R., Aitken, S., Goldsmith, M., Douglass,
    E., Clendennin, N., Nienhius, A., and Lippman, M.E. Dihydro-
    folate reductase gene amplification and possible rearrange-
    ment in estrogen-responsive methotrexate resistant human
    breast cancer cells. J. Biol. Chem. 257: 15079-15086, 1982.

21. Davidson, N.E., Bronzert, D.A., Chambon, P., Gelmann, E.P.,
    and Lippman, M.E. Use of two MCF-7 cell variants to evaluate
    the growth regulatory potential of estrogen-induced products.
    Cancer Res., 46: 1904-1908, 1986.

22. Davidson, N.E., Gelmann, E.P., Lippman, M.E., and Dickson,
    R.B. Expression of EGF receptor (EGF-R) and its MRNA in
    estrogen receptor (ER) negative human breast cancer cell
    lines. Proceedings of the Annual Meeting of the American
    Association for Cancer Research, Los Angeles, CA, 1986.

23. Delarco, J.E. and Todaro, G.J. Growth factors from murine
    sarcoma virus-transformed cells. Proc. Nat'l. Acad. Sci.
    (USA), 75: 4001-4005, 1978.

24. Derynck, R., Roberts, A.B., Winkler, M.E., Chen, E.Y. and
    Goeddel, D.V. Human transforming growth factor- : precursor
    structure and expression in E. coli. Cell, 38: 287-297, 1984.

25. Derynck, R., Jarrett, J.A., Chen, E.Y., Eaton, D.H., Bell,
    J.R., Assoian, R.K., Roberts, A.B., Sporn, M.B., and Goeddel,
    D.V. Human transforming growth factor :complementary DNA
    sequence and expression in normal and transformed cells.
    Nature, 316: 701-705, 1985.

26. Derynck, R., Roberts, A.B., Eaton, D.H., Winkler, M.C. and
    Goeddel, . Human transforming growth factor : precursor
    sequence, gene structure, and heterologous expression In
    Feramisco, J., Ozanne, B., and Stiles, C. (eds) Cancer Cells
    3: Growth factors and transformation. Cold Spring Harbor
    Laboratory, pp. 79-86, 1985.

27. Dickson, R.B., Smith, R., Brookes, S., and Peter, G. Tumorigenesis by mouse mammary tumor virus: proviral activation of a cellular gene in the common integration region int-2. Cell 37: 529-536, 1984.

28. Dickson, R.B. and Clark, C.R. Estrogen receptors in the male. Archives of Andrology, 7: 205-217, 1981.

29. Dickson, R.B., Bates, S.E., McManaway, M.E. and Lippman, M.E. Characterization of estrogen responsive transforming activity in human breast cancer cell lines. Cancer Res., 46: 1707-1713, 1986.

30. Dickson, R.B., Huff, K.K., Spencer, E.M., and Lippman, M.E. Induction of epidermal growth factor-related polypeptides by 17 -estradiol in MCF-7 human breast cancer cells. Endocrinology, 118: 138-142, 1986.

31. Dickson, R.B., McManaway, M., and Lippman, M.E. Estrogen induced growth factor activities from MCF-7 human breast cancer cells replace estrogen as in vivo stimuli of tumor formation. Science 232: 1540-1543, 1986.

32. Eidne, K.A., Flanagan, C.A., and Miller, R.P. Gonadotropin-releasing hormone binding sites in human breast carcinoma. Science, 229: 989-991, 1985.

33. Engle, L.W., and Young, N.W. Human breast carcinoma cells in continuous culture: a review. Cancer Res. 38: 4327-4339, 1978.

34. Fitzpatrick, S.L., Brightwell, J., Wittliff, J.L., Barrows, G.H., and Schultz, G.S. Epidermal growth factor binding by breast tumor biopsies and relationship to estrogen receptor and progesterone receptor levels. Cancer Res., 44: 3448-3453, 1984.

35. Freedman, V.H., and Shin, S. Cellular tumorigenicity in nude mice: correlation with cell growth in semi-solid medium. Cell 3: 355-359, 1974.

36. Freter, C.E., Lippman, M.E. and Gelmann, E.P. Hormonal effects of phosphatidyl inositol (P.I.) turnover in MCF-7 human breast cancer cells. Proceedings of the American Association for Cancer Research Annual meeting. Los Angeles, CA, 1986.

37. Furlanetto, R.W., and DiCarlo, J.N. Somatomedin C receptors and growth effects in human breast cells maintained in long-term culture. Cancer Res., 44: 2122-2128, 1984.

38. Gainsbury, J.R.C., Farndon, J.R., Sherbert, G.V., and Harris,

A.L. Epidermal growth factor receptors and oestrogen receptors in human breast cancer. The Lancet, Feb. 16, 364-366, 1985.

39. Gospodarowicz, D., Greenburg, G., Bialecki, H., and Zetter, B.R. Factors involved in the modulation of cell proliferation in vivo and in vitro: the role of fibroblast and epidermal growth factors in the proliferative response of mammalian cells. In Vitro, 14: 85-113, 1978.

40. Goustin, A.S., Leof, E.B., Shipley, G.D., and Moses, H.L. Growth factors and cancer. Cancer Res., 46: 1015-1029, 1986.

41. Hackett, A.J., Smith, H.S., Springer, E.L., Owens, R.B., Nelson-Rees, W.A., Riggs, J.L., and Gardner, M.B. Two syngeneic cell lines from human breast tissue: the aneuploid mammary epithelial (Hs578T) and the diploid myoepithelial (Hs578Bst) cell lines. J. Nat'l. Cancer Inst., 58: 1795-1806, 1977.

42. Halper, J., and Moses, H.L. Epithelial tissue-derived growth factor-like polypeptides. Cancer Res., 43: 1972-1979, 1983.

43. Heldin, C.H., and Westermark, B. Growth factors: mechanism of action and relations to oncogenes. Cell, 37: 9-20, 1984.

44. Horwitz, K.B., and McGuire, W.L. Estrogen control of progesterone receptor in human breast cancer. J. Biol. Chem. 253: 2223-2228, 1978.

45. Huff, K.K., Kaufman, D., Gabbay, K.H., Spencer, E.M., Lippman, M.E., and Dickson, R.B. Human breast cancer cells secrete an insulin-like growth factor-I-related polypeptide. Cancer Res., in press, 1986.

46. Huff, K.K., Knabbe, C., Kaufman, D., Gabbay, K.H., and Dickson, R.B. Hormonal regulation of insulin-like growth factor I (IGF-I) secretion from MCF-7 human breast cancer cells. Proceedings of the 68th Annual Meeting of the Endocrine Society, Anaheim, CA, 1986.

47. Huseby, R.A., Maloney, T.M., and McGrath, C.M. Evidence for a direct growth-stimulating effect of estradiol on human MCF-7 cell in vivo. Cancer Res., 44: 2654-2659, 1984.

48. Ikeda, T., Danielpour, D., and Sirbasku, B.A. Isolation and properties of endocrine and autocrine type mammary tumor cell growth factors (estromedins) in Bresciani, F., King, R.J.B., Lippman, M.E., Namer, M. and Raynaud, J.P. (eds). Progress in Cancer Research and Therapy. Vol 31. Raven Press, New York, pp. 171-186, 1983.

49. Ikeda, T., and Sirbasku, D.A. Purification and properties of a mammary-uterine-pituitary tumor cell growth factor from pregnant sheep uterus. J. Biol. Chem., 259: 4049-4064, 1984.

50. Jakesz, R., Smith, C.A., Aitken, S., Huff, K., Schuette, W., Shackney, S., and Lippman, M.E. Influence of cell proliferation and all cycle phase on expression of estrogen receptor in MCF-7 breast cancer cells. Cancer Res., 44: 619-625, 1984.

51. Jakolew, S.B., Breathnack, R., Jeltsch, J., and Chambone, P. Sequence of the pS2 mRNA induced by estrogen in the human breast cancer cell line MCF-7. Nucleic Acids Res., 12: 2861-2874.

52. Jansen, M., Van Schaik, F.M.A., Ricker, A.T., Bullock, B., Woods, P.E., Gabbay, K.H., Nussbaum, A.L., Sussenback, J.S., and Vander Branch, J.R. Sequence of cDNA encoding human insulin-like growth factor I precursor. Nature (London), 306: 609-611, 1983.

53. Jensen, E.V. Studies of growth phenomenon using tritium-labeled steroids. Proc. 4th Int. Congress of Biochem. Permagon Press, Vienna, p. 119

54. Jordan, V.C. Biochemical pharmacology of antiestrogen action. Pharmacological Reviews, 36: 245-276, 1984.

55. Kao, R.T., Hall, J., Engel, L., and Stern, R. The matrix of human breast tumor cells is mitogenic for fibroblasts. Amer. J. Path., 115: 109-116, 1984.

56. Kasid, A., Dickson, R., Huff, K., Bates, S., Lowy, D., Lippman, M., and Gelmann, E. V-ras[H] transfection mimics and bypasses estrogen-induced tumor phenotype of a human breast cancer cell line. Cold Spring Harbor Symposium on Viral Oncogenesis, 1985.

57. Kasid, A., Lippman, M.E., Papageorge, A.G., Lowy, D.R. and Gelmann, E.P. Transfection of v-ras[H] DNA into MCF-7 cells bypasses their dependence on estrogen for tumorigenicity. Science, 228: 725-728, 1985.

58. Kasid, A., Davidson, N., Gelmann, E., and Lippman, M.E. Transcriptional control of thymidine kinase gene expression by estrogens and antiestrogens in MCF-7 human breast cancer cells. J. Biol. Chem., 261: 5562-5567, 1986.

59. Kaufman, U., Zapf, J., Torretti, B., and Froesch, E.R. Demonstration of a specific serum carrier protein of nonsuppressible insulin-like activity in vivo. J. Clin. Endocrinol. Metab. 44: 160-166, 1977.

60. King, W.J. and Greene, G.L. Monoclonal antibodies localize estrogen receptor in the nuclei of target cells. Nature, 307: 745-749, 1984.

61. King, C.R., Kraus, M.H., and Aaronson, S. Amplification of a novel V-erb-B related gene in a human mammary carcinoma. Science, 229: 974-976.

62. Knabbe, C., Huff, K.K., Dickson, R.B., and Lippman, M.E. Transforming growth factor beta is a hormonally regulated negative growth factor in human breast cancer. Proceedings of the 68th Annual meeting of the Endocrine Society, Anaheim, CA, 1986.

63. Knabbe, C., Huff, K., Wakefield, L., Lippman, M.E., andn Dickson, R.B. Differential regulation of transforming growth factor β (TGFβ) and insulin-like growth factor I (IGF-I) in MCF-7 human breast cancer cells by growth inhibitory anti-esrogens and glucocorticoids. Proceedings of the 25th Annual Meeting of the America Society for Cell Biology, Atlanta, GA, 1985.

64. Knabbe, C.K., Lippman, M.E., Greene, G.L. and Dickson, R.B. Phorbol ester induced phosphorylation of the estrogen receptor in intact MCF-7 human breast cancer cells. Proceedings of the 77th Annual Meeting of the American Society of Biological Chemists, Washington, DC 1986.

65. Kraus, M.H., Yuasa, Y., and Aaronson, S.A. A position 12-activated H-ras oncogene in all Hs578T mammary carcino-sarcoma cells but not normal mammary cells of the same patient. Proc. Nat'l. Acad. Sci. (USA), 81: 5384-5388, 1984.

66. Kurachi, H., Okamoto, S., and Oka, T. Evidence for the involvement of the submandibular gland epidermal growth factor in mouse mammary tumorigenesis. Proc. Nat'l. Acad. Sci. (USA), 81: 5940-5943, 1985.

67. Kurachi, K., Davie, E.W., Strydom, D.J., Riordan, J.F., and Vallee, B.L. Sequence of the cDNA and gene for angiogenin, a human angiogenesis factor. Biochemistry, 24: 5494-5499

68. Liotta, L. Tumor invasion and metastases: role of the extra-cellular matrix. Proceedings of the American Association for Cancer Research. 26: 385-386, 1985.

69. Lippman, M.E., Bolan, G., and Huff, K. The effects of estrogens and antiestrogens on hormone-responsive human breast cancer cell line MCF-7. Cancer Res., 43: 1244-1249, 1983.

70. Lippman, M.E (1984). Definition of hormones and growth factors required for optimal proliferation and expression of

phenotypic responses in human breast cancer cells. In: <u>Cell Culture Methods for Molecular and Cell Biology</u>, edited by Barnes, D.W., Sirbasku, D.A., and Sato, G.H., pp. 183-200, Vol. 2, Alan R. Liss, New York.

71. Lippman, M.E., Buzdar, A., Tormey, D.C., and McGuire, W.L. Combining endocrine and chemotherapeutic any three benefits? <u>Breast Cancer Res. Treat.</u>, 4: 251-259, 1985.

72. Lipsett, M.B. and Lippman, M.E. Endocrine responsive cancers of man. In: Williams, R.H. (ed.) <u>Textbook of Endocrinology</u>, W.B. Saunders Co., Philadelphia, pp. 1213-1226, 1981.

73. Massague, J., Kelly, B. and Mottola, C. Stimulation by insulin-like growth factors is required for cellular transformation by type transforming growth factor. <u>J. Biol. Chem.</u>, 260: 4551-4554, 1985.

74. McGrath, C.M. Augmentation of the response of normal mammary epithelial cells to estradiol by mammary stroma. <u>Cancer Res.</u>, 43: 1355-1360, 1983.

75. Nishizuka, Y. Protein kinases in a signal transduction. <u>Trends Biochem. Sci.</u>, 9: 163-171, 1984.

76. Osborne, C.K., Boldt, D.H., Clark, G.M., and Trent, J.M. Effects of tamoxifen on human breast cancer cell cycle kinetics: accumulation of cells in early G_1 phase. <u>Cancer Res.</u>, 43: 3583-3585, 1983.

77. Osborne, C.K., Hobbs, K., and Clark, G.M. Effects of estrogens and antiestrogens on growth of human breast cancer cells in athymic nude mice. <u>Cancer Res.</u>, 45: 584-590, 1985.

78. Page, M.J., Field, J.K., Everett, N.P. and Green, C.D. Serum-regulation of the estrogen responsiveness of the human breast cancer cell line MCF-7. <u>Cancer Res.</u>, 43: 1244-1249, 1983.

79. Pastan, I. Regulation of cellular growth. <u>Adv. Metab. Dis.</u>, 8: 7-16, 1975.

80. Roberts, A.B., Anzano, M.A., Wakefield, L.M., Roche, N.S., Stern, D.F., and Sporn, M.B. Type transforming growth factor: a bifunctional regulator of cellular growth. <u>Proc. Nat'l. Acad. Sci. (USA)</u>, 82: 119-123, 1985.

81. Ross, G.T., Vande Wiele, R.L. and Frantz, A.G. The ovaries and the breasts. In: Williams R.H. (ed.) Textbook of Endocrinology, W.B. Saunders Co. Philadelphia, pp. 355-411, 1981.

82. Rozengurt, E., Sinnett-Smith, J., and Taylor-Papadimitriou, J. Production of PDGF-like growth factor by breast cancer cell lines. <u>Int. J. Cancer</u>, 36: 247-252, 1985.

83. Salomon, D.S., Zwiebel, J.A., Bano, M., Losonczy, I., Felnel, P., and Kidwell, W.R. Presence of transforming growth factors in human breast cancer cells. Cancer Res., 44: 4069-4077, 1984.

84. Schreiber, A.B., Kenney, J., Kowalski, J., Thomas, K.A., Gimenez-Gallego, G., Rios-Candelore, M., DiSalvo, J., Bamitault, D., Courty, J., Courtois, Y., Moemer, M., Loret, C., Burgess, W.H., Mehlman, T., Friesel, R., Johnson, W., and Maciag, T. A unique family of endothelial cell polypeptide mitogens: the antigenic and receptor cross-reactivity of bovine endothelial growth factor and eye-derived growth factor-II. J. Cell Biol., 101: 1623-1626, 1985.

85. Schuh, S., Yamemoto, W., Bragge, J., Bauer, V.J., Riehl, R.M., Sullivan, W.P., and Toft, D.O. A 90,000 dalton binding protein common to both steroid receptors and the rous sarcoma virus transforming protein $pp60^{v-src}$. J. Biol. Chem. 260: 14292-14296, 1985.

86. Shing, Y.W., and Klagsbran, M. Human and bovine milk contain different sets of growth factors. Endocrinology, 115: 273-282, 1984.

87. Slamon, D.J., deKernion, J.B., Verma, I.M., and Cline, M.J. Expression of cellular oncogenes in human malignancies. Science, 224: 256-262, 1984.

88. Smith, H.S., Scher, C.D., and Todaro, G.J. Induction of cell division in median lacking serum growth factor by SV40. Virology, 44: 359-370, 1971.

89. Soule, H.D., and McGrath, C.M. Estrogen responsive proliferation of clonal human breast carcinoma cells in athymic mice. Cancer Lett., 10: 177-189, 1980.

90. Sporn, M.B., and Todaro, G.J. Autocrine secretion and malignant transformation of cells. New England J. Med., 303: 878-880, 1980.

91. Stampfer, M.R., and Bartley, J.C. Induction of transformation and continuous cell lines from normal human mammary epithelial cells after cells after exposure to benzo[a]pyrene. Proc. Nat'l. Acad. Sci. (USA), 82: 2394-2398, 1985.

92. Stoscheck, C.M. and King, L.E. Role of epidermal growth factor in carcinogenesis. Cancer Res., 46: 1030-1037, 1986.

93. Sutherland, R.L., Hall, R.E. and Taylor, I.W. Cell proliferation kinetics of MCF-7 human mammary carcinoma cells in culture and effects of tamoxifen on exponentially growing and plateau phase cells. Cancer Res., 43: 3998-4006, 1983.

94. Swain, S., Dickson, R.B., and Lippman, M.E. Anchorage in-dependent epithelial colony stimulating activity in human breast cancer cell lines. Proceedings American Association for Cancer Research Annual Meeting, Los Angeles, CA, 1986.

95. Tasjian, A.H., Voelkel, E.F., Lazzaro, M., Singer, F.R., Roberts, A.B., Derynck, R., Winkler, M.E., and Levine, L. α and β human transforming growth factors stimulate prosta-glandin production and bone resorption in cultured mouse cal-varia. Proc. Nat'l. Acad. Sci. (USA), 82: 4535-4538, 1985.

96. Tucker, R.F., Shipley, G.D., Moses, H.L., and Holley, R.W. Growth inhibitor from BSC-1 cells closely related to platelet type transforming growth factor. Science, 226: 705-707, 1984.

97. Vignon, F., Capony, F., Chambon, M., Freiss, L., Garcia, M., and Rochefort, H. Autocrine growth stimulation of the MCF-7 breast cancer cell by the estrogen regulated 52K protein. Endocrinology, 118: 1537-1545, 1986.

98. Vignon, F., and Derocq, D.F., Chambon, M., and Rochefort, H. Estrogen induced proteins secreted by the MCF-7 human breast cancer cells stimulated their proliferation. C.R. Acad. Sci. Paris Endocrinol., 296: 151-157, 1983.

99. Watts, C.K.W., Murphy, L.C., and Sutherland, R.L. Microsomal binding sites for nonsteroidal antiestrogens in MCF-7 human mammary carcinoma cells. J. Biol. Chem. 259: 4223-4229, 1984.

100. West, D.C., Hampson, I.N., Arnold, F., and Kumar, S. Angio-genesis induced by degredation products of hyaluronic acid. Science, 228: 1324-1326, 1985.

101. Westley, B. and Rochefort, H. A secreted glycoprotein induced by estrogen in human breast cancer cell lines. Cell, 20: 353-362, 1980.

102. Williams, L.T., Daniel, T.O., Escobedo, J.A., Fried, U.A., and Coughlin, S.R. PDGF Receptors: Structural and functional studies. ICSU Short Reports 4: 168-171, 1986.

103. Zarbl, H., Sukumar, S., Arthur, A.V., Martin-Zanea, D., and Barbacid, M. Direct mutagenesis of Ha-ras-1 oncogenes by N-nitroso-N-methylurea during initiation of mammary carcino-genesis in rats. Nature, 315: 382-385, 1985.

104. Zwiebel, J.A., Buno, M., Nexo, E., Salomon, P., and Kidwell, W.R. Partial purification of transforming growth factors from human milk. Cancer Res., 46: 933-939, 1986.

Hormonal Manipulation of Cancer: Peptides, Growth Factors, and New (Anti) Steroidal Agents, edited by Jan G. M. Klijn et al. Raven Press, New York © 1987.

A 52 K ESTROGEN–INDUCED PROTEASE SECRETED BY BREAST CANCER CELLS WITH AUTOCRINE MITOGENIC ACTIVITY

H. Rochefort, F. Capony, G. Cavalié, M. Chambon, G. Freiss, M. Garcia, M. Morisset and F. Vignon

Unité d'Endocrinologie Cellulaire et Moléculaire (U 148 INSERM and University of Montpellier, 60 rue de Navacelles 34100 Montpellier France

Cancer cells acquire the ability to make and to respond to their own growth factors (autocrine mechanism) (7). In hormone responsive cancer, these growth factors may be induced by mitogenic hormones. The human mammary cancer cell lines (MCF7, T47D, etc...) are good systems to evaluate this hypothesis, since they contain estrogen and progesterone receptors and their proliferation is increased by estrogens and decreased by antiestrogens and progestins (4,6,15).

We have shown that glycoproteins present in conditioned media are able to stimulate the growth of resting MCF7 cells when prepared from estrogen–treated MCF7 cells but not from control cells (27). In this conditioned medium, there are several proteins and peptides which are putative autocrine mitogens in mediating the effect of estrogens on cell growth.

THE 52 K PROTEIN AND ITS MONOCLONAL ANTIBODIES

Seven years ago, we found a protein of Mr=52,000 (52 K protein) whose production in culture medium by estrogen–receptor–positive metastatic breast cancer cell lines was specifically increased by estrogens and inhibited by antiestrogens (29). The 52 K protein is produced in small amounts in culture medium ($5 ng/10^6$ cells/hour) by estrogen–treated MCF7 cells, and represents 20 to 40 % of all proteins released in the culture medium. This protein is specifically regulated by hormones (estrogens and high doses of androgens) that can bind to and activate the estrogen receptor.

Due to its low quantity, we used a three–step strategy to purify the 52 K glycoprotein and study its structure and function. First, using Concanavalin A Sepharose, we partially purified it from 22 µl of conditioned medium from MCF7 cells. Second, we obtained several monoclonal antibodies (12). Third, using these monoclonal antibodies on an immunoaffinity column, we purified the 52 K protein to apparent homogeneity (1,000–fold purification) both in its secreted and cellular form (1). We have used the monoclonal antibodies in clinical studies to determine the tissue distribution of the protein and its potential as a marker in breast cancer.

a. The 52 K protein is not a general marker of estrogen responsiveness, unlike the progesterone receptor or the 24 K protein (11,20), since it is not found in endometrium and it is present in some estrogen receptor negative cell lines.

b. The antibodies to the 52 K protein appear to be specific for the human protein.

c. The 52 K protein is a proliferation-associated marker. It is not detected in normal resting epithelial mammary cells but is produced by these cells when they proliferate in primary culture, fibrocystic disease and ductal hyperplasia (13,14). It may therefore help to define high-risk proliferative mastopathies (10).

We have developed double-determinant immunometric assays of the protein: one antibody is labeled with ^{125}I (IRMA) or coupled to an enzyme (IEMA) and the other antibody (site 1) adsorbed in plastic microwells. The concentration of the 52 K protein is determined by reference to a standard curve obtained with purified 52 K protein previously quantitated by silver staining of SDS-PAGE. We found that the protein is progressively accumulated in the MCF7 cell medium as a function of time. Other cell lines produce the 52 K protein, either under estrogen stimulation (ZR75-1) or constitutively (BT20, MDA-MB231), indicating that it is not restricted to hormone-dependent cancers (Derocq, Garcia et al., unpublished).

The assay of the 52 K protein in a large number of breast cancer cytosols by an immunoenzymatic metric assay (IEMA) (in collaboration with CLIN-MIDY/SANOFI and several cancer centers), combined with the assay of the estrogen and progesterone receptor content, may allow us to determine the value of this marker in predicting hormone responsiveness and its possible prognostic value as a function of the clinical development of these cancers.

Similar studies will be performed in parallel with a second series of antibodies more recently screened for their ability to interact exclusively with the precursor secreted 52 K protein and not with the mature cellular 34 K protein (Freiss et al., in preparation). The results may be different since the regulation, concentration and cellular localisation of the 52 K and cellular 34 K protein are different (see § Structure of the Protein).

AUTOCRINE ACTIVITY OF THE SECRETED 52 K PROTEIN

Six years ago, we proposed an autocrine-type mechanism (24,25) which was supported by studies showing that proteins from serum-free media conditioned by estrogen-stimulated MCF7 cells increased the growth of resting MCF7 cells, while the conditioned media from estrogen-withdrawn MCF7 cells were inactive (27). The mitogenic activity of the estrogen-induced conditioned media has now been confirmed by other groups (8,9,17). In these media however, several estrogen-regulated proteins have been described in addition to the 52 K protein. There is a 160 K protein (29) and a 65 K protein recently identified as being the α_1 antichymotrypsin (19). Moreover the pS2 protein of 6-10 K coded by the cloned pS2 mRNA (5) and more classical growth factors such as EGF-like peptides (9,26) have also been described by other laboratories. To determine which protein(s) is (are) responsible for the mitogenic activity of conditioned media, we used two approaches : One approach was the use of antiestrogen-resistant variants of MCF7 cells, cloned by their ability to grow in 1 μM tamoxifen. We found that with the R27 and RTx6 clones, tamoxifen became able, like an estrogen, to increase the production of the 52 K protein, whereas it remained unable, as in the wild type MCF7 cells, to stimulate the production of the estrogen-regulated 160 K secreted protein and of pS2 mRNA (30). In these cell lines, the 52 K protein was therefore a better candidate for being a mitogen than the pS2 or 160 K proteins. A possible mechanism for the resistance to antiestrogens of these clones was that tamoxifen became able to induce the production of autocrine growth factors.

A more direct approach was to purify a biologically active 52 K protein by immunoaffinity and to test it on estrogen-deprived recipient MCF7 cells (28). The dose-dependent stimulation of cell growth, as evaluated by DNA assay, ranged from 120 % to 240 %. A mean stimulation of 170 % was obtained in the 7 experiments performed. This stimulation represented 40 % of the effect obtained by estradiol and was observed at 52 K protein concentrations (1 to 10 nM) similar to those released into the culture medium. The growth stimulation was dose-dependent and not observed with ovalbumin, another control glycoprotein. The 52 K protein was also able, like estradiol, to stimulate the number and length of microvilli at the cell surface. This mitogenic activity of the purified 52 K protein could be due to a contaminant that we have not yet detected. However, we have excluded, by ^{35}S cysteine-labelling experiments, the possibility that it could be peptides containing cysteine residues such as TGF , pS2 protein or IGFI (28). The mitogenic activity of the purified 52 K protein was therefore in agreement with an autocrine mechanism. The study of the co- and post-translational modifications of the 52 K protein helped us to define the structure and enzymatic activity of the protein.

GLYCOSYLATION AND TRAFFIC OF THE 52 K PROTEIN

After exposure of cultured MCF7 cells to ^{32}P, the 52 K protein is heavily labelled. Most of this label can be removed by Endoglycosidase-H treatment which deletes two N-glycosylated chains of the protein. Mannose-6-P signals have been identified on these chains (2). Pulse-chase experiments and western blot analysis show that the 52 K protein is the precursor of a lysosomal enzyme which accumulates in lysosomes as a 34 K stable protein. About 40 % of the cellular 52 K precursor is secreted while 60 % is successively processed into a 48 K and a 34 K protein (22). Part of the secreted 52 K protein can be taken up and processed by the MCF7 cells, while this binding is specifically inhibited by Mannose-6-P receptors. It has however not yet been demonstrated that the autocrine mitogenic activity of the protein is mediated by this receptor.

THE 52 K PROTEIN, A LYSOSOMAL ACIDIC PROTEASE

The protein was shown to be different from plasminogen activator (18) and no enzymatic activity was found at neutral pH. By contrast, at acidic pH the purified secreted 52 K protein and the corresponding cellular proteins (52 K + 48 K + 34 K) displayed

FIGURE 1. Autocrine and paracrine control by estrogen-induced secreted proteins

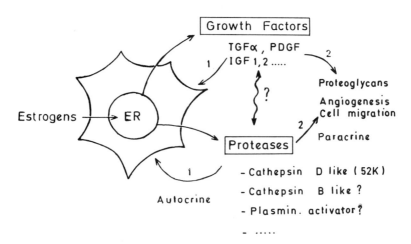

Estrogens, via their nuclear receptors (ER), induce several proteins which are secreted by breast cancer cells. One category (growth factors) may act as autocrine factors which stimulate the growth of these same cells (see Lippman contribution). Other proteins, such as proteases, have also the ability to facilitate cell migration, angiogenesis and possibly metastasis. The 52 K protein is the precursor of a cathepsin D-like protease which is also an autocrine mitogen in vitro. This property may stimulate the development of new therapeutic agents, since a means of selectively inhibiting its activity (antibodies, analogs, enzyme, inhibitors) might work in both hormone-responsive and resistant cancers.

a strong proteolytic activity which was mostly inhibited by pepstatin (21). There are similarties with the previously described cathepsin D (2) but also striking differences such as the hormonal regulation of the 52 K protein, the extent of its secretion by breast cancer cells, and its high concentration in proliferative ductal mammary cells (14). The relationship between the mitogenic and proteolytic activities of this protein is currently unknown. There are however previous examples such as thrombin, a protease with mitogenic activity (3). The proteolytic activity of the 52 K protein moreover strongly suggests that this protease may, at some step of mammary cancerogenesis, facilitate cell migration and metastasis, as this was suggested for other proteases (16,23). In vivo, the paracrine effect on adjacent cells, connective tissue and blood vessels, may be at least as equally important as the autocrine activity of this protein (Fig. 1). This protease is produced both by hormone-dependent and independent breast cancers cells in culture.

CONCLUSIONS

Estrogens may stimulate the growth of breast cancer cells in culture indirectly via the secretion of growth factors and/or of certain proteases, such as the 52 K protein which is able to act as an autocrine mitogen. The estrogen-induced secretion of an active protease such as the 52 K protein precursor, may also facilitate metastasis and tumor invasion. Cloning of the cDNA is in progress to specify the structure and possible function of this protein in carcinogenesis and/or growth control. These results on breast cancer may stimulate research on other hormone-regulated cancers (prostate, endometrium) where similar hormone-induced proteases may be found.

ACKNOWLEDGEMENTS

We are grateful to members of our laboratory and of CLIN-MIDY SANOFI Laboratory (B. Pau) (Grant INSERM/SANOFI n°81039.3) who have contributed to several parts of this work ; to D. Derocq, G. Salazar, C. Rougeot and C. Prébois for technical assistance and to E. Barrié for her skilfull preparation of the manuscript. We thank Drs M. Lippman, M. Rich, I. Keydar, and the Mason Research Institute, for their gifts of mammary cell lines and Pr P. Chambon for his gift of pS2 cDNA clone. Marker studies have been performed with the help of several clinical centers (Prs Pujol, Lamarque, Lasfargue and Pagès).

REFERENCES

1. Capony, F., Garcia, M., Capdevielle, J., Ferrara, P., and Rochefort, H. Submitted for publication.
2. Capony, F. et al, Submitted for publication.
3. Carney, D.H., and Cunningham, D.D. (1978): Cell, 15:1341-1349.
4. Chalbos, D., Vignon, F., Keydar, I., and Rochefort, H. (1982): J. Clin. Endocrin. Met., 55:276-283.

5. Chambon, P., Dierich, A., Gaub, M.P., Jakowlev, S., Jongstra, J., Krust, A., Lepennec, J.P., Oudet, P., and Reudelhuber, T. (1984): In: Recent Progress in Hormone Research, edited by O. Greep, Vol. 40, p. 1. Academic Press, New York.
6. Darbre, P., Yates, J., Curtis, S., and King, R.J.B. (1983): Cancer Res., 43:349–354.
7. DeLarco, J.E., and Todaro, G.J. (1978): Proc. Natl. Acad. Sci. USA, 75:4001–4005.
8. Dembinski, T.C., and Green, C.D. (1984): Lymphokine Res., 3.
9. Dickson, R.B., Huff, K.K., Spencer, E.M., and Lippman, M.E. (1986): Endocrinology, 118:138–142.
10. Dupont, W., and Page, D.L. (1985): N. Engl. J. Med., 312:146–151.
11. Edwards, D.P., Adams, D.J., Savage, N., and McGuire, W.L. (1980): Biochem. Biophys. Res. Commun., 93:804–811.
12. Garcia, M., Capony, F., Derocq, D., Simon, D., Pau, B., and Rochefort, H. (1985): Cancer Res., 45:709–716.
13. Garcia, M., Salazar-Retana, G., Richer, G., Domergue, J., Capony, F., Pujol, H., Laffargue, F., Pau, B., and Rochefort, H. (1984): J. Clin. Endocrin. Met., 59:564–566.
14. Garcia, M., Salazar-Retana, G., Pagès, A., Richer, G., Domergue, J., Pagès, A.M., Cavalié, G., Martin, J.M., Lamarque, J.L., Pau, B., Pujol, H., and Rochefort, H. (1986): Cancer Res., in press (July/August).
15. Lippman, M.E., Bolan, G., and Huff, K. (1976): Cancer Res., 36:4595–4601.
16. Liotta, L.A. (1986): Cancer Res., 46:1–7.
17. Manni, A., Wright, C., Feil, P., Baranao, L., Demers, L., Garcia, M., and Rochefort, H. (1986): Cancer Res., 46: 1594–1598.
18. Massot, O., Capony, F., Garcia, M., and Rochefort, H. (1984): Mol. Cell. Endocrinol., 35:167–175.
19. Massot, O., Baskevitch, P.P., and Rochefort, H. (1985): Mol. Cell. Endocrinol., 42:207–214.
20. McGuire, W.L. (1980): In: Recent Progress in Hormone Research, Vol. 36, p. 135, Academic Press, New York.
21. Morisset, M., Capony, F., and Rochefort, H. (1986): Biochem. Biophys. Res. Commun., in press.
22. Morisset, M., Capony, F., and Rochefort, H., Submitted for publication.
23. Poole, A.R. (1979): In: Lysosomes in Biology and Pathology, edited by J.T. Dingle, and Fell. pp. 304–337. American Elsevier Publications Co., New York.
24. Rochefort, H., Coezy, E., Joly, E., Westley, B., and Vignon, F. (1980): In: Hormones and Cancer, edited by S. Iacobelli et al. Vol. 14, pp. 21–29. Raven Press, New York.
25. Rochefort, H., Chalbos, D., Capony, F., Garcia, M., Veith, F., Vignon, F., and Westley, B. (1984): In: Hormones and Cancer, edited by E. Gurpide et al. Vol. 142, pp. 37–51.
26. Salomon, D.S., Zwiebel, J.A., Bano, M., Losonczy, L., Fehnel, P., and Kidwell, W.R. (1984): Cancer Res., 44:4069–4077.

27. Vignon, F., Derocq, D., Chambon, M., and Rochefort, H. (1983): C. R. Acad. Sci. Paris, 296:151–156.
28. Vignon, F., Capony, F., Chambon, M., Freiss, G., Garcia, M., and Rochefort, H. (1986): Endocrinology, 118:1537–1545.
29. Westley, B., and Rochefort, H. (1980): Cell, 20:353–362.
30. Westley, B., May, F.E.B., Brown, A.M.C., Krust, A., Chambon, P., Lippman, M.E., and Rochefort, H. (1984): J. Biol. Chem., 259:10030–10035.

Hormonal Manipulation of Cancer: Peptides, Growth Factors, and New (Anti) Steroidal Agents, edited by Jan G. M. Klijn et al. Raven Press, New York © 1987.

EPIDERMAL GROWTH FACTOR RECEPTORS IN PRIMARY HUMAN BREAST
AND BLADDER CANCER: RELATION TO TUMOUR DIFFERENTIATION,
INVASION AND PATIENT SURVIVAL

Professor Adrian L. Harris[*ς], J.R.C. Sainsbury[+], K. Smith[*],
D.E. Neal[+], R.R. Hall[+], J.R. Farndon[+]

[*]Department of Clinical Oncology, Cancer Research Unit,
Royal Victoria Infirmary, Newcastle upon Tyne and
[+]University Department of Surgery, Newcastle upon Tyne.

[ς]To whom reprint requests should be directed

INTRODUCTION

Epidermal growth factor (EGF) is a 53 amino acid peptide of
molecular weight 6045 daltons which contains 3 intra-chain disulphide bridges. Originally, it was isolated by Cohen from the
submaxillary gland of the immature male mouse and was found to
cause premature eye opening and eruption of the incisor teeth (2).
Independently, Gregory isolated a peptide from human urine (urogastrone) that inhibited gastric acid secretion (12): urogastrone
is human EGF (30).

EGF is found in human tissues including Brunner's glands of the
duodenum, the anterior pituitary, certain cells in the bone marrow, the skin and its appendages, the kidney and male genital
tract and it is secreted in milk (6,7,13,18). Large quantities
of EGF are found in human urine and are probably the result of
secretion by renal tubular cells. A 4,700 nucleotide sequence
messenger RNA has been found in kidney which codes for a large
molecular weight precursor of EGF - prepro-EGF (24). Prepro-EGF
consists of around 1,200 amino acids and part of it is similar to
the EGF receptor. It is possible that prepro-EGF is the source
of urinary EGF which is released by a processing enzyme on the
plasma membrane of the renal tubular cell (23).

The physiological role of EGF has not yet been clarified. In
addition to its effects on the newborn mouse, it induces maturation of the foetal lung (11) and may play a role in the normal
regeneration of the epithelial surfaces of the gut and urinary
tract. For instance, EGF given intravenously to an infant with
microvillous atrophy was recently reported to result in increased
crypt cell proliferation (32).

The EGF Receptor

The actions of EGF are mediated by binding to a specific membrane bound receptor. EGF receptors have been identified on cells of different origins including fibroblasts, corneal cells, kidney cells, breast cells and cells derived from tumours of different types (3,9,10,19,20,21,26,29).

The EGF receptor has been identified by several methods, including chemical cross linking and immuno-affinity purification, its molecular weight is between 160,000 d and 180,000 d. Much of the recent work on the EGF receptor has been carried out on A431 human epidermoid tumour cells which were derived originally from a vulval squamous tumour and which express a high concentration of EGF receptors (31), although these cells are stimulated to grow only by low concentrations of EGF. Human placenta is also a rich source of EGF receptor. The EGF receptor has two main parts - an external domain of 621 amino acids which is responsible for binding of EGF and other ligands (including TGF-α) and a cytoplasmic part of 542 amino acids which contains a tyrosine specific protein kinase (5), linked by a short transmembrane section (31).

EGF receptor and the erb-B oncogene

The structure of the EGF receptor has recently been shown to be similar to the oncogene product of erb-B of the avian erythroblastosis virus (5). The cytoplasmic and transmembrane portion of the EGF receptor showed 90% homology with the gp65v-erb-B protein. Thus, the erb-B oncogene protein may represent a truncated EGF receptor which lacks the external binding site for EGF. Initially, it was thought that erb-B lacked a tyrosine specific protein kinase. However, in the absence of the external binding site, stimulation of activity is difficult to detect and recent evidence suggests that erb-B may contain a tyrosine specific protein kinase which is self-activated (5,14).

Transforming growth factor-alpha (TGF-α)

TGFs have been classified on the basis of their interaction with the EGF receptor (25). TGF-α binds to the EGF receptor whereas TGF-β does not. TGF-α has been found in the conditioned medium of several transformed and malignant cell lines (28).

TGF-α exhibits competitive binding to the EGF receptor, although differences were observed in the optimum conditions for binding. TGF-α has molecular weight of 7,000 d and despite a similar action to EGF on the EGF receptor, no immunological cross-reactivity was demonstrated between the two and TGF-α has only limited sequence homology with EGF. TGF-α is secreted as a 160 amino acid precursor (TGF-α is 50 amino acids in length) and has 3 pairs of cysteine residues like EGF (4) but has only about 40% homology with EGF (15,16). m-RNA encoding TGF-α is correspondingly long and the gene is found on chromosome 2. The similar affinity of TGF-α to EGF for the EGF receptor is due to homology over part of the polypeptide chain. Binding of TGF-α also stimulates the EGF receptor tyrosine kinase.

Increased expression of mRNAs encoding TGF-α has been

identified in several human tumours including cells from the A431 line and other mainly solid primary human tumours such as renal, breast and squamous tumours (4).

TGF-β do not bind to the EGF receptor (EGFr) but can act synergistically with TGF-α to stimulate cell growth. Under some circumstances, TGF-β may be a growth inhibitor.

EGFr provide a final common pathway by which tumours that secrete growth factors as the result of several different transformation mechanisms cause autocrine growth stimulation.

Because variations in normal EGFr expression may modify response to local tumour growth factors and hence biological behaviour of human tumours, we have evaluated quantitative EGFr assays in primary breast and bladder tumours. The prognostic importance has been followed prospectively and in all cases immunohistochemistry has been performed, as well as ligand binding assays, in order to control for the problem of endogenous ligands blocking the receptors.

METHODS

Primary tumour membranes were prepared by homogenisation in 10 mM tris 50 mM NaCl buffer, pH 7.4, at 4°C. Sequential centrifugations at 100 G for 10 minutes and 100,000 G for 45 minutes produced a cell pellet enriched in plasma membranes, as shown by 5' nucleotidase assay. ^{125}I-EGF was prepared by the iodogen method (label specific activity 50 - 80 µCi/µg). Incubations were for 2 hours at 26°C with shaking. Total reaction volume was 400 µl, with 100 µg protein. Non-specific binding was assessed at 1 nM labelled EGF by using 100-fold excess unlabelled EGF. The reaction was terminated by adding cold buffer and centrifugation. Non-specific binding was 0.5 - 1% of added counts and specific binding was defined as binding detectable above 95% confidence limits for the non-specific binding in triplicate (19,26,27).

The EGF receptor was also identified on frozen sections by an indirect immunoperoxidase technique with a murine monoclonal antibody (EGFR1, donated by Dr. M. Waterfield). After blocking with normal rabbit serum, EGFR1 was added and rabbit anti-mouse immunoglobulin conjugated with peroxidase was used as the second antibody. The positive control in each run was human placenta, and negative controls included omission of EGFR1, use of mouse immunoglobulin of the same class and preincubation of the antibody with purified EGFr receptors. Oestrogen receptors were measured by a dextran-coated charcoal method, in the National Quality Control Scheme.

Human Breast Cancer

To compare EGFr with other known prognostic variables, oestrogen receptors (ER), both "nuclear" and "cytoplasmic", were also measured in all primary tumours. Although it is clear that ER is nuclear in location, there is a more easily extractable component, the "cytoplasmic receptor".

EGF receptor was detected in the range of 4 - 43 fmol/mg membrane protein. Two binding sites were identified by Scatchard analysis, the higher affinity having a Kd range of 0.7 - 2.3 nM. Non-specific binding accounted for less than 10% of binding. Steady state binding was reached in 2 hours at 26 °C and was similar to that observed at 37 °C.

In 183 primary tumours, there was a striking inverse correlation of EGFr with ER (Table 1) (p < .001). For the purposes of statistical analysis, EGF binding < 5 fmol/mg membrane proteins was considered to be EGFr negative and ER binding < 5 fmol/mg cytosol protein was ER negative.

TABLE 1
EGFr in Primary Breast Carcinoma

	EGFr		
	+	−	
ER +	8	74	82
−	56	45	101
	64	119	183

The ER negative tumours can thus be split into two groups, those which are EGFr +ve and those which are EGFr -ve.

The ligand binding results were compared with semiquantitative grading of EGFr by immunohistochemistry and there was a significant correlation (27). EGFr measured by ligand binding is more sensitive than immunochemistry, accounting for EGFr +ve tumours that are negative in histochemistry. These results suggest that endogenous ligands are not interfering with the EGFr assay, since $EGFR_1$ antibody reacts with a peptide external domain of the EGFr and does not interfere with the binding site for EGF.

To correlate EGFr with other prognostic variables, Bloom and Richardson grading was carried out on 108 primary tumours (Table 2).

TABLE 2.   Bloom and Richardson
Grading v. EGF Receptor

	I	II	III	
EGFr +	2	11	32	45
−	10	25	28	63
	12	36	60	108

p < 0.002

EGFr were correlated with poorly differentiated tumours. The inverse correlation of EGFr with ER also occurred in regional lymph node metastases, 3 ER +ve metastases were EGFr -ve and 10 EGFr +ve

metastases were ER -ve (p < 0.02). No EGFr +ve metastases arose
from primary tumours that were EGFr -ve. To assess serial changes in EGFr status, we are now using fluorescence activated cell
sorting of needle aspirates stained with $EGFR_1$ antibody.

Both the monoclonal antibody and EGF ligand studies only detect
the external domain of the receptor, but do not give information
on the activity of the receptor. Therefore, immunoprecipitation
studies were carried out to detect autophosphorylation of the
EGFr. Membranes were incubated with or without 100 nM unlabelled
EGF and ^{32}ATP and the labelled receptor precipitated with $EGFR_1$
antibody after solubilization. Autoradiography showed that EGFr
were functional and that in some cases EGFr undetectable by ligand
binding or immunochemistry could be detected by enhancement of
autophosphorylation with EGF. However, for prognostic purposes
and correlation with other variables, ligand binding results have
been used.

None of these methods would detect EGFr analogous to erb-B,
which lacks the external domain and shows much less autophosphorylation than EGFr. We therefore used a polyclonal antibody raised
to a synthetic peptide homologous to a region of the internal
EGFr domain (gift of Dr. W. Gullick). 42 primary tumours were
studied and the particular immunochemical pattern that would show
an erbB type protein would be negative staining with $EGFR_1$ but
positive staining with the internal antibody. The control for
the internal antibody consisted of preincubation with the synthetic peptide to which it was raised. Only 2 tumours showed this
pattern and they were also EGFr negative by ligand binding. Unfortunately, there was insufficient material for molecular biological studies - so this remains to be confirmed. However, it is
clear that this is not a common finding in breast cancer (< 5%
of cases).

Two other groups have confirmed the reciprocal relationship of
EGFr to ER, although in the case of Fitzpatrick et al. (9,22) the
results did not reach significance. Their EGFr values ranged
from 1 - 121 fmol/mg membrane protein in 137 tumours. Perez et
al. (22) found a range of 1 - 64 fmol/mg membrane protein and a
significant inverse relationship in 95 human breast cancers. The
Kd mean was 3.7×10^{-9}M, and in pooled samples Fitzpatrick et al.
found a value of 2 nM. Thus a total of 415 breast tumours have
been described with good agreement of Kd and binding capacity.
However, the cut-off point for correlating EGFr with other variables is different in each series - for example, Fitzpatrick et
al. had a background binding of 54% to membrane filters used to
separate bound from free EGF. They considered specific binding
greater than 15% of total binding minus filter binding to be
EGFr +ve. They probably estimated tumours to be EGFr +ve which we
would not have done on statistical grounds. Thus, they found 48%
of tumours were positive and we found 35% positive. Perez et al.
found 42% of tumours positive but did not describe how they decided on EGFr +ve status, or what their background non-specific
binding was.

Since we have shown a highly significant association of EGFr status with ER -ve and poorly differentiated tumours, it would appear that our definition of EGFr +ve can be justified on the usefulness of the clinical correlation as well as the grounds of analysis of counting reliability.

The prognostic significance of EGFr status as defined above has now been analysed on the first 125 patients followed prospectively. As expected, there is a slower relapse initially with ER +ve tumours but by three years from first diagnosis, the relapse-free survival (RFS) curves come together again. Nevertheless, the curves for RFS and overall survival (OS) are both significantly different for ER +ve and ER -ve tumours.

Of particular interest is the result for ER -ve tumours stratified by EGFr status. There is a highly significant difference in OS as well as RFS, with EGFr +ve patients having a much higher mortality (RFS is 76% vs. 39% at 3 years and OS is 82% vs. 41%). The difference between ER +ve tumours and ER -ve tumours is not significant. Thus the early separation of survival curves for ER -ve and ER +ve tumours can be accounted for by the rapid demise of ER -ve EGFr +ve patients, and the coming together of the survival curves is related to the better prognosis of ER -ve EGFr -ve patients. These results provide an explanation for a major controversy in the literature on the effect of ER status on RFS. Studies following patients for over 5 years generally do not show a significant effect on RFS, but those analysing at 1 - 2 years do. An early relapsing poor prognosis subgroup would account for these results. We have defined such a subgroup by EGFr status.

There are other known prognostic factors such as tumour size and Bloom and Richardson grading, so we analysed these factors in our patients. There was no significant separation of survival (OS or RFS) using these criteria. Stratifying for these variables, EGFr +ve tumours always had the worst survival.

The separation of a poor prognostic subgroup in a relatively low number of patients followed up for 3 years suggests that EGFr status is a powerful discriminator and could be used for prospective trials of adjuvant therapy.

The expression of EGFr and poor prognosis suggests that the initial hypothesis that tumours expressing higher EGFr could be more responsive to endogenous growth factors is correct. This therefore provides new therapeutic options for this group of patients. Monoclonal antibodies to EGFr could be used to target drugs or radioisotopes. Since the third thiol disulphide loop of EGF and TGF-α appears critical for binding to EGFr, and is highly conserved, synthetic peptides homologous to this region have been synthesised. They antagonise the actions of EGF and hence there is the possibility of peptide hormone therapy in this group of tumours.

Because EGFr are detectable on the basal proliferative layers of several epithelia, it was of interest to see if in other common epithelial neoplasms there was a correlation of EGFr with tumour behaviour.

EGFr and Human Bladder Cancer

An important factor in predicting survival after treatment of patients with bladder cancer is the pathological stage of the tumour. In the long term, 70 - 80% of superficial bladder tumours can be controlled satisfactorily by means of regular cystoscopic treatment (8). In 10 - 15% of patients, invasive tumours will develop during follow-up and in 10 - 15% the superficial tumours will become difficult to control. Survival of patients with invasive bladder cancer is poor; only about 30% of patients are alive 5 years after radical local treatment (1).

We studied 48 patients with bladder cancer; 40 were male, 8 female. The median age was 62 years (range 35 - 90). 24 patients had superficial transitional cell carcinoma (15 pTa, 9 pT1); 5 were poorly differentiated (2 pTa, 3 pT1) and 19 moderately differentiated. 24 patients had invasive transitional cell carcinoma (pT3); 16 were poorly differentiated and 8 moderately differentiated.

Bladder biopsy samples were taken from 12 control patients with no evidence of bladder carcinoma (median age 64 years, range 30 - 70), 10 of whom had bladder outflow obstruction and underwent prostatectomy.

Urothelium from the 12 control patients did not stain positively for the EGF receptor. Weak staining, of insufficient intensity to be graded positive, was identified in the basal layers of the urothelium of 4 control patients. In another control patient weak staining was noted in an area of cystitis cystica. Weak background staining of the detrusor muscle was observed both in controls and in patients with bladder tumours.

7 of the 24 superficial tumours (29%) were graded positive for EGF receptors, 3 were pTa and 4 were pT1 tumours; 4 were moderately and 3 poorly differentiated. In 4 of the remaining 17 tumours, weak staining, of similar intensity to the background, was observed.

21 of the 24 invasive tumours (87.5%) were positively stained for EGF receptors. Thus the proportion of patients positive for EGF receptors was significantly greater for those with invasive than for those with superficial tumours (X^2 = 14.49; $p < 0.001$). The stain in positive tumours, invasive or superficial, was in the cytoplasm in all but 2; in these the stain was membranous. The distribution of the positively stained cells throughout the tumours was not uniform, but focal positivity was observed in only 4 of the 28 positive tumours.

Significantly more of the poorly differentiated tumours (18 of 21) than the moderately differentiated tumours (10 of 27) were positively stained (X^2 = 9; $p < 0.01$). Thus in another common epithelial cancer there is a correlation of EGFr expression with invasion and poor differentiation.

The above studies were carried out using immunohistochemistry and semiquantitative grading. We have now assessed 24 primary tumours by ligand binding with ^{125}I-EGF. The maximum binding occurred by 2 hours at 26°C and the range of positive binding was

8.5 - 1020 fmol/mg membrane protein. The Kd ranged from 0.23 -
1.78 nM. [11]/24 tumours were positive for EGFr by ligand binding.
The results of histochemistry and ligand binding were concordant
in [19]/24 cases (85%). The discrepancies were due to 4 tumours
positive by ligand binding but negative by immunochemistry -
suggesting that ligand binding is more sensitive. One tumour
stained strongly for EGFr, but the biopsy was mainly muscle and
stroma - thus accounting for low ligand binding. [5]/16 superficial
tumours were EGFr +ve by ligand binding, compared with [6]/8 invasive tumours. Thus the results of histochemistry were confirmed.

There was a marked difference in the amount of EGFr expressed
in positive superficial compared with positive invasive tumours
(Table 3).

TABLE 3. EGFr Binding to Bladder Cancers
(fmol/mg membrane protein) ([11]/24 positive)

Invasive	Superficial
n = 6	n = 5
23.4 - 1020	8.5 - 32.4
median 67	median 11.4
[4]/6 > 50 fmol/mg	all < 50 fmol/mg

Whether expression of EGFr is relative to local invasive recurrence in superficial bladder cancer or to particularly bad
prognosis in invasive bladder cancer is not yet known but these
patients are being followed prospectively.

Relevance of EGFr to Malignant Behaviour

Although EGFr is homologous to the erb-B oncogene, we have
shown that the receptor is essentially normal in ligand binding
and functional properties, in contrast to erb-B which lacks the
external ligand binding domain. Also, erb-B leads to erthro-
leukaemia in chickens, whereas the EGFr is expressed in epithelial
malignancies. EGFr was related to tumour stage and differentiation, suggesting that it is not a directly acting transforming
gene. Our interpretation is therefore that concomitant increased
expression of EGFr modifies the biological behaviour but is not
per se related to transformation.

These results show the importance of applying the fundamental
knowledge on oncogenes developed from molecular biology to the
clinical situation. The oncogenes may interact very differently
in common human epithelial malignancies - as shown for EGFr.

This work was supported by the North of England Cancer Research
Campaign.

REFERENCES

1. Bloom, H.J.G., Hendry, W.F., Wallace, D.M., and Skeet, R.G. (1982): Br. J. Urol., 54: 136-151.
2. Cohen, S. (1962): J. Biol. Chem., 237: 1555-1562.
3. Cohen, S. (1983): Cancer, 51: 1787-1791.
4. Derynck, R., van Tilburg, A., Rhee, L., and Chen, E. (1986): J. Cell Biochem., Suppl. 10C: 105.
5. Downward, J., Yarden, Y., Mayes, E. et al. (1984): Nature, 307 521-527.
6. Elder, J.B., Williams, G., Lacey, E. and Gregory, H. (1978): Nature, 217: 466-467.
7. Elson, S.D., Brown, C.A., and Thorburn, G.D. (1984): J. Clin. Endocrinol. Metab., 58: 589-594.
8. England, H.R., Paris, A.M.I., and Blandy, J.P. (1981): Br. J. Urol., 53: 593-597.
9. Fitzpatrick, S.L., LaChance, M.P., and Schultz, G.S. (1984a): Cancer Res. 44: 3442-3447.
10. Fitzpatrick, S.L., Brightwell, J., Wittliff, J.L., Barrows, G.H., and Schultz, G.S. (1984b): Cancer Res., 44: 3448-3453.
11. Goldin, G.V., and Opperman, L.A. (1980): J. Embryol. Exp. Morphol., 60: 235-243.
12. Gregory, H. (1975): Nature, 257: 325-327.
13. Kasselberg, A.G., Orth, D.N., Gray, M.E., and Stahlman, M.T. (1985): J. Histochem. Cytochem., 33: 315-322.
14. Kris, R.M., Lax, I., Gullick, W. et al. (1985): Cell, 40: 619-625.
15. Marquardt, H., Hunkapiller, M.W., Hood, L.E. et al. (1983): Proc. Natl. Acad. Sci. USA, 80: 4684-4688.
16. Marquardt, H., Hunkapiller, M.W., Hood, L.E. and Todaro, G.J. (1984): Science, 223: 1079-1081.
17. Messing, E. (1984): J. Urol., 131: 111A.
18. Nanney, L.B., Magid, M., Stoschek, C.M., and King, L.E. (1984) J. Invest. Dermatol., 83: 385-393.
19. Neal, D.E., Marsh, C., Bennett, M.K. et al. (1985): Lancet, i: 366-368.
20. Osborne, C.K., Hamilton, B., Titus, G., and Livingstone, R.B. (1980): Cancer Res., 40: 2361-2366.
21. Osborne, C.K., Hamilton, B., and Nover, M. (1982): J. Clin. Endocrinol. Metab., 55: 86-93.
22. Perez, R., Pascual, M., Macias, A., and Lage, A. (1984): Breast Cancer Res. Treat., 4: 189-193.
23. Pfeffer, S., and Ullrich, A. (1985): Nature, 313: 184.
24. Rall, L.B., Scott, J., and Bell, G.I. (1985): Nature, 313: 228-231.
25. Roberts, A.B., Frolik, C.A., Anzano, M.A., and Sporn, M.B. (1983): Fed. Proc., 42: 2621-2626.
26. Sainsbury, J.R.C., Sherbet, G.V., Farndon, J.R. and Harris, A.L. (1985): Lancet, i: 364-366.
27. Sainsbury, J.R.C., Malcolm, A.J., Appleton, D.R., Farndon, J.R., and Harris, A.L. (1985): J. Clin. Path., 38: 1225-1228

28. Saloman, D.S., Zwiebal, J.A., Bano, M., Losonczy, I., Fehnel, P., and Kidwell, W.R. (1984): Cancer Res., 44: 4069-4077.
29. Sherwin, S.A., Minna, J.D., Gazdar, A.F., and Todaro, G.J. (1981): Cancer Res., 41, 3538-3542.
30. Starkey, R.H., Cohen, S., and Orth, D.N. (1975): Science, 189: 800-802.
31. Ullrich, A., Coussens, L., Hayflick, J.S. et al. (1984): Nature, 309: 418-425.
32. Walker-Smith, J.A., Phillips, A.D., Walford, N. et al. (1985): Lancet, ii: 1239-1240.

Hormonal Manipulation of Cancer: Peptides, Growth Factors, and New (Anti) Steroidal Agents, edited by Jan G. M. Klijn et al. Raven Press, New York © 1987.

POSSIBLE ROLE OF GASTRO-INTESTINAL HORMONES IN GASTRIC AND PANCREATIC CARCINOGENESIS

C.B.H.W. Lamers

Department of Gastroenterology and Hepatology, University Hospital, Leiden, The Netherlands

Gastro-intestinal hormones have trophic effects on the gastrointestinal tract (12). Recent studies in animals have shown that gastro-intestinal hormones may also stimulate development and growth of benign and malignant gastro-intestinal tumours, including stomach and pancreatic cancer. Two types of studies have been performed to demonstrate the effect of gastro-intestinal hormones on tumour growth. First, studies on the promotion by exogenous or endogenous gastro-intestinal hormones on carcinogenesis induced by chemical carcinogens and, second, studies on the effect of hormones on growth of tumour cells in vitro or transplanted into animals.

Effect of gastrointestinal hormones on gastric carcinogenesis.
Studies on the promotion of gastric carcinogenesis by gastro-intestinal hormones are mainly restricted to the effects of gastrin. Gastrin, a peptide-hormone produced by G-cells in the gastric antrum and the upper small intestine, is a powerful stimulus of gastric acid secretion. Furthermore, the peptide has a trophic effect on the gastrointestinal tract, especially on the stomach (12). In 1975, Tahara and Haizuka (27) reported that prolonged administration of gastrin resulted in a remarkable increase in the production of scirrhous gastric cancer in rats produced by N-methyl-N'-nitro-N-nitrosoguanidine (MNNG). Some years later, Kurihara at al (15) also succeeded in producing scirrhous carcinoma of the dog stomach by combined treatment of N-ethyl-N'-nitro-N-nitrosoguanidine and gastrin. Subsequently, Tahara et al (28) showed that in the rat gastrin promotes the development not only of gastric cancer but also of gastric carcinoids induced by administration of MNNG in the drinking water. Kishimoto et al (13) studied the effect of endogenous hypergastrinaemia on carcinogenesis by MNNG in rats. These workers induced atrophic gastritis in rats by immunization using homologous gastric mucosal homogenate as antigen. Six of the 10 rats developed gastric cancer. Serum gastrin concentrations in these 6 rats (168.5 ± 25.6 pg/ml) were significantly higher than the gastrin levels in the rats that did not develop gastric cancer (64.5 ± 20.0 pg/ml). These studies suggest that hypersecretion of endogenous gastrin may also stimulate gastric carcinogenesis by MNNG. It has recently been suggested that type I cAMP-dependent protein kinase is involved in the enhancement

by gastrin of gastric carcinogenesis induced by MNNG (30).

Growth promoting effects of gastro-intestinal hormones have also been demonstrated using rat stomach cancer cells in vitro. In this model not only gastrin, but also cholecystokinin, caerulein, glucagon and secretin were shown to possess tumour growth stimulating properties, whereas insulin, vasoactive intestinal polypeptide, thyroxin, epinephrine and steroid hormones were devoid of any effect on tumour growth in this model (14). It is interesting to note that the peptides of the gastrin-cholecystokinin family (gastrin, cholecystokinin, caerulein) had a more powerful effect on tumour growth than those of the secretin family (secretin, glucagon). The stimulating effect of gastrin on tumour growth has also been shown in the xenotransplantable human gastric cancer in the nude mouse model (25).

It has recently been shown that endogenous hypergastrinaemia is also involved in the development of gastric carcinoid tumours in rats (4). Since these tumours arise from ECL-cells in the gastric body they are also named ECL-oma's. In these experiments marked hypergastrinaemia was induced by long-term administration of very high doses of omeprazole. Omeprazole, a substituted benzimidazol, inhibits the enzyme H^+/K^+ ATPase in the parietal cell. High doses of the drug induce achlorhydria and secondary hypergastrinaemia. The development of gastric carcinoids was accompanied by ECL-cell hyperplasia (4). When hypergastrinaemia was prevented by antrectomy, omeprazole did not induce ECL-cell hyperplasia or carcinoid tumours (26).

At present it is not known whether gastrin is also involved in gastric carcinogenesis and tumour growth in man. Patients with hypergastrinaemia due to atrophic gastritis have an increased incidence of gastric adenocarcinoma and carcinoids (5), but the exact contribution of gastrin to the development of these tumours is poorly understood. On the other hand, in patients with hypergastrinaemia due to gastrin-producing tumours (Zollinger-Ellison syndrome) gastric carcinoids may be present, but gastric cancer is extremely rare.

Effect of gastrointestinal hormones on pancreatic carcinogenesis
Two animal models of pancreatic carcinogenesis have been used to study the effects of possible promotors or inhibitors of tumour growth. First, the acinar cell-type adenocarcinoma induced by azaserine in rats (Longnecker model; 18) and, second, the ductal/ductular cell-type adenocarcinoma induced by certain nitrosamines in hamsters (Pour model; 22). Histologically, human pancreatic adenocarcinoma resembles the ductular adenocarcinoma in hamsters (7). However, there is no agreement as to the origin

of human gastric cancer. It has recently been suggested that ductular carcinoma may originate not only from ductular cells, but also by dedifferentiation from acinar cells (10,24). Therefore, both the rat acinar cell tumour model and the hamster ductular cell tumour model may contribute to our understanding of pancreatic carcinogenesis in man.

Rat acinar cell tumour model.
Administration of azaserine induces acinar cell tumours (adenoma and carcinoma) in rats (18). The development of azaserine-induced tumours can be greatly enhanced by feeding raw soya flour (20). It is noteworthy that in rats a raw soya flour diet alone has potent pancreatic growth stimulating actions, resulting in hypertrophy, hyperplasia, adenoma's and adenocarcinoma's (19).Heating the soya flour reduces but does not abolish the trophic effect of the diet on the pancreas. It is suggested that the trypsin-inhibiting potency of raw soya flour interferes with a postulated luminal trypsin/plasma cholecystokinin feedback mechanism, resulting in increased plasma cholecystokinin concentrations (9,21). Cholecystokinin, a peptide hormone produced in the upper small intestine, stimulates gallbladder contraction and pancreatic enzyme secretion. In addition, cholecystokinin has trophic effects on the gastrointestinal tract, especially on the pancreas (12). In fact, long-term administration of cholecystokinin is reported to have similar growth stimulating properties as raw soya flour (8,16). Furthermore, increased plasma concentrations of cholecystokinin during a raw soya flour diet in rats have been demonstrated by gallbladder bioassay (3) and radioimmunoassay (1). The promoting effect of a high fat diet on azaserine-induced pancreatic tumours may also be mediated by cholecystokinin, because fat is a potent stimulus of cholecystokinin release (23). Interestingly, a combination of di(2-hydroxy-propyl)nitrosamine and raw soya flour induces acinar-cell tumours in the rat, while the nitrosamine alone does not produce pancreatic tumours in these animals (16).

Hamster ductal/ductular cell tumour model
Administration of several nitrosamines induces ductal/ductular cell adenocarcinoma in hamsters. Three studies on a possible promoting effect of cholecystokinin on the induction of ductular cell carcinoma by nitrosamines have been performed with contrasting results. Johnson et al (11) reported that cholecystokinin inhibits pancreatic carcinogenesis induced by di-isopropanol nitrosamine in hamsters, while Andrén-Sandberg et al (2) were unable to demonstrate any effect of caerulein, a synthetic cholecystokinin-analogue, on the development of pancreatic cancer by N-nitrosobis(2-hydroxypropyl)amine in hamsters. On the other hand, Howatson and Carter (10) found a marked enhancement by cholecystokinin of pancreatic carcinogene-

sis induced by N-nitrosobis(2-oxopropyl)amine. Several differences in the design of the three studies may be responsible for the contrasting results.

Townsend et al (29) have studied the effect of cholecystokinin and secretin on a tissue culture cell line of pancreatic ductal adenocarcinoma from Syrian golden hamster injected into hamster cheek pouches. In this model cholecystokinin had a modest tumour growth promoting effect, which was greatly enhanced by the addition of secretin.

It has also been demonstrated that epidermal growth factor, another regulatory peptide, promotes pancreatic carcinogenesis by N-nitrosobis(2-oxopropyl)amine in hamsters (6). Furthermore, epidermal growth factor stimulates tumour growth of a human pancreatic adenocarcinoma cell line in vitro (17). Interestingly, the stimulatory effect of epidermal growth factor in this model is inhibited by somatostatin (17).

Conclusion

Several studies in experimental animals have shown that gastro-intestinal hormones may influence development and growth of gastric and pancreatic cancer. Obviously, more studies have to be performed to allow definite conclusions about the effects of various peptide hormones on gastro-intestinal tumours. Furthermore, studies have to be performed to determine whether hormonal manipulation is helpful in influencing tumour growth in both animals and man.

REFERENCES

1. Adrian, T.E., Pasquali, C., Pescosta, F.,
   Bacarese-Hamilton, A.J., and Bloom, S.R. (1982): Gut,
   23:A889.
2. Andrén-Sandberg, Å., Dawiskiba, S., and Ihse, I. (1984):
   Scand. J. Gastroenterol., 19:122-8.
3. Brand, S.J., and Morgan, R.G.H. (1981): J. Physiol.,
   319:325-43.
4. Carlsson, E., Larsson, H., Mattsson, H., Ryberg, B., and
   Sundell, G. (1986): Scand. J. Gastroenterol., 21 (suppl
   118):39-45.
5. Carney, J.A., Go, V.L.W., Fairbanks, V.F., Moore, S.B.,
   Alport, E.C., and Nora, F.E. (1983): Ann. Intern. Med.,
   99:761-6.
6. Chester, J.F., Gaissert, H.A., Ross, J.S., and Malt, R.A.
   (1985): Proc. AACR, 26:121.
7. Cubilla, A.L., and Fitzgerald, P.J. (1975): Cancer Res.,
   35:2234-48.
8. Fölsch, U.R., Winckler, K., and Wormsley, K.G. (1978):
   Scand. J. Gastroenterol., 13:663-71.

9. Green, G.M., and Lyman, R.L. (1972): Proc. Soc. Exp. Med., 140:6-12.

10. Howatson, A.G., and Carter, D.C. (1985): Br. J. Cancer, 51:107-14.

11. Johnson, F.E., LaRegina, M.C., Martin, S.A., and Bashiti, H.M. (1983): Cancer Detect. Prev., 6:389-402.

12. Johnson, L.R. (1981): Cancer, 47:1640-5.

13. Kishimoto, S., Kunita, S., Shimizu, S., Koh, H., Yamamoto, M., Kajiyama, G.,and Miyoshi, K. (1983): Hir. J. Med. Sci., 32:213-8.

14. Kobori, O., Vuillot, M.T., Martin, F. (1982): Int. J. Cancer, 30:65-7.

15. Kurihara, M., Shirakabe, H., Yamaya, F., Miyasaka, K., Mariyama, T., Izumi, T., Yasui, A., and Kamano, T. (1979): Acta Pathol. Jpn., 29:171-6.

16. Levison, D.A., Morgan, R.G.H., Brimacombe, J.S., Hopwood, D., Coghill, G., and Wormsley, K.G. (1979): Scand. J. Gastroenterol., 14:217-24.

17. Liebow, C., Hierowski, M., and duSapin, K (1986): Pancreas, 1:44-8.

18. Longnecker, D.S., and Curphey, T.J., (1975): Cancer Res., 35:2249-58.

19. McGuinness, E.E., Morgan, R.G.H., Levison, D.A., Frape, D.L., Hopwood, D., and Wormsley K.G. (1980): Scand. J. Gastroenterol., 15:497-502.

20. McGuinness, E.E., Morgan, R.G.H., Levison, D.A., Hopwood, D., and Wormsley, K.G. (1981): Scand. J. Gastroenterol., 16:49-56.

21. McGuinness, E.E., Morgan R.G.H., and Wormsley, K.G. (1984): Environ. Health Perspect., 56:205-12.

22. Pour, P., Krueger, F.W., Althoff, J., Cardesa, A., and Mohr, U. (1974): Am. J. Pathol., 76:349-58.

23. Roebuck, B.D., O'Connor, T.P., and Campbell, T.C. (1985): Fed. Proc., 44:769.

24. Scarpelli, D.G., and Rao, M.S. (1978) Fed. Proc., 37:232.

25. Sumiyoshi, H., Yasui, W., Ochiai, A., and Tahara E. (1984): Cancer Res., 44:4276-80.

26. Sundler, F., Carlsson, E., Hakanson, R., Larsson, H., and Mattsson, H. (1986): Scand. J. Gastroenterol., 21 (suppl. 118):39-45.

27. Tahara, E., and Haizuka, S. (1975): Gann, 66:421-6.

28. Tahara, E., Shimamoto, F., Taniyama, K., Ito, H., Kosako, Y, and Sumiyosih, H. (1982): Cancer Res., 42: 1781-7.

29. Townsend, C.M., Franklin, R.B., Watson, L.C., Glass, E.J., and Thompson, J.C. (1981): Surg. Forum, 32:228-9.

30. Yasui, W., and Tahara, E. (1985): Cancer Res., 45:4763-7.

Hormonal Manipulation of Cancer: Peptides, Growth Factors, and New (Anti) Steroidal Agents, edited by Jan G. M. Klijn et al. Raven Press, New York © 1987.

SOMATOSTATIN ANALOGS IN THE TREATMENT

OF VARIOUS EXPERIMENTAL TUMORS

Andrew V. Schally, Tommie W. Redding, Ren-Zhi Cai, Jose I. Paz, Menashe Ben-David, and Ana-Maria Comaru-Schally

VA Medical Center and
Tulane University School of Medicine
1601 Perdido Street, New Orleans, LA 70146 U.S.A.

Various experimental approaches for the treatment of hormone-dependent tumors based on the use of analogs of LH-RH, analogs of somatostatin and other peptides, alone or in combination, are being investigated in animal tumor models and human cancer lines transplanted to nude mice (38,40). Our findings that some of the early analogs of somatostatin-14 (S-S-14) inhibited tumor growth in animal models of breast cancer, prostate cancer, chondrosarcomas, osteosarcomas, pituitary tumors, and pancreatic cancer (10,33,34,37,38,40), led us to synthesize more than 200 modern octapeptide analogs of somatostatin (5,6). These analogs were designed for selective, enhanced and prolonged activities (6). Among these octapeptides, some contained N-terminal D-Phe, followed by hexapeptide sequences Cys-2, Phe-3, D-Trp-4, Lys-5, Thr-6, Cys-7 or Cys-2, Tyr-3, D-Trp-4, Lys-5, Val-6, Cys-7 and Thr-8-NH_2 or Trp-8-NH_2 as C-Terminal residues. Analog RC-121, D-Phe-Cys-Tyr-D-Trp-Lys-Val-Cys-Thr-NH_2 and RC-160, D-Phe-Cys-Tyr-D-Trp-Lys-Val-Cys-Trp-NH_2 were 158-177 times and 113-134 times more potent, respectively, than somatostatin in inhibiting growth hormone (GH) release and showed a prolonged duration of action (6). In tests in animal tumor models, various analogs of both Phe-3, Thr-6, and Tyr-3, Val-6 series were shown to possess significant antitumor activity. In this article we will review some studies with the earlier analogs and report our recent investigations of antitumor activities of the new selective superactive and long-acting somatostatin analogs.

Prostate Cancer

Combination of LH-RH agonists with somatostatin analogs, may lead to a greater inhibition of prostate tumors, than that which can be obtained with LH-RH agonists alone (37). This hypothesis is based on the evidence that prolactin may be a promoter of prostate growth and could be involved in prostate

cancer as a co-factor (2,4,8,12,13,16,19,28,30,37,43). It has
been shown that prolactin enhances metabolic and proliferative
processes in the prostate and may potentiate the action of
5-dihydrotestosterone (DHT) (2,4,8,13,16,19,28,43).
Somatostatin analogs and peptides with PIF (prolactin inhibiting
factor) activity inhibit prolactin release (37,38,40).
Somatostatin analogs also suppress growth hormone release and
have direct antiproliferative effect on cells resulting in
growth inhibition (6,14,24,37). One of the major mechanisms by
which GH acts is by inducing hepatic production of the
somatomedins (Sm/IGF-1) (9,11). Recently, GH has been shown,
both in vitro and in vivo, to increase local production of
SM/IGF-1 in multiple tissues (9,11). This suggests that GH may
be involved in paracrine or autocrine mechanisms of cell growth.
Somatomedin C/IGF.1 is one of the important growth factors found
in serum and plasma and is active in stimulating the
proliferation of a large number of cultured cells (9,11). The
reduction in prolactin levels produced by the administration of
a suitable somatostatin analog or a peptide with PIF activity,
combined with the decrease in serum testosterone, which results
from chronic treatment with LH-RH agonists, may inhibit prostate
tumors better than LH-RH agonists alone. Decrease in GH levels
induced by somatostatin analogs might also contribute to an
additional inhibition of tumor growth.

Evidence obtained so far in animal models of prostate
tumors is in agreement with this view. In Dunning R-3327H model
of prostate adenocarcinoma in Copenhagen-Fisher rats, twice
daily s.c. administration of 25µg D-Trp-6-LH-RH or L-5F-Trp-8,
D-Cys-14 somatostatin significantly reduced the percent change
in tumor volume (37). The combination of somatostatin analog
with LH-RH agonist resulted in even greater reduction in tumor
volume than that which was obtained with either peptide given
alone (37).

Modern superactive octapeptide analogs of somatostatin,
including D-Phe-Cys-Tyr-D-Trp-Lys-Val-Cys-Thr-NH$_2$ (analog
RC-121), in doses of 2.5µg b.i.d., significantly decreased the
weight and volume of Dunning R-3327H prostate cancers and when
given in combination with once-a-month D-Trp-6-LH-RH microcapsules potentiated the effects of the latter. Microcapsules
of analog D-Phe-Cys-Tyr-D-Trp-Lys-Val-Cys-Trp-NH$_2$ (RC-160),
designed for a controlled release of this analog over a 15-30
day period, inhibited the growth of Dunning prostate tumors when
given alone. When the microcapsules of this somatostatin analog
were combined with injectable microcapsules of D-Trp-6-LH-RH,
they potentiated the effect of the latter. Continued
investigations are in progress in the Dunning model and in human
lines of prostate carcinoma transplanted into nude mice. The
aim of these studies is to determine whether the combination of
D-Trp-6-LH-RH with one of somatostatin analogs could result in

an increase in the therapeutic response in prostate cancer. It is possible that delayed delivery systems of somatostatin analogs could be used as adjuncts to microcapsules of Decapeptyl in the treatment of prostate cancer in man.

Breast Cancer

Various studies support the concept that prolactin may play a role in the growth of breast cancer in rodents as well as in humans (1,23,31,37). The presence of prolactin receptors in mammary tumors, including human breast cancer cells, also lends support to the theory that a certain proportion of mammary tumors can be prolactin-dependent (3). Growth hormone and somatomedins may also be involved in the growth of human breast cancer (29). Thus, the reduction in prolactin and GH levels induced by administration of a somatostatin analog, combined with the decrease in estrogen values that results from chronic treatment with LH-RH agonists, could lead to a greater inhibition of mammary tumors than that which can be obtained with LH-RH agonists alone. (Fig. 1.)

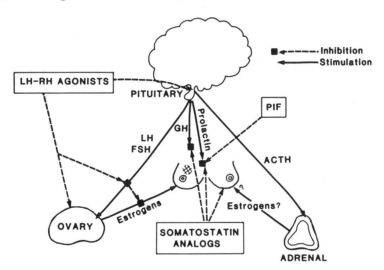

FIG. 1. Highly simplified schematic representation of how somatostatin analogs (or PIF) could be used alone or together with LH-RH agonists for the treatment of breast cancer. The selection of the rational therapy would be based on the status of the receptors for prolactin and sex steroids. Prolactin enhances metabolic and proliferative processes in the breast. Somatostatin analogs and/or PIF inhibit prolactin release. Somatostatin analogs also suppress growth hormone and have direct antiproliferative effect on cells. About 1/3 of all breast cancers are estrogen-dependent. LH-RH agonists create a state of estrogen deprivation.

Currently, the prediction of the response to endocrine therapy (anti-estrogen-Tamoxifen or LH-RH agonists) in human breast cancer is made according to the status of receptors for estrogen and progesterone only (27). The status of the receptors for prolactin was not evaluated as it was incorrectly considered to be of no value. This view stemmed from conflicting reports regarding the correlation between basal plasma prolactin levels and human breast cancer (45). The presence of prolactin receptors may decrease the amount of prolactin in the circulation, which in turn may account for the inconsistency of various reports on the correlation between plasma prolactin levels and human breast cancer. It is more likely that the presence of prolactin receptors in breast tissue, rather than circulating prolactin, is the determining factor in assessing the involvement of prolactin in breast cancer. Ben-David, et al. (3) have recently demonstrated the presence of specific binding sites for prolactin in human breast cancer specimens. Future hormonal treatment for breast cancer may be based on the status of both nuclear (steroid) and membrane (prolactin) receptors in any one patient. Breast tissue specimens, taken from women with breast cancer, are being assessed for the presence of binding sites for prolactin, estrogen and progesterone. The appropriate therapy could be given according to the presence (or absence) of binding sites for the respective hormone. After receptor evaluation, patients who are eligible for hormonal treatment would be divided into groups. In the case of the established estrogen dependency of their cancers, the patients would receive LH-RH analogs (21,38,40). Patients showing high levels of prolactin receptors would be treated with agents inhibiting prolactin secretion--such as somatostatin analogs or PIF. The therapy would therefore be more rational because it would be based on the status of the individual receptors. A combination of LH-RH analogs and somatostatin analogs could be used to treat women showing both high steroid and prolactin receptors (37,38,40).

Our own studies in Wistar/Furth rats bearing estrogen- and prolactin-dependent MT/W9A mammary adenocarcinoma showed that once-a-month administration of microcapsules releasing 25µg/day of D-Trp-6-LH-RH or twice daily injection of 3µg somatostatin analog Ac-p-Cl-D-Phe-Cys-Phe-D-Trp-Lys-Thr-Cys-Thr-NH$_2$ (RC-15) can inhibit the growth of this tumor (6,37). In another study, microcapsules releasing 5µg of analog (RC-160) D-Phe-Cys-Tyr-D-Trp-Lys-Val-Cys-Trp-NH$_2$ or 25µg D-Trp-6-LH-RH per day significantly inhibited the growth of the MT/W9A mammary tumor. When both types of microcapsules were given together, a significant synergism between the LH-RH agonists and the somatostatin analog was demonstrated in the inhibition of tumor growth. If these results can be confirmed and extended to human breast cancer lines, somatostatin analogs could be tried alone or as adjuncts together with agonistic analogs of LH-RH in the treatment of breast cancer in women, depending on the status of the receptors.

Osteosarcomas and Chondrosarcomas

The incidence of osteosarcomas may be influenced by growth hormone (17,38,40). Hormonal factors also play an important role in the growth of malignant cartilage tissue. Swarm rat chondrosarcoma is a tumor dependent upon GH, somatomedins, glucocorticoids and insulin (25,26,35). Somatostatin analogs, by inhibiting the GH secretion, could have potential therapeutic implications in treatment of this neoplasm. Our studies showed that in male Sprague-Dawley rats bearing transplanted Swarm chondrosarcoma, chronic administration of pNH_2-Phe-4-S-S-14, D-5F-Trp-8-S-S-14 or D-5-Methoxy-Trp-8-S-S-14 significantly reduced tumor weights and/or volume (33). D-Trp-6-LH-RH administered alone or with somatostatin analogs also reduced the weight and/or volume of chondrosarcomas (33). GH and prolactin levels were significantly decreased in rats treated with D-5F-Trp-8-S-S (33). Several experiments were also carried out in mice with Dunn osteosarcomas. L-5F-Trp-8,D-Cys-14-S-S prolonged the survival rate by 86%, L-5Br-Trp-8,D-Cys-14-S-S by 73% and D-Trp-6-LH-RH by 29%-37% (37,38,40). The analogs Ac-p-Cl-Phe-Cys-Phe-D-Trp-Lys-Thr-Cys-Thr-NH_2 (RC-15) and D-Phe-Cys-Tyr-D-Trp-Lys-Val-Cys-Trp-NH_2 (RC-160-2H) in doses of 2-5µg b.i.d. also appeared to have antitumor activities as shown by an increased survival rate in mice bearing the Dunn osteosarcoma. At these dosages, tumor weight and volume were not significantly changed from routine values, but the survival rates were doubled by the administration of RC-15 and increased by 25% by RC-160-2H (6,37).

The Dunn murine model is similar, in many aspects, to human osteosarcoma including the elevation of alkaline phosphatase levels during tumor growth (15). There is a positive correlation between pulmonary metastatic tumors and serum alkaline phosphatase values (15). Somatostatin analogs that increased survival rates also appeared to decrease serum alkaline phosphatase levels in mice treated with those analogs. The inhibitory effect of somatostatin analogs on the growth of chondrosarcomas and osteosarcomas can most likely be explained by suppression of GH levels (33,37). It is also possible that some somatostatin analogs have a direct antiproliferative effect on tumor tissue (37). The mechanism of suppression of these tumors by D-Trp-6-LH-RH is not clear, but the state of sex-hormone deprivation, induced by therapy with D-Trp-6-LH-RH may affect estrogen- or testosterone-dependent proteins in bone and cartilage (33,36,40). Inhibition of the Swarm chondrosarcomas and Dunn osteosarcomas by analogs of somatostatin and LH-RH agonists raises some hope that they might lead to a new endocrine therapy for chondrosarcomas, osteosarcomas and related hormone-dependent neoplasms, which could be of value in patients with osteogenic malignancies where conventional therapy had failed (37,38,40).

Pancreatic Carcinoma

Malignant exocrine tumors arise most frequently from the ducts and thus most carcinomas are in the head of the pancreas (7,20,41). Carcinoma of the pancreas has a very poor prognosis and causes 20,000 deaths per year in the U.S. (7,20,41,42). Somatostatin and some of its analogs inhibit secretion and/or action of gastrin, secretin, cholecystokinin (CCK) and VIP (vasoactive intestinal polypeptide) (32,39). Gastrin, cholecystokinin and secretin produce hyperplasia and hypertrophy of the exocrine pancreas (18) and might influence the growth of the malignant cells of the pancreas as well (44). Clinical studies have demonstrated that somatostatin or its analogs can inhibit the secretion of insulin in patients with insulinomas, glucagon in cases of glucagonoma as well as the secretion of ectopic endocrine tumors of the pancreas (22,32,37,40).

Using animal models of pancreatic cancer, we investigated the effect of analogs of hypothalamic hormones on the growth of pancreatic tumors (34). In Wistar/Lewis rats bearing the acinar pancreatic tumors DNCP-322, chronic administration of L-5Br-Trp-8-Somatostatin significantly decreased tumor weights and volume. D-Trp-6-LH-RH also decreased tumor weight and volume. In Syrian hamsters with a ductal form of pancreatic cancer, administration of L-5-Br-Trp-8-S-S for 21-30 days, diminished tumor weights and volume. D-Trp-6-LH-RH, given twice daily or injected in the form of constant-release microcapsules, significantly decreased tumor weight and volume and suppressed serum levels of testosterone (34). These findings suggest that pancreatic adenocarcinoma may be sensitive to both gastrointestinal and sex hormones. D-Trp-6-LH-RH might decrease the growth of pancreatic carcinomas by creating a state of sex-hormone deprivation (34). Somatostatin analogs reduce the growth of pancreatic ductal and acinar cancers, probably by inhibiting the release and/or stimulatory action of gastrointestinal hormones and other growth factors on tumor cells (34,40). It is also possible that some somatostatin analogs act directly on tumor tissue since somatostatin-14 has been shown to have antiproliferative effects on cells and to nullify the growth stimulation produced by Epidermal Growth Factor (EGF) (14,24,37).

Modern analogs, D-Phe-Cys-Tyr-D-Trp-Lys-Val-Cys-Thr-NH$_2$ (RC-121) and D-Phe-Cys-Tyr-D-Trp-Lys-Val-Cys-Trp-NH$_2$ (RC-160), in doses of 2.5µg b.i.d. inhibited the growth of W.D. ductal pancreatic tumors in golden hamsters in agreement with results obtained earlier with less potent analogs of somatostatin

(6,37). Some analogs of somatostatin could also be useful in the treatment of gastric and colon cancer. The inhibition of the growth of ductal and acinar pancreatic tumors by D-Trp-6-LH-RH or analogs of somatostatin reported by us appears to be the first attempt at endocrine management of these tumors (34). These observations could be of clinical significance. Somatostatin analogs and D-Trp-6-LH-RH should be considered for the development of a new hormonal therapy for cancer of the pancreas (34,37,40).

Summary and Conclusion

Some superactive and long-acting octapeptide analogs of somatostatin possess antitumor activities as shown by the inhibition of growth of animal models of prostate and mammary cancer, tumors of bone and cartilage, and ductal pancreatic cancer. The clinical efficacy of these compounds remains to be demonstrated. However, theoretical considerations and collective data from the animal tumor models appear to support our contention that an approach based on modern somatostatin analogs could become a useful addition to the present methods of treatment of certain endocrine-dependent or hormone-sensitive tumors.

Acknowledgements

We thank the National Hormone and Pituitary Program (NHPP) for the gifts of materials used in radioimmunoassays.

The experimental work described in this paper was supported by National Institutes of Health Grants AM07467, CA 40003, CA 40077 and CA 40004 and by the Medical Research Service of the Veterans Administration. We thank Ms. Nancy Meadows for the preparation of figures.

References

1. Arafah, B.M., Manni, A., and Pearson, O.H. (1980): Endrocrinology, 107:1364-1369.

2. Assimos, D., Smith, C., Lee, C., and Grayhack, J.T. (1984): Prostate, 5:589-595.

3. Ben-David, M., Dror, Y., and Biran, S. (1981): Israel J. Med. Sci., 17:965-969.

4. Blankenstein, M.A., Bolt-de Vries, J., Coert, H., Nievelstein, H., and Schroder, F.H. (1985): Prostate, 6:277-283.

5. Cai, R.-Z., Szoke, B., Fu, D., Redding, T.W., Colaluca, J., Torres-Aleman, I., and Schally, A.V. (1986): In: Synthesis and Evaluation of Activities of Octapeptide Analogs of Somatostatin: Ninth American Peptide Symposium, Toronto, edited by V.J. Hruby, K.D. Koppel, and C.M. Deber, pp. 627-630. Pierce Chemical, Rockford, IL.

6. Cai, R.-Z., Szoke, B., Lu, R., Fu, D., Redding, T.W., and Schally, A.V. (1986): Proc. Natl. Acad. Sci. U.S.A., 83:1896-1900.

7. Carbone, J.V., Lloyd, L., Brandborg, L.L., Silverman, S. Jr., (1976): In: Current Medical Diagnosis and Treatment, edited by M.A. Krupp, and M.J. Chatton, pp. 321-398. Lange, Los Altos, Calif.

8. Coert, A., Nievelstein, H., Kloosterboer, H.J., Loonen, P., and Van der Vries, J. (1985): Prostate, 6:269-276.

9. Davoren, J.B., and Hsueh, A.J.W. (1986): Endocrinology, 118:888-890.

10. deQuijada, M.G., Redding, T.W., Coy, D.H., Torres-Aleman, I., and Schally, A.V. (1983): Proc. Natl. Acad. Sci. U.S.A., 80:3485-3488.

11. Goustin, A.S., Leof, E.B., Shipley, G.D., and Moses, H.L. (1986): Cancer Res., 46:1015-1029.

12. Grayhack, J.T. (1963): Natl. Cancer Inst. Monogr., 12:189-199.

13. Grayhack, J.T., Bunce, P.L., Kearns, J.W., and Scott, W.W. (1955): Bull. Johns Hopkins Hosp., 96:154-163.

14. Hierowski, M.T., Liebow, C., du Sapin, K., and Schally, A.V. (1985): FEBS Lett., 179:252-256.

15. Hiramoto, R.N., Ghanta, V.K., Soong, S.-J., and Hurst, D.C. (1977): Cancer Res., 37:365-368.

16. Holland, J.M., and Lee, C. (1980): Biol. Reprod., 22:351-355.

17. Johnson, L.C. (1953): Bull. N.Y. Acad. Med., 29:164-171.

18. Johnson, L.R. (1981): Cancer, 47:1640-1645.

19. Johnson, M.P., Thompson, S.A., Lubaroff, D.M. (1985): J. Urol., 133:1112-1120.

20. Jordan, G.L. Jr. (1976): In: Brief Textbook of Surgery, edited by C.P. Artz, I. Cohn, and J.H. Davis, pp. 278-293. Saunders, Philadelphia.

21. Klijn, J.G.M., and DeJong, F.H. (1982): Lancet, i:1213-1216.

22. Long, R.G., Barnes, A.J., Adrian, T.E., Mallinson, C.N. Brown, M.R., Vale, W., Rivier, J.E., Christofides, N.D., and Bloom, S.R. (1979): Lancet, ii:764-767.

23. Malarkey, W.B., Kennedy, M., Allred, L.E., and Milo, G. (1983): J. Clin. Endocrinol. Metab. 56:673-677.

24. Mascardo, R.N., and Sherline, P. (1982): Endocrinology, 111: 1394-1396.

25. McCumbee, W.D., and Lebovitz, H.E. (1980): Endocrinology, 106:905-910.

26. McCumbee, W.D., McCarty, K.S. Jr., and Lebovitz, H.E. (1980): Endocrinology, 106:1930-1940.

27. McGuire, W.L. (1979): Proc. Soc. Exp. Biol. Med., 162:22-25.

28. Muntzing, J., Kirdani, R., Murphy, G.P., and Sandberg, A.A. (1977): Invest. Urol. 14:492-495.

29. Myal, Y.C., Shiu, R.P.C., and Bhaumick, B. (1983): Program Annual Meeting, Endocrine Society, Abstract No. 170, p. 123. San Antonio, Texas.

30. Negro-Vilar, A., Saad, W.A., and McCann, S.M. (1977): Endocrinology, 100:729-737.

31. Pearson, O.H., Murray, R., Mozaffarian, G., and Pensky, J. (1972): In: Prolactin and Carcinogenesis. Proceedings of the Fourth Tenovus Workshop on Prolactin and Carcinogenesis, edited by A.R. Boyns and K. Griffiths, pp. 154-157. Alpha Omega Alpha, Cardiff, Wales.

32. Raptis, S., Rosenthal, J., and Gerich, J.E. (eds.) (1984): In: 2nd International Symposium on Somatostatin, Athens (Greece), Attempto Verlag Tubingen GMBH, Germany.

33. Redding, T.W., and Schally, A.V. (1983): Proc. Natl. Acad. Sci. U.S.A., 80:1078-1082.

34. Redding, T.W., and Schally, A.V. (1984): Proc. Natl. Acad. Sci., U.S.A., 81:248-252.

35. Salomon, D.S., Paglia, L.M., and Verbruggen, L. (1979): Cancer Res., 39:4387-4395.

36. Schally, A.V. (1984): In: LHRH and Its Analogues, edited by F. Labrie, A. Belanger, and A. Dupont, pp. 3-15. 1984 Elsevier Science Publishers B.V., Amsterdam-New York.

37. Schally, A.V., Cai, R.-Z., Torres-Aleman, I., Redding, T.W., Szoke, B., Fu, D., Hierowski, M.T., Colaluca, J., and Konturek, S. (1986): In: Neural and Endocrine Peptides and Receptors, edited by T.W. Moody, (in press). Plenum, New York.

38. Schally, A.V., Comaru-Schally, A.M., and Redding, T.W. (1984): Proc. Soc. Exp. Biol. Med., 175:259-281.

39. Schally, A.V., Coy, D.H., and Meyers, C.A. (1978): In: Annual Review of Biochemistry, edited by E.E. Snell, pp. 89-128. Annual Reviews, Palo Alto, California.

40. Schally, A.V., Redding, T.W., and Comaru-Schally, A.M. (1984): Cancer Treat. Rep., 68-281-289.

41. Snodgrass, P.J. (1977): In: Harrison's Principles of Internal Medicine, edited by G.W. Thorn, R.D. Adams, E. Braunwald, K.J. Isselbacher, and R.G. Petersdorf, pp. 1643-1645. McGraw-Hill, New York.

42. Theve, N.O., Pousette, A., and Carlstrom, K. (1983): Clin. Oncol., 9:193-197.

43. Thomas, J.A., and Keenan, E.J. (1976): In: Cellular Mechanisms Modulating Gonadal Hormone Action, Advances in Sex Hormone Research, edited by R.L. Singhal, and J.A. Thomas, Vol. 2, pp. 425-470. University Park Press, Baltimore.

44. Townsend, C.M., Franklin, R.B., Watson, L.C., Glass, E.J., and Thompson, J.C. (1981): Surg. Forum, 32:228-229.

45. Wilson, R.G., Bachan, R., Roberts, M.M., Forrest, A.P.M., Boyns, A.R., Cole, E.N., and Griffiths, K. (1974): Cancer, 33:1325-1327.

Hormonal Manipulation of Cancer: Peptides,
Growth Factors, and New (Anti) Steroidal
Agents, edited by Jan G. M. Klijn et al.
Raven Press, New York © 1987.

SOMATOSTATIN ANALOG TREATMENT OF PITUITARY TUMORS

S.W.J. Lamberts

Department of Medicine,Erasmus University,Rotterdam,the Netherlands

INTRODUCTION

Somatostatin, a cyclic peptide consisting of 14 amino acids, was originally characterized as a growth hormone (GH)-release inhibiting factor in the hypothalamus (3). It has become more and more clear, however, that Somatostatin-containing cells are also present throughout the body (16,17). The name Somatostatin is therefore now considered to be inappropriate because the compound is involved in physiological actions in cells that have nothing to do with GH regulation, including an extensive distribution within the nervous system and in the gastro-intestinal tract (16,17). These multiple simultaneous actions of Somatostatin and its short duration of action after intravenous injection (half-life of 3 min) made its clinical use impractical (5). In addition,the post-infusion rebound hypersecretion of hormones, as for example present in acromegalic patients, greatly hampered the initial enthusiasm for the clinical use of this peptide. Recently Bauer et al. (1) succeeded in synthesizing a Somatostatin analog by step by step modification of a conformationally stabilized part of Somatostatin which was thought to be the central essential active moiety of the molecule. This analog, codenamed SMS 201-995 (Sandostatin; Sandoz, Basel, Switzerland) was at least 45 times more active than natural Somatostatin in its inhibitory effect on GH secretion in monkeys, while it was less powerful in its inhibitory actions on glucagon and especially insulin release. The reason for these differential effects on hormone release are currently unknown.SMS 201-995 is highly resistent to degradation by enzymes and tissue homogenates, which explains its much longer and stronger inhibitory action on GH release in vivo (1). Indeed natural Somatostatin and SMS 201-995 were shown on an equimolar base to exert a similar inhibitory effect on GH release by cultured human GH-secreting pituitary tumor cells (6,7). After a single subcutaneous injection of 50 μg SMS 201-995 to normal subjects, peak plasma SMS levels of 2.0 - 3.0 ng/ml (1.6 - 2.5 pM) were found 15 and 30 min. after injection. Del Pozo et al. (12) calculated the elimination half-life of SMS 201-995 after subcutaneous administration to be 113 min.

ACROMEGALY

Subcutaneous injection of 50 μg SMS 201-995 suppressed circulating GH levels in 7 acromegalic patients from 1 till 10 h after the drug from 30 ± 5 μg/l on a control day to 10.7 ± 4 μg/l (mean ± SEM; 7). The course of plasma GH levels in one of our patients on a control day and on the next day after the subcutaneous injection of 50 μg SMS 201-995 is shown in Fig. 1. A most important observation was the absence of rebound hypersecretion of GH after

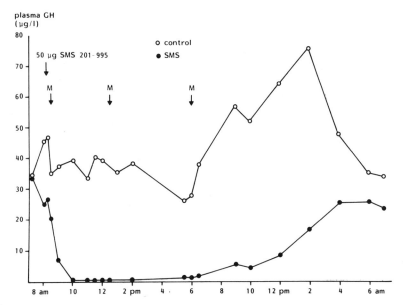

FIG. 1. The course of plasma GH levels on a control day (o—o) in an untreated acromegalic patient. On the next day 50 μg SMS 201-995 was injected subcutaneously at 9.15 am and plasma GH levels were measured (●—●).

SMS 201-995 administration. Apart from a transient post-prandial increase in circulating glucose concentrations, which was caused by the acute inhibitory effect of SMS 201-995 on insulin release, no side-effects were observed.

Five acromegalic patients were treated over a period of 8-24 weeks with SMS 201-995. These patients received daily subcutaneous doses of 100 to 300 μg in 2 to 3 injections (8). A rapid and outspoken improvement of the clinical picture occurred during SMS 201-995 treatment, while there was also evidence of a minor shrinkage of pituitary tumor size in 3 of these 5 patients. Plasma GH (measured in 18-20 samples over 24 h) fell from 59 ± 12 μg/l initially to 5.6 ± 3 μg/l at the end of the investigational period. Circulating Somatomedin-C levels, which were greatly elevated in all patients before the start of SMS 201-995 therapy, normalized after several weeks of treatment in 4 of these 5 patients (Fig. 2).

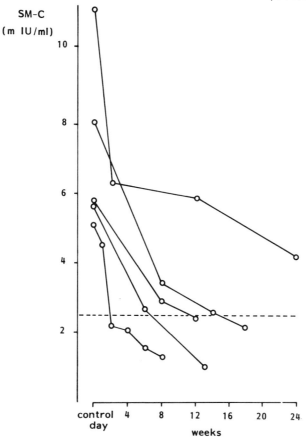

FIG. 2. The course of the plasma Somatomedin -C (SM-C) concentrations of 5 acromegalic patients during chronic therapy with 200-300 μg SMS 201-995 daily.

No important side effects were recorded throughout the treatment period of these patients. Two patients observed minor steatorrhea. The suppression of insulin secretion and the resulting hyperglycemia observed at the beginning of treatment became less marked as SMS 201-995 therapy progressed.

Similar preliminary beneficial results of the acute effects and chronic therapy in acromegaly with SMS 201-995 were also observed by Plewe et al. (11) and Ch'ng et al. (4) and suggest that SMS 201-995 represents an additional option for the management of acromegaly, especially in those patients who do not benefit sufficiently from surgery or radiotherapy, and who do not or incompletely respond to dopaminergic drugs.

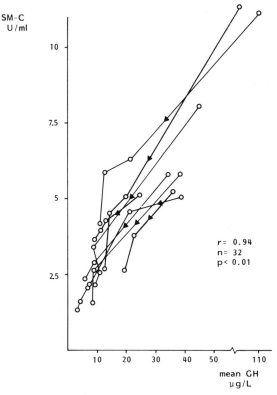

FIG. 3. The course of the plasma Somatomedin-C (SM-C) concentrations and the mean plasma GH levels (mean of 20 samples collected over a 24 hr-period) in 8 acromegalic patients treated for 6-48 weeks with 200-300 μg SMS 201-995 daily.

EXPERIMENTAL TUMORS.

Somatostatin and its analogs have been shown to exert an inhibitory effect on tumor growth in several experimental tumor models. The chronic subcutaneous administration of 3 different Somatostatin analogs significantly reduced tumor volume and/or weight as compared with control tumors in rats bearing the Swarm chondrosarcoma (14), in hamsters bearing a ductal type of pancreatic carcinoma (15) and the transplantable prolactin-secreting rat pituitary tumor 7315a (13). Reubi (19) showed that chronic administration of SMS 201-995 (1.25 mg/kg once a day for 25 days, 5 days per week) also inhibited the growth of chondro-sarcomas and insulinomas in rats and hamsters.

A matter of discussion is at present whether the Somatostatin analogs exert their inhibitory action on tumor growth in these experimental models via 1, 2 or all 3 of the following mechanisms: 1) inhibition of GH and insulin secretion; 2) direct or indirect (via GH) inhibition of Somatomedin-C production or of other tumor growth factors or 3) direct inhibitory effect on the tumor via specific Somatostatin receptors. No definitive answers can be given as yet with regard to the mechanism(s) of these anti-tumor effects of Somatostatin. No or only moderate inhibitory effects on plasma GH levels were reported at the end of the treatment period by Redding and Schally (14,15), and Reubi (19). No Somato-medin-C measurements were carried out by these investigators. Reubi (19) detected specific high affinity receptors for both Somatostatin and SMS 201-995 in hamster insulinoma tumor tissue, but not in the chondrosarcomas used in the studies mentioned above.

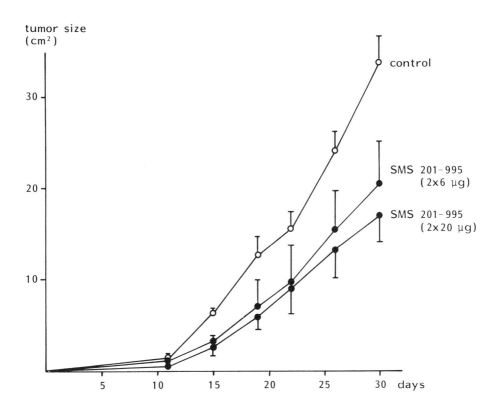

FIG. 4. The effect of the subcutaneous administration of SMS 201-995 (2 x 6 or 2 x 20 μg daily) from day 1 until day 30 after tumor implantation on the growth of the transplantable PRL/ACTH-secreting rat pituitary tumor 7315a (mean of 6 rats/group; mean ± SEM).

We showed in preliminary experiments that SMS 201-995 (2 x 6 or 2 x 20 μg daily for 30 days) inhibited the growth of the transplantable prolactin (PRL) (ACTH-secreting rat pituitary tumor 7315a by 36 % and 48 %, respectively (9). A biphasic curve of the inhibitory effect of the Somatostatin analog tumor growth was recognized : the actual tumor growth-inhibitory effect occurred during the first 15 days, after which the tumors grew during the following 15 days in parallel with the control tumors despite SMS 201-995 treatment. At the end of the 30 days SMS 201-995 therapy plasma GH and Somatomedin-C levels were similar to those in the control tumor-bearing rats. In separate experiments (Fig. 5) we showed that tachyphylaxis of the GH-inhibitory effect of 3 different doses of SMS 201-995 occurs in normal rats already within 6-10 days in a dose-dependent manner.

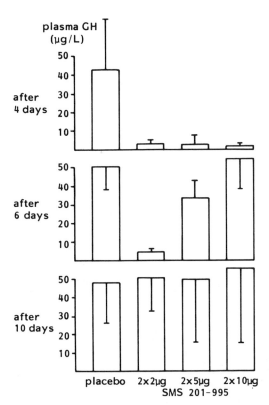

FIG. 5. The effect of the twice daily subcutaneous administration of SMS 201-995 or placebo for 4, 6 or 10 days on plasma GH levels in normal female rats. Blood was collected 30 min. after the last injection; 8 animals per group; mean ± SEM.

The studies mentioned above show that the dose and the scheme of administration of Somatostatin analogs and also the presence or absence of specific receptors for Somatostatin on different tumors play an important role in determining the ultimate effect of therapy with the analogs on tumor growth. These factors have hardly been studied in man and should be investigated further in detail before clinical studies with Somatostatin analogs can be carried in different oncological indications.

CLINICAL PHARMACOLOGY AND TOXICOLOGY OF SOMATOSTATIN ANALOGS : POTENTIAL PROBLEMS

1. Desensitization or tachyphylaxis

It was discussed that repeated administration (2-10 µg twice daily subcutaneously)of SMS 201-995 rapidly induces desensitization or tachyphylaxis of its inhibitory effects on GH secretion in the rat in a dose-dependent manner (Fig. 5). Prolonged Somatostatin pre-treatment was also shown to desensitize its inhibitory effect on ACTH release by cultured mouse anterior pituitary tumor cells (18). Märki et al. (10) reported that multiple subcutaneous injections of a Somatostatin analog in rats rapidly induces tachyphylaxis of the suppression of insulin release, but not of glucagon secretion. Chronic treatment of one of our patients with a metastasized VIPoma with SMS 201-995 resulted in a rapidly occurring desensitization. In contrast, however, we observed that the GH-secretion-inhibitory effect of SMS 201-995 in acromegalic patients did not show a tendency towards desensitization. After chronic therapy with SMS 201-995 (200-300 µg daily in 3 divided doses) for up till 70 weeks no signs of the development of tachyphylaxis for the powerful inhibitory effects on tumorous GH-secretion and also on Somatomedin-C production were observed in any of 10 patients. In conclusion, desensitization both of tumoral and normal hormone secretion seems to occur in some instances during chronic treatment with SMS 201-995. The frequency of administration and the amount of the analog used probably play a role, but these factors have not been studied in depth yet.

2. Duration of action

Our studies on the effects of therapy with SMS 201-995 of acromegalic patients show that the duration of action of the analog on GH-secretion varies considerably between patients. A typical example of the effect of different doses of administration of SMS 201-995 in an acromegalic patient is shown in Fig. 6. This figure shows that 50 µg SMS 201-995 three-times daily resulted in an important suppression of GH secretion, but GH tended to increase towards the next injection, which was again followed by an inhibition of GH release. An increase in the dose of SMS 201-995 to 100 µg three times daily prolonged the inhibitory effect on GH release slightly, but did not prevent this tendency of GH secretion to "escape" towards the next injection. These observations suggest the need for a Somatostatin analog which can be given orally or

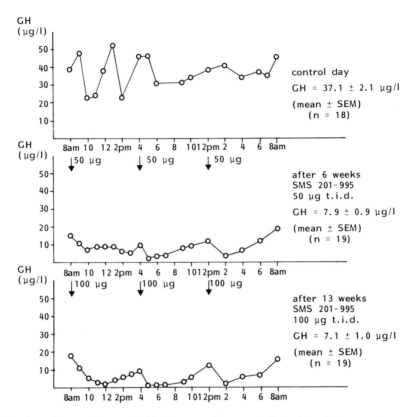

FIG. 6.   The effect of different doses of SMS 201-995 on circula-
           ting GH levels in an acromegalic patient.

which can be given intramuscularly in a slow-release formulation.
However, such more frequent oral or a continuous intramuscular
application might result in earlier desensitization or tachyphylaxis than the currently used twice or three times daily subcutaneous administration.

     A new and not well studied observation is, that pathological
hormone secretion by human tumors seems to be more sensitive to
the inhibitory effects of SMS 201-995 than "normal" hormone secretion. The inhibitory effect of the subcutaneous SMS 201-995 administration was effective on normal GH release for 3-5 h and on
GH secretion in acromegalics for 6-12 h, on normal insulin release
for 2-3 h and on insulin release in insulinoma patients for 6-12
h, on normal gastrin release for 3-4 h and on gastrin release by
a gastrinoma patient for 12 h. These preliminary observations
suggest a differential mechanism of action of Somatostatin on normal and tumorous endocrine cells.

3. Side effects
SMS 201-995 is a synthetic compound. No problems of allergy or

the production of antibodies with cross-reactivity inducing inactivation of natural Somatostatin have been observed sofar. The analog is very well tolerated and caused in our patients no local changes in the subcutaneous administration depots in the upper legs.

Side-effects of SMS 201-995 treatment of great clinical importance are also not to be expected on the basis of the observation that the model of chronic hyper-Somatostatinemia as caused by Somatostatin-producing pancreatic tumors is also very uneventful. A relatively small number of Somatostatinomas has been reported in the literature. Bloom and Polak(2)summarized the clinical picture of the Somatostatinoma Syndrome. It consists of an impaired carbohydrate tolerance (varying from mild, fasting hyperglycemia to more outspoken signs and symptoms of diabetes mellitus, malabsorption (steatorrhea) and symptoms of a- or hypochlorhydria. Unexpectedly, many patients with Somatostatinomas were found to have multiple gall stones. This may be due to the inhibitory effect of Somatostatin on the choledochus duct or on bile salt metabolism. So, deterioration of carbohydrate tolerance and steatorrhea are expected to be the main side-effects of chronic therapy with Somatostatin analogs like SMS 201-995, while achlorhydria and gall stone formation eventually can be expected.

REFERENCES

1. Bauer, W., Brimer, U., Doepfner, W., Hall, R., Huguenin, R., Marbach, P., Petcher T.J., and Pless, J. (1982) : Life Sci. 31 : 1133-1141.
2. Bloom, S.R. and Polak, J.M. (1980) : Clin. Endocrinol. Metab. 9 : 285-297.
3. Brazeau, P., Vale, W., Burgus, R., Ling, N., Butcher, M., Rivier, J., and Guillemin, R. (1973) : Science 179 : 77-79.
4. Ch'ng, L.J.C., Sandler, L.M., Kraenzlin, M.E., Burrin, J.M., Joplin, G.F., and Bloom, S.R. (1985) : Br. Med. J. 290 : 284-285.
5. Guillemin, R. (1978) : Science 202 : 390-402.
6. Lamberts, S.W.J., Verleun, T., and Oosterom R. (1984) : J. Clin. Endocrinol. Metab. 58 : 250-255.
7. Lamberts, S.W.J., Oosterom, R., Neufeld, M., and del Pozo, E. (1985) : J. Clin. Endocrinol. Metab. 60 : 1161-1165.
8. Lamberts, S.W.J., Uitterlinden, P., Verschoor, L., van Dongen, K.J., and del Pozo, E. (1985) : New Engl. J. Med. 313: 1576-1580.
9. Lamberts, S.W.J., Reubi, J-C., Uitterlinden, P., Zuiderwijk, J., vd Werff, P., and van Hal, P. (1986): Endocrinology (in press) .
10. Märki, F., Bucher, U.M., and Richter, J.C. (1982) : Regul. Pept. 4 : 333-338.
11. Plewe, G., Beyer, J., Krause, U., Neufeld, M. , and del Pozo, E. (1984) : Lancet ii : 782-784.

12. del Pozo, E., Schlüter, K., Neufeld, M., Tortosa, F., Marbach, P., Wendel, L., and Kerp, L. (1986) : Acta Endocrinol : (in press) .

13. de Quijada, M.G., Redding, T.W., Coy, D.H., Torres-Aleman, I., and Schally, A.V. (1983) : Proc. Natl. Acad. Sci. USA 80 : 3485-3488.

14. Redding T.W., and Schally A.V. (1983) : Proc. Natl. Acad. Sci. USA 80 : 1078-1082.

15. Redding T.W., and Schally, A.V. (1984) : Proc. Natl. Acad.Sci. USA 81 : 248-252.

16. Reichlin, S. (1983) : New. Engl. J. Med. 309 : 1495-1501.

17. Reichlin, S. (1983) : New. Engl. J. Med. 309 : 1556-1563.

18. Reisine, T., and Axelrod, J. (1983) : Endocrinology 113 : 811-813.

19. Reubi, J.C. (1985) : Acta Endocrinol. 109 : 108-114.

Hormonal Manipulation of Cancer: Peptides, Growth Factors, and New (Anti) Steroidal Agents, edited by Jan G. M. Klijn et al. Raven Press, New York © 1987.

SOMATOSTATIN ANALOGUE TREATMENT OF ENDOCRINE TUMOURS

S R Bloom

Department of Medicine, Royal Postgraduate Medical School, Hammersmith Hospital, Du Cane Road, London, W12 OHS, U.K.

It is now known that many tumours produce agents (hormones) that act at a distance. Endocrine tumours differ in that they are derived from recognised endocrine tissue and frequently present clinically with the results of the excess hormone production rather than the effects of tumour mass per se. In general they are slow growing and therefore if they cannot be ablated, for example by surgery, long-term palliation is a worthwhile goal. Where the main clinical problems arise from the excess hormone production, as is often the case, palliation may involve suppression of hormone output or blockade of the effects of excess hormone.

Somatostatin is a polypeptide hormone which was first isolated from the hypothalamus as a factor which inhibited growth hormone release from the anterior pituitary. It was subsequently found to be widely distributed in the body and to be present both in neurones and peripheral endocrine cells. For example, the D cell of the islet of Langerhans, whose product had previously been unknown, was shown to be producing somatostatin (15). The peptide is also produced by a specific type of mucosal endocrine cell of the gastrointestinal tract. Several molecular forms of somatostatin have now been isolated, but all have the last 14 amino acids in common which contains the active sequence of somatostatin itself (Fig. 1). Synthetic manipulation of this sequence has resulted in a range of biologically active analogues. Soon after the demonstration that somatostatin could inhibit growth hormone, it was found also to potently inhibit the release of other hormones including gastrin, insulin and glucagon (2,5,13). Subsequently somatostatin has been shown to suppress the release of gastric inhibitory peptide, motilin, neurotensin and a number of other gut peptides. Its effect is powerful, and a total inhibition of release is achieved at quite moderate concentrations. In addition somatostatin frequently has a direct effect on the target tissue of the hormone it inhibits. Thus, it suppresses gastric acid secretion even during an infusion of exogenous gastrin (3). On account of these actions somatostatin was early considered for therapy of endocrine tumours. It had two major disadvantages, however. Firstly its breadth of action was a significant disadvantage, for example unwanted obligatory suppression of insulin meant that somatostatin treatment was likely to result in the "side-effect" of carbohydrate intolerance. Secondly it had to be administered intravenously as it has a half life of only a few minutes.

Thus, shortly after its isolation somatostatin was tried in a number of endocrine tumour syndromes and found to be successful at inhibiting the relevant hormone, for example growth hormone in acromegaly, gastrin in gastrinomas etc., and it was also acutely successful in the treatment of endocrine syndromes where the hormone was less well recognised, for example,medullary carcinoma of the thyroid and the carcinoid syndrome (12).

The development of analogues of somatostatin that were both selective and long-acting was the desired goal. Such an agent would then provide practical therapy. A number of different compounds were synthesized which, in the rat, were relatively selective in the inhibition of insulin, glucagon or growth hormone. Unfortunately when these analogues were tested in man no such selectivity was demonstrated (1). Thus, at the present time there is no indication that sub-families of somatostatin receptors exist in man which could be exploited to produce differential hormone inhibition. Early work also failed to result in any long acting analogue, though some preparations of low solubility could be used to produce a subcutaneous depot with subsequent slow release into the circulation (11).

Somatostatin (SRIF)

H-Ala-Gly-Cys-Lys-Asn-Phe-Phe-Trp-Lys-Thr-Phe-Thr-Ser-Cys-OH

SMS 201-995

H-(D)Phe-Cys-Phe-(D)Trp-Lys-Thr-Cys-Thr-ol, acetate

FIG. 1.   Amino acid sequence of somatostatin and SMS 201-995.

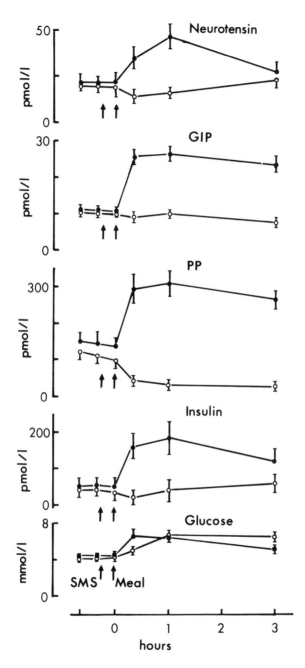

FIG. 2. Plasma hormonal and glucose concentrations in healthy
volunteers after a meal with SMS 201-995 O——O
and without SMS 201-995 ●——●

Recently a new long-acting analogue was developed by the Sandoz Company (4) and this has become available for the treatment of patients. In healthy volunteers it suppressed both basal and meal stimulated secretion of gut hormones and significantly lowered pancreatic polypeptide, secretin, motilin, pancreatic glucagon, gastric inhibitory peptide and insulin (8) (Fig. 2). However, it showed little evidence of selectivity in its inhibition of growth hormone, insulin or gastrointestinal hormones. SMS 201-995 is administered by subcutaneous injection and is associated with local discomfort lasting a few minutes. The technique is very similar to that used by a diabetic for the administration of insulin and appears acceptable to patients who are able to administer it at home. The initial dosage used for endocrine tumour suppression was 50 µg, twice daily, but this may be associated with a considerable period of escape prior to the subsequent injection. An 8 hourly regimen (breakfast, mid afternoon and last thing at night) is therefore probably preferable. Larger doses are associated with a longer time period of hormone suppression and doses of 200 ug 8 hourly are well tolerated. Indeed the upper limit of dosage has not yet been established.

Side-effects may include the development of nausea within a few minutes of the injection, which may last for an hour or more and is the most likely dose limiting symptom. Suppression of gastrointestinal adsorption, particularly in patients who already have impaired pancreatic exocrine secretion due to the presence of a pancreatic tumour, may lead to steatorrhoea. Acute abdominal pain may occur during initiation of therapy and dosage should therefore be built up over a few days. The inhibition of insulin secretion is nearly always associated with impaired glucose tolerance and occasionally may result in the development of overt diabetes mellitus.

The first clinical situation in which SMS 201-995 was tested was in acromegaly (14). It was found to be highly successful therapy (6,9,10). In a recent series of nine acromegalic patients, six previously untreated, who were studied between 3 and 15 months on SMS 201-995 100 µg three times daily, the mean growth hormone concentration was found to have fallen from 82 ± 21 mIU/l to 32 ± 13 (p<0.001). Eight of the nine patients showed a reduction of at least 50% in growth hormone levels in the fasting state, and there was a 30% fall in the serum concentrations of insulin-like growth factor. There was a rapid clinical improvement in all patients, with loss of sweating and headache and a significant reduction in skin fold thickness, hand volume and finger size. In contrast, however, there was no change in the CAT appearance of the pituitary tumour. In this respect treatment with SMS 201-995 is strikingly different from the treatment of prolactinomas with bromocriptine where tumour shrinkage is the rule. Interestingly the fasting plasma glucose concentrations did not change during treatment (initial 5.4 ± 0.3, final 5.5 ± 0.3 mmol/l). However, the postprandial glucose rise was greater and insulin output was considerably reduced. From this and other studies it can be concluded that SMS is a safe and effective long-term treatment for patients with acromegaly in whom more conventional treatment is not indicated or has failed.

Treatment of pancreatic endocrine tumours was similarly successful. In a series of 7 patients with gut and pancreatic endocrine tumours treated with twice daily subcutaneous SMS for 3 days, a dramatic improvement in endocrine related symptoms occurred in association with a fall in circulating tumour peptides. The most dramatic effect was abolition or reduction of diarrhoea in patients with VIPoma. The diarrhoea was also reduced in patients with gastrinoma, perhaps in part consequent on inhibition of gastric acid secretion (16). A patient with carcinoid syndrome had a marked reduction in stool frequency and symptomatic relief. In a series of 5 patients followed up for between 3 and 6 months, it was noted that a significant reduction in tumour related hormone concentrations was seen in 4 patients, although in none did the values return to normal. All 5 patients noted a major symptomatic improvement, however, and this suggests that SMS may act in part through its direct effect on the effector tissue. It was particularly notable in this study that there was no deleterious effect on fasting blood glucose and the patients accepted the home injections of SMS without complaint. Indeed because of the remissions of symptoms they all volunteered to continue with the therapy after the trial had stopped. One of the earliest VIPoma patients treated has now been on SMS for over 3 years. He was initially confined to hospital due to persistent severe diarrhoea and severe hypokalemia. He was unable to spend more then a few hours without intravenous infusion of fluids. The administration of SMS produced a dramatic improvement and within a day his diarrhoea had remitted so that he was able to leave hospital, return to full-time employment and indeed even achieved a promotion. An otherwise fit young man he had always indulged in long distance running and while on his SMS therapy he was able to participate again in the London Marathon. There was some suggestion that his hepatic metastases were reduced in size (7). In the last year his course has been less satisfactory with regrowth of the tumour and occasional escape of diarrhoea which did not respond to further increase of the dose of SMS. He is now again under control with a combination of SMS and low dose steroid therapy. Clearly the period of palliation is coming to an end.

In conclusion the newly available long-acting somatostatin analogue SMS 201-995 offers a very useful new therapeutic tool in the treatment of patients with endocrine tumours not amenable to surgery or other conventional treatment. It appears safe and is well tolerated with minimal side-effects. Early enthusiasm that it might cause tumour shrinkage has turned out to be misplaced though it is possible that the rate of growth is reduced.

REFERENCES

1. Adrian, T.E., Barnes, A.J., Long, R.G., O'Shaughnessy. D.J., Brown, M.R., Rivier, J., Vale, W., Blackburn, A.M. & Bloom, S.R. (1981): The effect of somatostatin analogues on secretion of growth, pancreatic and gastrointestinal hormones in man. J. Clin. Endocrinol. Metab., 53:675-681.

2. Alford, F.P., Bloom, S.R., Nabarro, J.D.N., Hall, R., Besser, G.M., Coy, D.H., Kastin, A.J. & Schally, A.V. (1974): Glucagon control of fasting glucose in man. Lancet 2:974.

3. Barros D'Sa, A.A.J., Bloom, S.R. & Baron, J.H. (1975): Direct inhibition of gastric acid by growth hormone release inhibiting hormone in dogs. Lancet 1:886-887.

4. Bauer, W., Briner, U., Doepfner, W., Haller, R., Huguenin, R., Marbach, P., Petcher, T.J. & Pless, J. (1982): SMS 201-995 a very potent and selective octa-peptide analogue of somastatin with prolonged action. Life Sciences Vol 31: pp 1131-1140.

5. Bloom, S.R., Mortimer, C.H., Thorner, M.O., Besser, G.M., Hall, R., Gomez-Pan, A., Roy, V.M., Russell, R.C.G., Coy, D.H., Kastin, A.J. & Schally, A.V. (1974): Inhibition of gastrin and gastric-acid secretion by growth hormone release-inhibiting hormones. Lancet 2:1106-1109.

6. Ch'ng, L.J.C., Sandler, L.M., Kraenzlin, M.E., Burrin, J.M., Joplin, G.F. & Bloom, S.R. (1985): Long-term treatment of acromegaly with a long acting analogue of somatostatin. Br. Med. J., 290:284-285.

7. Kraenzlin, M.E., Ch'ng, J.L.C., Wood, S.M., Carr, D.H. & Bloom, S.R. (1984): Long-term treatment of a VIPoma with somatostatin analogue resulting in remission of symptoms and possible shrinkage of metastases. Gastroenterology 88:185-187.

8. Kraenzlin, M.E., Wood, S.M., Neufeld, M., Adrian, T.E. & Bloom, S.R. (1985): Effect of long acting somatostatin analogue, SMS 201-995, on gut hormone secretion in normal subjects. Experientia 41:738-748.

9. Lamberts, S.W.J., Oosterom, R., Neufeld, M. & Del Pozo, E. (1985): The somatostatin analogue SMS 201-995 induces long-acting inhibition of growth hormone secretion without rebound hypersecretion in acromegalic patients. J. Clin. Endocrinol. Metab. 60:1161-1165.

10. Lamberts, S.W.J, Uitterlinden, P., Verschool, L., Van Dongen,K.J. & Del Pozo, E. (1985): Long-term treatment of acromegaly with the somatostatin analogue SMS 201-995. N.Engl. J. Med. 313:1579-1580.

11. Long, R.G., Barnes, A.J., Adrian, T.E., Mallinson, C.N., Brown, M.R., Vale, W., Christofides, N.D. & Bloom, S.R. (1979): Suppression of pancreatic endocrine tumour secretion by long-acting somatostatin analogue. Lancet 2:764-767.

12. Long, R.G., Peter, J.M., Bloom, S.R., Brown, M.R., Vale, W.,Rivier, J.E. & Grahame-Smith, D.G. (1981): Somatostatin gastrointestinal peptides, and the carcinoid syndrome. Gut 22:549-553.

13. Mortimer, C.H., Carr, D., Lind, T., Bloom, S.R., Mallinson,C.N., Schally, A.V., Turnbridge, W.M.G., Yeomans, L., Coy, D.H., Kastin, A. & Besser, G.M. (1974): Growth hormone rlease-inhibiting hormone: effects on circulating glucagon, insulin and growth hormone in normal, diabetic, acromegalicand hypopituitary patients. Lancet 1:697-701.

14. Plewe, G., Beyer, J., Krause, U., Neufeld, M. & Del Pozo, E. (1984): Long-acting and selective suppression of growth hormone secretion by somatostatin analogue SMS 201-995 in acromegaly. Lancet II: 782-784.

15. Polak, J.M., Pearse, A.G.E., Grimelius, L., Bloom, S.R. & Arimura, A. Growth hormone release-inhibiting hormone in gastrointestinal and pancreatic D cells. Lancet 1:1220-225.

16. Wood, S.M., Kraenzlin, M.E., Adrian, T.E. & Bloom, S.R. (1985): Treatment of patients with pancreatic endocrine tumours using a new long-acting somatostatin analogue symptomatic and peptide responses. Gut 26:438-444.

Hormonal Manipulation of Cancer: Peptides, Growth Factors, and New (Anti) Steroidal Agents, edited by Jan G. M. Klijn et al. Raven Press, New York © 1987.

EFFECTS OF SOMATOSTATIN ANALOG (SANDOSTATIN) TREATMENT IN EXPERIMENTAL AND HUMAN CANCER

J.G.M. Klijn, B. Setyono-Han, G.H. Bakker, M.S. Henkelman, H. Portengen, and J.A. Foekens

Depts. of Endocrine Oncology (Endocrinology and Biochemistry) The Dr Daniel den Hoed Cancer Center, P.O.Box 5201, Rotterdam, The Netherlands

INTRODUCTION

New approaches to the therapy for some known hormone-dependent but also unknown "hormone-dependent" tumors are being developed on the basis of experimental studies in animal models. For instance such a new approach is the use of recently produced analogs of hypothalamic hormones, especially of Luteinizing-Hormone-Releasing-Hormone (LHRH) and somatostatin (30,31). In the last few years the value of LHRH analog treatment has been established by a number of clinical studies concerning metastatic breast and prostate cancer (see this book). However, only a few studies are reported about the application of somatostatin analogs in the treatment of malignant tumors (2,24,25,28,31,36).

Somatostatin is a cyclic tetradecapeptide and was first isolated by Brazeau et al. (1973) from the hypothalamus (5). It is believed that somatostatin acts primarily locally, with paracrine effects, but it can act also endocrine, autocrine and as a lumone (9,26,27). The natural hormone has a short half-life and a short duration of action. To circumvent this short duration of action and to develop organ-selective compounds, extensive attempts to synthesize analogs have been made (1,24-28, 31). Several somatostatin analogs have been shown in experimental animals to possess greater potency, longer duration of action and a different spectrum of biological actions compared to the parent somatostatin molecule. They appeared to suppress the secretion of pituitary hormones (GH, PRL, TSH), insulin, glucagon and several other gastrointestinal hormones, some of which (gastrin, secretin, cholecystokinin) being involved in the growth regulation of gastrointestinal tumor cells (15,20, 25,27,34,35, Lamers this book). Furthermore, plasma concentrations of some growth factors as somatomedin C (IGF-1) (16, 17) and epidermal growth factor (EGF) (10), which factors stimulate the growth of some types of tumor cells (mammary, pancreatic), may decrease during chronic treatment. On the basis of the mechanism of actions as mentioned above, it is conceivable that somatostatin analogs may have direct and indirect inhibiting actions even on the growth of unknown "endocrine-related" tumors as showed by Redding and Schally (24,25,31). Very recently, sufficient quantities of somatostatin analogs came available for long-term (pre)clinical studies. In this article we will summarize our results of chronic somatostatin analog treatment in various tumor models using the analog Sandostatin (SMS-201-995), kindly provided by Sandoz, Basel. Furthermore we will present preliminary data of a clinical study in patients with malignant gastrointestinal tumors.

RESULTS

Pancreatic tumors

A number of pancreatic tumors appears to contain high levels of steroid hormone receptors and enzymes involved in steroid metabolism (14, Johnson this book) indicating potential hormone dependency. Furthermore the secretion of some gastrointestinal hormones, which are involved in the growth regulation of pancreatic (tumor) cells, can be suppressed by somatostatin. These data and those reported by Redding and Schally (25) prompted us to examine the effects of Sandostatin, a new potent somatostatin analog, in rats with a transplantable pancreatic acinar tumor (Prof. Longnecker). We have investigated the characteristics of this tumor(model) and the mechanism of action of Sandostatin. Furthermore we have compared the effects of different dosages of Sandostatin on tumor growth and plasma concentrations of some hormones and growth factors with those of other endocrine measures.

Tumors were kindly provided by Dr. A.G. Bogden, E.G. and Mason Research Institute. About 100 microliter of tumor suspension was injected subcutaneously (s.c.) in the left- and right side of male inbred Lewis rats. Two weeks after the tumor transplantation 95% of the rats already had a detectable tumor mass. With respect to other tumor characteristics we have demonstrated in these tumors the presence of EGF receptors and low levels of progesterone receptors (PgR) in the absence of estradiol receptors (ER), while Reubi and Maurer (Sandoz, Basel) were able to show the presence of specific binding sites for the somatostatin analog by autoradiography.

Subcutaneous treatment was usually started right from tumor transplantation (prophylactic treatment) or 2 weeks after transplantation (treatment groups). The treatment groups (n=8) were compared with control groups with tumor and supercontrols without tumor. The rats were treated twice daily with 5 dosages of Sandostatin (0.05, 0.2, 1.0, 5.0, and 20 µg), the LHRH agonist buserelin (5 µg), and the aromatase inhibitor aminoglutethimide (0.5 and 2.0 mg).

Tumor bearing control rats showed lower body weight than rats without transplanted tumors (32). Somatostatin analog treatment had no or minor effect on the body weight of tumor bearing rats. Untreated tumor bearing rats had lower plasma concentrations of GH, IGF-1 and EGF compared to rats without tumors. This might be explained by the worse condition of rats with tumors accompanied by delayed body growth. In tumor bearing rats treatment with Sandostatin decreased plasma concentrations of GH (+40%), IGF-1 (+15%), EGF (20-80%), and tumor PgR levels (30-50%). Rats treated right from time of tumor inoculation showed pronounced inhibition of tumor growth after 2 weeks (4.1. +6.6 mm2 (s.d.) vs. 45.8 + 34.4 mm2 in controls) and 55% inhibition after 6-9 weeks. In the average a growth inhibition of 35% was reached in the non-prophylactic treatment groups after 6-9 weeks of treatment with the different dosages of Sandostatin used. A dose of 1.0 µg twice daily seems slightly more effective than the other dosages when used prophylactically, but we did not observe a difference in growth inhibiting effects between the 5 different dosages of Sandostatin used in the treatment groups with tumors. Treatment with 2x2 mg aminoglutethimide caused comparable tumor growth inhibition (50%) while buserelin appeared somewhat less effective (Fig.1).

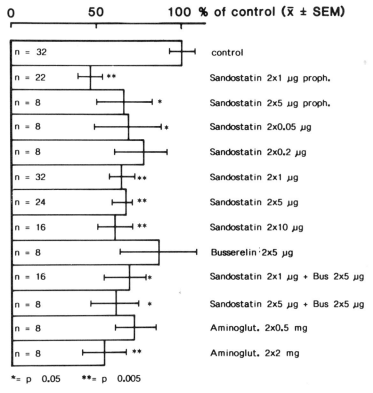

FIG.1. Tumor growth inhibiting effects of different kinds of treatment in rats with transplantable pancreatic tumors.

Rhabdomyosarcomas

The observation that some sarcomas can produce growth factors as insulin-like growth factor II (IGF-2) and secondly that IGF-1 is involved in the growth regulation of muscle cells, led us to study the effect of Sandostatin treatment on the growth of transplantable rhabdomyosarcomas in WAGRIJ rats. However, no growth inhibiting effect could be observed (Fig.2).

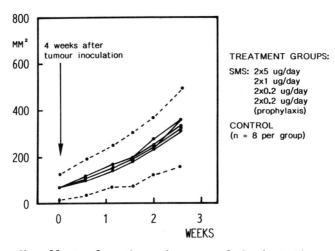

FIG.2.   No effect of various dosages of Sandostatin on tumor load in rats bearing rhabdomyosarcoma on the back (results are mean values with indication of the maximal S.D. values calculated).

DMBA rat mammary tumors

Rats with DMBA induced mammary tumors were treated twice daily with the same 5 dosages of Sandostatin as described before (i.e. 0.05, 0.2, 1.0, 5.0, and 20 µg) for 3 weeks. We observed a bell-shaped curve of dose-response relationship for single Sandostatin treatment (Fig.3, Table 1). Maximal tumor growth inhibition (82% as compared to controls i.e. 10% vs. 57% growth) was reached with a dose of 2 x 0.2 µg per day. Lower and higher dosages of Sandostatin appeared to cause less or no growth inhibition. There was even a tendency to an increased tumor growth rate in rats treated with the highest dose.

Treatment with buserelin showed equal results as ovariectomy causing clear tumor regression, while single somatostatin analog treatment caused only inhibition of tumor growth. The best results were obtained with the combination of LHRH and somatostatin agonists i.e. 77% regression (Table 1).

Sandostatin treatment with the highest dosages caused no

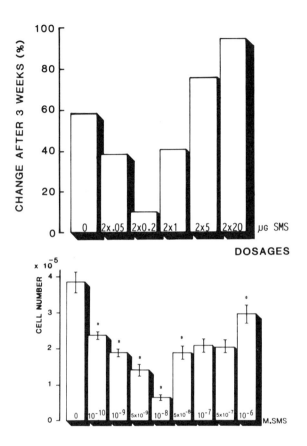

FIG.3. Effects of different dosages of Sandostatin on rat mammary tumor growth in vivo (upper part) and on MCF-7 tumor cell growth in vitro (lower part).

effects on the weight of the pituitary, adrenals, ovaries and uterus. Using the lowest dosages sometimes a small but significant decrement of the weight of these organs was observed. Treatment with Buserelin caused highly significant decrement of the weight of the uterus and ovaries. Plasma hormone studies are in progress. No binding sites for Sandostatin could be demonstrated by autoradiography (Maurer and Reubi, Basel) using a technique described in detail before (29).

Human breast cancer cells (MCF-7)

Looking for possible direct effects at the level of tumor cells we have studied the effects of 9 different concentrations

TABLE 1. Comparison of the relative effects on rat mammary tumor load of various doses of Sandostatin compared to those of other endocrine treatments

	CHANGE (%)
CONTROL	+57/+57
2x 0.05µg SMS	+38
2x 0.2µg SMS	+10
2x 1µg SMS(L)	+38/+42
2x 5µg SMS	+76
2x 20µg SMS(H)	+94
2x 5µg Buserelin	-40/-49
Buserelin + SMSL	-77
Buserelin + SMSH	-27
ovariectomy	-51

of Sandostatin between 10^{-6} and 10^{-10} M in cultures of MCF-7 tumor cells both in the absence and presence of estradiol and/or insulin. The known stimulating effects of estradiol and insulin were confirmed. But, we showed for the first time that a somatostatin analog directly inhibits the growth of breast cancer cells in vitro. In all four conditions tested Sandostatin appears to inhibit tumor cell growth. Based on 3 consecutive experiments the most profound inhibition (73 $\pm$ 18%; x $\pm$ SEM) measured by cell number (Fig.3), DNA and protein content of the cultures was observed in cultures with insulin and without added estradiol (p < 0.005). With respect to dose-response relationship, strikingly again a bell-shaped curve was observed as in the in vivo experiments with rat mammary tumors. Maximal suppression of the growth of the cultures was obtained at a sharply defined amount of Sandostatin (10^{-8} mol); at lower and higher dosages the inhibition of cell growth was less striking.

The observation that Sandostatin had a direct inhibitory effect in vitro on MCF-7 cell growth prompted us to investigate the possible presence of somatostatin receptors. We have measured the kinetics of uptake of the Sandostatin derivative ^{125}I-SMS 204-090 in MCF-7 cell cultures and indeed specific binding was observed namely 3 x 10^4 molecules per cell (32).

Patients with pancreatic and gastrointestinal adenocarcinomas

Patients with metastatic pancreatic (n=7), gastric (n=2) and colorectal tumors (n=9) were chronically treated with 3 x 200 µg Sandostatin s.c. per day. Plasma IGF-I decreased in nearly all patients. IGF-1 concentrations in plasma (measured directly and by acid extraction) decreased both in patients with pancreatic tumors and colorectal tumors but an increase occurred to pretreatment levels after 8-13 weeks of treatment (Fig.4).

Acid-extracted IGF-1 concentrations were much lower in pancreas carcinoma patients than in colorectal carcinoma patients and appeared in the first group not different from direct assayable IGF-1 plasma concentrations. This might be explained by the fact that most patients with (liver) metastases of pancreatic cancers were cachectic and had no appetite.

With respect to possible antitumor effects, no objective remissions were observed but 3 patients with metastatic colorectal tumors showed stable disease during 3-9 months. No serious side effects were observed. Nearly all patients had increased fecal fat loss, but significant loss of body weight did not occur.

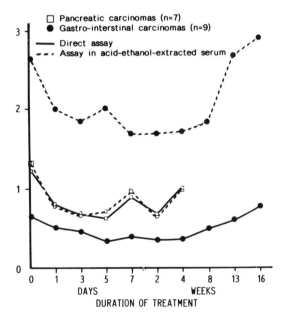

FIG. 4. Mean serum IGF-1 concentrations during chronic treatment with Sandostatin in patients with metastatic pancreatic and gastrointestinal carcinomas.

DISCUSSION AND CONCLUSIONS

Somatostatin analog treatment appeared to cause clear (dose dependent) growth inhibiting effects in experimental pancreatic and breast cancer. From our experience the dose used appeared very critical. Higher dosages than the optimally suppressive dose are less effective, maybe as a consequence of desensitization of the cells during treatment.

With regard to mechanism of action somatostatin analogs have direct and indirect effects on tumor cells. In Lewis rats with pancreatic tumors growth inhibition might be caused both via the demonstrated somatostatin receptors and/or decrement of hormone and growth factor secretion especially of EGF.

Sandostatin can act on mammary tumor cells also by different ways. Based on our observation of growth inhibition in vitro of tumor cells (MCF-7) bearing binding sites for Sandostatin and of mammary tumors in vivo without somatostatin receptors the presence of direct and indirect effects is probable. Somatostatin and analogs may exert their action directly by interacting with its specific receptor or by modulation of other hormone receptors, and indirectly by a decrease in the secretion of pituitary hormones (GH, PRL) and growth factors such as IGF-1 and EGF. With respect to indirect actions Murphy et al. (23) described that human GH may be a potent ligand for the lactogenic receptor in human breast cancer cells, while Shiu and Iwasiow (33) observed induction of specific proteins by GH and prolactin (PRL) in human breast cancer cells. The observations that increased plasma GH levels in breast cancer patients occur (8) and that hyperprolactinemia is an unfavorable prognostic factor (6) might be of importance.

In addition somatostatin may act as a paracrine or autocrine regulator of tumor cell proliferation by influencing secretion of autocrine or paracrine growth factors. Recently IGF-1 appeared to be one of the autocrine growth factors for various breast tumor cell lines and to stimulate the growth of MCF-7 tumor cells (18,19). The interaction of mammogenic peptide hormones (GH, PRL, insulin), steroids and EGF with modulation of their respective receptors (7,11-13,22,23) in addition to the possible inhibiting effects of Sandostatin on the secretion of EGF and IGF-1, suggests a very complex mechanism through which somatostatin and its analogs act in vivo and in vitro. It is interesting to note that analogs of LHRH (3,4,21) and somatostatin (this report) have direct inhibitory effects on tumor cell growth antagonizing in vitro biological effects of those steroid (estradiol) and peptide hormones (GH, insulin) which secretion in vivo is suppressed by pharmacological doses of the same neuropeptide analogs.

In conclusion

1. In experimental pancreatic and breast cancer models somatostatin analog treatment appears to cause clear tumor growth inhibitory effects in vivo and in vitro.

2. With respect to dose-response relationship a bell-shaped curve was observed.

3. Specific binding sites for a iodinated derivative of Sandostatin appear to be present in MCF-7 cells and pancreatic tumors.

4. No antitumor effect was observed in rats with rhabdomyosarcomas.

5. In the majority of patients with gastro-intestinal tumors chronic Sandostatin treatment decreased plasma IGF-1 levels; the clinical data with respect to tumor growth inhibition are thus far too scarce for definite conclusions.

6. More studies are needed to define the optimal dose and mode of administration in patients with carcinomas.

REFERENCES

1. Adrian, T.E., Barnes, A.J., Long, R.G., O'Shaughnessy, Brown, M.R., Rivier, J., Vale, W., Blackburn, A.M., and Bloom, S.R. (1981): J.Clin.Endocrinol.Metab., 53:675-681.
2. Bonfils, S. (1985): Gut, 26:433-437.
3. Blankenstein, M.A., Henkelman, M.S., and Klijn, J.G.M. (1983): J.Steroid Biochem., 19 Suppl., 95 S.
4. Blankenstein, M.A., Henkelman, M.S., and Klijn, J.G.M. (1985): Eur.J.Cancer Clin.Oncol., 21:1493-1499.
5. Brazeau, P., Vale, W., Burgus, R., Ling, N., Butscher, M., Rivier, J., and Guillemin, R. (1973): Science, 179:77-79.
6. Dowsett, M., McGarrick, G.E., Harris, A.L., Coombes, R.C., Smith, I.E., and Jeffcoate, S.L. (1983): Br.J.Cancer, 47:763-769.
7. Edery, M., Imagawa, W., Larson, L., and Nandi, S. (1985): Endocrinol., 116:105-112.
8. Emerman, J.T.,Leahy, M., Gout, P.W., and Bruchovsky, N. (1985): Horm.Metabol.Res., 17:421-424.
9. Fenoglio, C.M., and King, D.W. (1983): Human Pathology, 14:475-479.
10. Ghirlanda, G., Uccioli, L., Perri, F., Altomonte, L., Bertoli, A., Manna, R., Frati, L., and Greco, A.V. (1983): Lancet, 1:65.
11. Hilf, R., and Crofton, D.H. (1985): Endocrinol., 116:154-163.
12. Horwitz, K.B., and Freidenberg, G.R. (1985): Cancer Res., 45:167-173.
13. Imagawa, W., Tomooka, Y., Hahamoto, S., and Nandi, S. (1985): Endocrinol., 116:1514-1524.
14. Iqbal, M.J., Greenway, B., Wilkinson, M.L., Johnson, P.J., and Williams, R. (1983): Clin.Science, 65:71-75.
15. Kobori, O., Viullot, M.T., and Martin, F. (1982): Int.J.Cancer, 30:65-67.

16. Lamberts, S.W.J., Uitterlinden, P., Verschoor, L., van Dongen, K.J., and Del Pozo, E. (1985): New Engl.J.Med. 313:1576-1579.
17. Lamberts, S.W.J., Zweens, M., Klijn, J.G.M., van Vroonhoven, C.C.J., Stefanko, S.Z., and Del Pozo, E. (1986): Clin.Endocrinol., in press.
18. Lippman, M.E. (1985): Clin.Res., 83:375-382.
19. Lippman, M.E., Dickson, R.B., Bates, S., Knabbe, C., Huff, K., Swain, S., McManaway, M., Bronzert, D., Kasid, A., and Gelmann, E.P. (1986): Breast Cancer Res.Treat., 7:59-70.
20. Lupulescu, A. (1983): J.Steroid Biochem., 19 (Suppl.) : 63 S.
21. Miller, W.R., Scott, W.N., Morris, R., Frazer, H.M., and Sharpe, R.M. (1985): Nature, 313:231-233.
22. Mukku, V.R., and Stancel, G.M. (1985): J.Biol.Chem., 260:9820-9824.
23. Murphy, L.J., Sutherland, R.L., and Lazarus, L. (1985): Biochem.Biophys.Res.Commun., 131:767-773.
24. Redding, T.W., and Schally, A.V. (1983): Proc.Natl.Acad. Sci.USA, 80:1078-1082.
25. Redding, T.W., and Schally, A.V. (1984): Proc.Natl.Acad. Sci.USA, 81:248-252.
26. Reichlin, S. (1983): New Engl.J.Med., 309:1495-1501.
27. Reichlin, S. (1983): New Engl.J.Med., 309:1556-1563.
28. Reubi, J.C. (1985): Acta Endocrinol., 109:108-114.
29. Reubi, J.C., Maurer, R., Klijn, J.G.M., Stefanko, S.Z., Foekens, J.A., Blaauw, G., Blankenstein, M.A., and Lamberts, S.W.J. (1986): J.Clin.Endocrinol.Metab. 63: 433-438.
30. Schally, A.V., Redding, T.W., and Comaru-Schally, A.M. (1984): Cancer Treatm.Rep., 68:281-289.
31. Schally, A.V., Redding, T.W., Cai, R.Z., Paz, J.I., Ben-David, M., and Comaru-Schally, A.M. (1986): EORTC Monograph Series, Raven Press, New York, this book.
32. Setyono-Han, B., Henkelman, M.S., Foekens, J.A., and Klijn, J.G.M. (1986): Cancer Res., in press.
33. Shiu, R.P.C., and Iwasiow, B.M. (1985): J.Biol.Chem., 260: 11307-11313.
34. Townsend, C.M., Franklin, R.D., Watson, L.C., Glass, E.J., and Thompson, J.C. (1981): Surg.Forum, 32:228-229.
35. Viullot, M.T., Kobori, O., and Martin, F. (1983): J.Steroid Biochem., 19 (Suppl.): 56 S.
36. Wood, S.M., Kraenzlin, M.E., Adrian, T.E., and Bloom, S.R. (1985): Gut, 26:438-444.

Hormonal Manipulation of Cancer: Peptides, Growth Factors, and New (Anti) Steroidal Agents, edited by Jan G. M. Klijn et al. Raven Press, New York © 1987.

HORMONAL MANIPULATION OF TUMOR CELLS

IN COMBINATION WITH CHEMOTHERAPY

C. Kent Osborne

Department of Medicine
University of Texas Health Science Center
San Antonio, Texas 78284, USA

INTRODUCTION

Except for the promising results of adjuvant therapy, the treatment of breast cancer with drugs has not witnessed a significant advance since the development of combination chemotherapy in the early 1960s (7). Although new, less toxic endocrine treatments are now available, still only about one-third of patients with breast cancer have hormonally-responsive tumors. Combination chemotherapy induces partial remissions in 50-60% of patients with advanced breast cancer, but the complete response rate is less than 20% with standard regimens, and response durations are short. Thus, there is a clear need for the development of new treatment strategies.

One approach has been to empirically combine an endocrine treatment with cytotoxic chemotherapy with the hope of increasing cell kill in a heterogeneous tumor that is composed of mixtures of cells variably sensitive and resistant to the two modalities. If no interaction occurs between the two treatments administered simultaneously, and if one assumes a simple additive effect on cell kill, then a modest increase in cell kill reflected by an increased response rate and duration might be expected with combined therapy (11). The impact of this approach would theoretically be greater in the subset of patients with estrogen receptor positive tumors where the response to endocrine therapy is highest. Numerous trials attempting to evaluate chemoendocrine therapy have been published (11). The study design of many of these trials is not optimal; nevertheless, the overall results are disappointing. A trend for an increased response rate is evident in certain trials. Response duration and survival, however, are not improved. One large adjuvant therapy trial comparing chemotherapy with or without the antiestrogen tamoxifen even shows a deleterious effect on survival with the addition of tamoxifen in certain subgroups (6).

The explanation for these disappointing results is not clear, but there are several potential problems. One modality could interact with host tissues in such a way as to alter the net effect of the other modality.   For instance, estrogens and antiestrogens are known to influence hepatic drug metabolism and to influence immune function. Second, the two modalities could interact pharmacologically resulting in antagonism.   Third, antagonism could result on a cell kinetic basis, thereby altering net cell kill.   There is a growing body of evidence to suggest that the predominant effect of endocrine therapy is cytostatic rather than cytocidal.   Endocrine therapy may slow the transit of breast cancer cells through the cell cycle, or may actually block the cells in G_0 G_1, rendering them less vulnerable to cycle active or S-phase-specific drugs.

The ability to perturb the cell cycle of hormone dependent tumor cells by endocrine manipulation may actually be used to advantage by offering a new treatment strategy.   In the case of breast cancer, the inhibition of cell cycle transit imposed by endocrine therapy is reversible with the administration of estrogen.   In experimental model systems, estrogen therapy can increase the rate of proliferation and synchronize a large fraction of cells in S-phase, where they may be more vulnerable to cytotoxic therapy.   Theoretically, a similar approach could be utilized with antiandrogen and androgen manipulation of prostate cancer, or with other cancers for which growth factors regulating cell proliferation have been identified.   Clinical trials have now been initiated in patients with advanced breast and prostate cancers.

In this paper I will review the scientific data providing the rationale and justification for investigating this approach and, using breast cancer as a model, I will discuss problems and pitfalls that need to be considered in current and future clinical trials.

EFFECTS OF HORMONE MANIPULATION ON
BREAST CANCER CELL PROLIFERATION

Effects of Antiestrogens

Data from Lippman et al. (12) provided the initial suggestion that estrogens and antiestrogens have potent effects on breast cancer cell kinetics.   These studies used the estrogen receptor-positive MCF-7 human breast cancer cell line.   Over an eight day period in tissue culture, cell proliferation was increased above control by estradiol while growth was inhibited by the antiestrogen tamoxifen.   It is important to note that cell number did not decline in the presence of tamoxifen, but, rather, increased slowly compared to controls.   Thymidine incorporation was also stimulated by estradiol and inhibited by tamoxifen.   However, this reduction in DNA synthesis by tamoxifen was reversible by the later addition of estradiol indicating that the cells were not lethally arrested by the antiestrogen.   Interestingly, DNA synthesis in these "estrogen-rescued" cells increased at a rapid rate and peaked at a rate higher than cells treated with estradiol alone.   Synchronization of the cells by the tamoxifen block and estrogen rescue was suggested as a mechanism for these observations.

These results sparked a series of studies by other investigators who examined the cell cycle kinetic effects of estrogens and antiestrogens in more detail (16,20). Using the autoradiographic technique of thymidine labeling of cells as an estimate of the S-phase fraction and the technique of flow cytometry of cells stained with a DNA fluorochrome to identify S-phase cells as well as cells in G_0G_1 and G_2 + M phases, Lippman's hypothesis of cell synchronization by antiestrogens and estrogens was proven correct. Antiestrogens reduced the fraction of cultured breast cancer cells in S and G_2 + M phases and increased the fraction in G_0G_1. In fact, after several days of exposure to tamoxifen, more than 90% of MCF-7 breast cancer cells were in G_0G_1 phase, compared to 60-70% of control cells. Cytogenetic mapping of the G_0G_1 phase revealed that antiestrogen-treated cells were accumulating in early to mid G_1 phase, in contrast to control cells which accumulate at the G_1/S interface when they reach a confluent density (15). Other studies showed that the major effects of tamoxifen could be achieved by a brief exposure of the cells to the drug in mid G_0G_1; drug exposure outside this time frame had markedly fewer effects (21). These studies demonstrate that a major effect of antiestrogen treatment of human breast cancer may be a cell kinetic alteration with inhibition of cell cycle progression in G_0G_1 phase.

This reduction in S-phase cells with a concomitant increase in G_0G_1 cells might be expected to reduce the effects of cycle specific cytotoxic agents. Hug et al. (8) found that tamoxifen attenuates the toxicity of doxorubicin and 5-fluorouracil in cultured human breast cancer cell lines regardless of estrogen receptor status. It is doubtful that this antagonism was due to a cell cycle alteration, since cells were pretreated with tamoxifen for only two hours prior to exposure to the cytotoxic agent, insufficient time for cells to accumulate in G_0G_1 phase. Furthermore, tamoxifen would not alter the cell cycle kinetics of the estrogen receptor-negative cell line. Benz et al. (2) reported a synergistic effect of tamoxifen combined with 5-fluorouracil on cultured human breast cancer cells. These studies were performed under conditions in which an accumulation of cells in G_0G_1 was observed. The synergism was explained on the basis of increased RNA-directed toxicity from 5-fluorouracil which is greater in G_1 phase cells.

We have recently examined the effects of tamoxifen pretreatment on the toxicity of 5-fluorouracil for MCF-7 human breast cancer cells (Table 1). A 72 hour pretreatment with 1 μM tamoxifen resulted in an antagonistic interaction with 5-fluorouracil.

TABLE 1. Interaction of tamoxifen and 5FU

Drug	Colonies Surviving Fraction
5FU*	.16
Tamoxifen	.63
Tamoxifen + 5FU	.30
Tamoxifen + 5FU (expected)	.10

*3 μg/ml, 1 hour exposure

The discrepancies among these studies remain to be explained, but they may be due to differences in drug dose or scheduling, or to differences among breast cancer cell lines. In any event, it is clear that interactions which may have clinical relevance between tamoxifen and cytotoxic agents do occur in these experimental model systems.

Effects of Estrogen Rescue

Although antiestrogen treatment inhibits cell proliferation and causes a block in G_1 transit, this block is reversible with the addition of estrogen (16). Within 24 hours after the addition of estradiol to tamoxifen-treated MCF-7 cells, the majority of cells have resumed transit through G_1 phase into S-phase. Eventually this synchronous cohort of cells passes through S-phase and into G_2 + M phase and rapidly resumes asynchronous growth. By this technique 60% to 70% of MCF-7 cells can be synchronized in S-phase where, theoretically, they would be more vulnerable to S-phase-specific agents. The cytotoxicity of arabino-furanosylcytosine (20) and doxorubicin (9) has been reported to be enhanced by the addition of estradiol to MCF-7 cells. The ability to manipulate breast cancer cell cycle kinetics with hormones in this fashion provides the rationale for the new treatment strategy discussed later.

Studies in the Nude Mouse Model

The effects of estrogens and antiestrogens on human breast cancer cell proliferation have also been studied using an in vivo model system, the athymic nude mouse. Growth of estrogen receptor-positive cell lines such as MCF-7 requires estrogen. Receptor-negative cells form tumors in castrated mice. We have studied the effects of endocrine therapy with estrogen withdrawal and antiestrogen therapy on MCF-7 tumors growing subcutaneously in female nude mice (17). Endocrine therapy reduces tumor growth but causes little or no tumor regression of MCF-7 or ZR75-1 cells. Prolonged endocrine therapy for up to four months reduces the mitotic index but does not cause necrosis or histologic evidence for cell death. Furthermore, continued viability of the tumor cells even after several months of therapy has been demonstrated by successful in vitro cloning of cells from treated tumors, by transplantation of tumor fragments into fresh mice, and by the ability of estrogen replenishment to restore tumor growth in vivo. These results support the in vitro studies described above and suggest that a major action of antiestrogens and estrogens is to regulate transit through the cell cycle. The nude mouse studies also demonstrate the feasibility of "estrogen rescue" of cell proliferation in an in vivo model system.

HORMONE MANIPULATION AND CHEMOTHERAPY IN PATIENTS

The idea of hormone "priming" combined with a cytotoxic agent to increase the effectiveness of cancer treatment is not new. More than 40 years ago radiotherapists used estrogen administration in patients with breast cancer and other tumors in an attempt to improve the cytocidal effects of irradiation. Androgen priming combined with ^{32}P therapy has been used for many years in patients with metastatic prostatic and breast cancer involving bone, to enhance uptake of the radioisotope into the tumor and adjacent bone.

In the past few years several clinical trials using hormonal manipulation to theoretically alter tumor cell cycle kinetics, thereby increasing the effectiveness of chemotherapy, have been initiated in breast and prostate cancer.

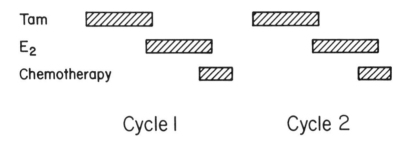

FIG. 1. Treatment strategy for studies of hormone synchronization and chemotherapy in breast cancer

Several of these trials are reviewed elsewhere in this book. Although there are some differences in the doses, schedules, and agents used in these studies, the basic treatment strategy for breast cancer is shown in Figure 1. Patients are first given the antiestrogen tamoxifen to block cell cycle progression in $G_0 G_1$ phase. Estrogen replenishment is given next to reverse the cell cycle block allowing a cohort of cells to leave G_1 and enter S-phase simultaneously. Chemotherapy is given after estrogen rescue, hopefully at a time when many cells are actively synthesizing DNA and are sensitive to cytotoxic drugs. Similar strategies have been used in prostate cancer using androgen depletion followed by short-term androgen priming. Although the results of some of these trials generate cautious optimism, several questions and problems require consideration.

It is clear that hormones can synchronize a large fraction of cultured cancer cells in G_1 or S-phase. This high degree of synchronization is possible in part due to the large growth fraction (non-G_0 cells) present in cells in culture. However, the cell cycle distribution of human solid tumors in vivo is considerably different. The median growth fraction of a series of human breast cancers has been reported to range from 4% to 24%, much lower than that for cultured cells, indicating that the majority of cells are in G_0 (3,18). The median S-phase fraction has been reported to range from 2% to 5% (3,14,18). Thus, even if 50% of the cycling cells could be synchronized in S-phase, in a tumor with a growth fraction of 20%, only 10% of the total tumor cells would be appropriately affected. On the other hand, if estrogen administration also resulted in recruitment of G_0 cells into the proliferating pool, the degree of synchronization might be improved substantially. If the growth fraction was increased to 50%, then 25% of the total cell population might be synchronized in the desired cell cycle phase under these circumstances.

There are few published trials evaluating the effects of hormone priming on the growth fraction or S-fraction of human breast cancer. In one study using the thymidine labeling index (TLI) to estimate the S-fraction, administration of estrogen and progesterone increased the TLI in 7 of 10 patients within three days, regardless of tumor estrogen receptor status (4). However, the maximum TLI observed in these patients even after treatment was 10.1%. In another study, the primer-dependent DNA polymerase assay was used to estimate the growth fraction and the TLI was used to measure S-phase cells after three days of DES therapy (3). An increase in the TLI was observed in 8/16 patients, but the median TLI in these patients went from 1.6% before DES to only 3.8% after. Furthermore, although the growth fraction increased in 13/16 patients, the increase was modest with a median growth fraction of 4.6% before DES and 9.1% after. These cell kinetic changes are of questionable biological significance when one considers the much higher growth and S-phase fractions routinely observed in other more rapidly proliferating tumors that are curable with cytotoxic agents.

The strategy to recruit or synchronize human tumor cells with hormones is confronted with several other potential problems. First, for maximal anti-tumor effect, the clonogenic fraction of the tumor is the major population of interest, since these cells have the capacity for continued replication and self-renewal. Whether the hormone synchronization scheme described above affects the clonogenic fraction of the tumor or only the more differentiated nonclonogenic cells is unknown. Clonogenic cells may have fewer estrogen receptors compared to their more differentiated non-clonogenic offspring, theoretically rendering them less hormonally responsive (10). Second, human tumors in vivo may be composed of cells quite heterogeneous with regard to cell cycle kinetic parameters such as cell cycle time. This heterogeneity could make synchronization of a large fraction of the tumor very difficult, even if the cells responded appropriately to the hormonal manipulation. Third, optimal timing of cell synchronization could vary significantly among different patients. Proper timing of the chemotherapy would then require serial tumor cell kinetic analyses during estrogen priming for each patient. Patients without easily accessible tumor for repeated biopsy would then be ineligible for this approach.

The optimal dose and schedule of tamoxifen and estrogen required for synchronization in vivo have not been rigorously determined. Two studies gave intermittent cycles of tamoxifen for several days at the usual maintenance dose of 10-20 mg Bid (1,13). Therapeutic drug levels are reached very slowly with this dose, and levels may be insufficient to cause the G_1 transition delay (5). The prolonged half-life of seven days after withdrawal of tamoxifen and its conversion to more active metabolites further complicate the sequence and makes intermittent "pulsing" of the antiestrogen difficult.

The dose of estrogen required for reversal of the antiestrogen block is also problematic. Premarin at the total dose of 1.25 mg/day for one to four days has been used in two studies (1,13). However, even after three weeks blood levels of estradiol only reach 0.3 nM with this dose and there is significant conversion to the less potent estrone (23). Although the affinity of estradiol for the estrogen receptor is about 50-fold greater than tamoxifen, these estrogen concentrations would be insufficient to reverse the effect of tamoxifen, the concentration of which reaches more than 1000-fold higher (about 1000 nM) in patients during chronic adminstration, and may reach more than 100-fold higher after only one week of therapy (5). Additional pharmacologic studies of tamoxifen block and estrogen rescue are required to define the appropriate dose and schedule. Since the majority of cells in a human breast cancer in vivo are already in G_0G_1 phase, administration of tamoxifen may not be necessary to achieve the desired cell kinetic alteration. Deletion of tamoxifen would greatly simplify this therapeutic strategy.

Finally, two other problems related to deliberate hormone stimulation of tumor cell proliferation require consideration. The first is the possible adverse effect on the patient due to a transient increase in tumor growth. The "tumor flare" phenomenon occasionally associated with additive hormone therapy can result in significant morbidity. Patients with metastatic breast or prostate cancer involving bone may have severe bone pain with estrogen or androgen priming. Life-threatening hypercalcemia may also occur in patients with metastatic breast cancer receiving estrogen therapy. More critical, however, is the possibility of inducing spinal cord compression in patients with vertebral metastases. This catastrophic complication occurred in 4% of nearly 200 patients receiving androgen priming and ^{32}P therapy for metastatic prostate cancer, and it occurred in one of 21 patients reported by our group who received only four days of androgen stimulation with fluoxymesterone (19). Clearly, careful patient selection and close monitoring during therapy are required if this approach is to be used safely in patients with metastatic disease.

Hormone priming could also adversely influence patient survival. Even transient stimulation of tumor cell proliferation would have a negative impact if a large fraction of the tumor was genetically, rather than kinetically, resistant to the cytotoxic agents. These considerations demand that carefully designed pilot studies testing the feasibility and optimizing the dose and schedule of the agents used precede large scale evaluation of this new approach. When feasibility has been demonstrated, larger randomized trials will be required to confirm the utility of this strategy. As other hormone growth factors are identified, this approach may be applied to other solid tumors in the future.

REFERENCES

1. Allegra, J. C., Woodcock, T. M., Richman, S. P., Bland, K. I., and Wittliff, J. L. (1982): Breast Cancer Res. Treat., 2:93-99.
2. Benz, C., Cadman, E., Gwin, J., Wu, T., Amara, J., Eisenfeld, A., and Dannies, P. (1983): Cancer Res., 43:5298-5303.
3. Conte, P. F., Fraschini, G., Alama, A., Nicolin, A., Corsaro, E., Canavese, G., Rosso, R., and Drewinko, B. (1985): Cancer Res., 45:5926-5930.
4. Dao, T. L., Sinha, D. K., Nemoto, T., and Patel, J. (1982): Cancer Res., 42:359-362.
5. Fabian, C., Sternson, L., El-Serafi, M., Cain, L., and Hearne, E. (1981): Cancer, 48:876-882.
6. Fisher, B., Redmond, C., Brown, A., Wickerham, L. D., Wolmark, N., Allegra, J., Escher, G., Lippman, M., Savlov, E., Wittliff, J., and Fisher, E. R., with the contributions of Plotkin, D., Bowman, D., Wolter, J., Bornstein, R., Desser, R., Frelick, R., and other NSABP investigators (1983): J. Clin. Oncol., 1:227-241.
7. Greenspan, E. M., Fieber, M., Lesnick, G., and Edelman, S. (1963): J. Mount Sinai Hosp., 30:246-267.
8. Hug, V., Hortobagyi, G. N., Drewinko, B., and Finders, M. (1985): J. Clin. Oncol., 3:1672-1677.
9. Hug, V., Johnston, D., Finders, M., and Hortobagyi, G. (1986): Cancer Res., 46:147-152.
10. Kodama, F., Greene, G. L., and Salmon, S. E. (1985): Cancer Res., 45:2720-2724.
11. Lippman, M. E. (1983): Breast Cancer Res. Treat., 3:117-127.
12. Lippman, M., Bolan, G., and Huff, K. (1976): Cancer Res., 36:4595-4601.
13. Lippman, M. E., Cassidy, J., Wesley, M., and Young, R. C. (1984): J. Clin. Oncol., 2:28-36.
14. Meyer, J. S., McDivitt, R. W., Stone, K. R., Prey, M. U., and Bauer, W. C. (1984): Breast Cancer Res. Treat., 4:79-88.
15. Osborne, C. K., Boldt, D. H., Clark, G. M., and Trent, J. M. (1983): Cancer Res., 43:3583-3585.
16. Osborne, C. K., Boldt, D. H., and Estrada, P. (1984): Cancer Res., 44:1433-1439.
17. Osborne, C. K., Hobbs, K., and Clark, G. M. (1985): Cancer Res., 45:584-590.
18. Schiffer, L. M., Braunschweiger, P. G., Stragand, J. J., and Poulakos, L. (1979): Cancer, 1707-1719.
19. Suarez, A. J., Lamm, D. L., Radwin, H. M., Sarosdy, M., Clark, G., and Osborne, C. K. (1982): Cancer Chemother. Pharmacol., 8:261-265.
20. Sutherland, R. L., Hall, R. E., and Taylor, I. W. (1983): Cancer Res., 43:3993-4006.
21. Taylor, I. W., Hodson, P. J., Green, M. D., and Sutherland, R. L. (1983): Cancer Res., 43:4007-4010.
22. Weichselbaum, R. R., Hellman, S., Piro, A. J., Nove, J. J., and Little, J. B. (1978): Cancer Res., 38:2339-2342.
23. Whitaker, P. G., Morgan, M. R. A., and Dean, P. D. G. (1980): Lancet, 1:14-16.

Hormonal Manipulation of Cancer: Peptides,
Growth Factors, and New (Anti) Steroidal
Agents, edited by Jan G. M. Klijn et al.
Raven Press, New York © 1987.

CHEMOTHERAPY WITH ESTROGENIC RECRUITMENT

IN BREAST CANCER

EXPERIMENTAL STUDIES. R.J. Paridaens (1), R. Kiss
(2), Y. de Launoit (2) and G. Atassi (3).
CLINICAL STUDIES. R.J. Paridaens (4), J.G.M. Klijn
(4), A. Clarysse (4), N. Rotmentz (4) and
R.J. Sylvester (5).

(1) Service de Médecine. Inst. J. Bordet, Brussels.
(2) Lab. d'Histologie, Faculté de Médecine, ULB, Brussels. (3) Lab. de Chimiothérapie Expérimentale et
Screening. Inst. J. Bordet. Brussels. (4) Members of
the EORTC Breast Cancer Cooperative Group. (5) EORTC
Data Center. Brussels - Belgium.

INTRODUCTION

During the last two decades, the therapeutic
results obtained in breast cancer, at any stage of the
disease, have improved because of the use of systemic
treatments consisting of either endocrine manipulations (HT), chemotherapy (CT), or both modalities
together. The mechanisms of antitumor action of HT
and of CT, although not entirely elucidated, seem very
different. It is well known that endocrine manipulations are effective almost exclusively in tumors containing steroid-hormone receptors, i.e. estrogen receptors (ER) and/or progesterone receptors (PgR).
Endocrine ablative modalities (castration, adrenalectomy, adrenal blocking agents and aromatase inhibitors) deprive the tumors from the endogenously produced hormones (mainly estrogens) deemed to exert a
promoting effect on their growth. Antihormones (antiestrogens) and pharmacological doses of steroids (androgens, estrogens, progestins) compete for the binding of natural hormones to their receptors, inhibit
receptors resynthesis, and sometimes exert multiple
endogenous blockades of hormone metabolism at various
levels, including the neoplastic cell itself. All
these maneuvers, when effective, reduce the proliferative index in hormone-sensitive tumors, leading to the
death of the most hormone-dependent part of the neop-
lastic-cell population, and putting the remaining part
in a quiescent, non-dividing status, outside of the

cell cycle (GO). On the other hand, cytotoxic drugs
are known to kill predominantly the cell engaged in
the mitotic cycle, several agents being more specifically active during one or another phase of this
cycle. Thus, the lack of true synergism between HT and
CT on neoplastic cells may be ascribed to their different, possibly mutually exclusive mechanisms of action. Moreover, one possible mechanism of resistance
of cancer cells in chemo-sensitive tumors may operate
through the temporary reversible shift of one part of
the cell population (theoretically, one single cell
may suffice) to the GO state, in which they are prote-
cted towards cytotoxic agents, leading later to the
regrowth of the tumor.

Recently, new perspectives arose from experiments
showing that hormones might be used for modulating the
cell cycle kinetics of neoplastic target cells, providing a means to obtain synergistic hormonochemotherapeutic conditions (2, 6, 8, 10, 12). Our contribution
in this field was to show, in a murine model, that one
brief estrogenic stimulus could transiently force
quiescent estrogen-dependent neoplastic cells, chronically deprived of estrogens, to re-enter the mitotic
cycle, rendering them vulnerable to cycle-active cytotoxic drugs. This manipulation, "estrogenic recruitment" might allow to eradicate all progenitor neoplastic cells in ER-positive tumors. Furthermore, it might
also induce partial synchronisation of the dividing
cell population, which could then be killed by a
phase-specific agent, given at the appropriate time.
This concept has now reached the step of clinical
testing.

The first part of this paper will summarize our
experimental data, obtained with an ovarian-dependent
mammary tumor of the mouse (MXT model); the second
part will be the report of a pilot clinical study,
based on the concept, which was conducted by the
E.O.R.T.C. (European Organization for Research and
Treatment of Cancer) Breast Cancer Cooperative Group.
The results of a few comparable clinical trials will
be reviewed briefly, before discussing the limitations
and the potential developments of this new therapeutic
approach in oncology.

EXPERIMENTAL STUDIES

Description of the MXT model

These studies were performed on an hormone-dependent mouse mammary tumor (MXT model) initially developed by Watson et al. in 1977 (11), and kindly provided to our laboratory by Dr. A.E. Bogden (Mason Research Institute, Mass.). This tumor, maintained by serial transplantations on intact adult female mice, displays the microscopic features of a well-differentiated adenocarcinoma, and contains significant amounts of estrogen receptors (ER).

Effects of hormones on the MXT tumor

We analyzed first the effects of a brief in vivo estrogenic stimulation in MXT tumors (8). Therefore, we castrated a series of animals bearing fully grown tumors, 4 weeks after their implantation. This operation, which was done in order to suppress the influence of endogenously produced ovarian hormones, never induced the regression of tumors, but rather slowed their growth compared to that observed in intact subjects. A few days later, a near physiologic dose of estradiol (E2, 0.25 mcg) was injected intraperitoneally, and the animals were sacrificed by lots of 5 at 12 h intervals, i.e. 12, 24, 36 and 48 hours thereafter. Controls received a placebo injection of saline and were killed 24 h later. Just one hour prior to sacrifice, 25 uCi 3H-thymidine was injected i.p. After killing, mammary tumors were removed and processed histologically for autoradiography. Uteri were also removed and handled similarly, as control normal estrogen-target organs. Both on uteri and on tumors, the proportions (%) of cells of each given morphologic type with labeled nuclei were determined by counting, providing an index (TLI = thymidine labeling index), which is a measure of the proportion of cells engaged in the DNA synthetic phase, and thus also a means to evaluate cell proliferation.

The results of this first experiment clearly indicated that the neoplastic cells were very sensitive to the mitogenic action of E2, as was the uterine epithelium. A transient increase of the MXT TLI was observed, lasting from the 12th to the 36th hour after E2 administration, and reaching its maximum ($\pm$ 3 times the basal TLI) at the 24th hour. Subsequent experiments confirmed the finding, exploring more in details the cell kinetic parameters (S phase duration, cell cycle duration, growth fraction) under influence of E2. We then studied the effects of higher doses of E2, and found that a greater mitogenic stimulation could even be obtained with 2.5 mcg E2. Higher dosages were not better in this regard. Finally, very recently, we looked at the effects of Progesterone (Pg) and of Prolactin (PRL). Both hormones were found to be potent mitogens on MXT tumors, but not on the uterus. Experiments are in progress, which investigate the effects of multiple hormonal injections, and the interactions between E2 and Pg, or E2 and PRL at the MXT level.

Effects of cytotoxic drugs on the MXT tumor

Among various cytotoxic drugs tested on the model, only Cyclophosphamide (CPA), and also, with a lesser efficiency, Doxorubicin (ADM), were able to slow down significantly the growth of the MXT tumors. Methotrexate, 5-Fluorouracil and Cytosine-arabinoside had no detectable effects.

Estrogen plus chemotherapy in the MXT model

These experiments aimed at testing the hypothesis that estrogenic recruitment might amplify the antineoplastic action of a cycle-active cytotoxic agent. Therefore, 90 mice underwent bilateral s.c. transplantation with 2 small pieces of MXT on day 1 and were randomly allocated into 9 groups of equal size (groups A to I). Group A was left intact, while all others underwent bilateral oophorectomy on day 10. On day 15, 8 cycles of treatment with either placebo, and/or cyclophosphamide (CPA 30 mg/kg) and or E2 (0.25 or 2.5 mcg) given according to various schedules were administered at 72h intervals and tumors were measured weekly. Treatments given to the nine experimental groups were as follows: (A) placebo; (B) placebo; (C) E2 0.25 mcg; (D) E2 2.5 mcg; (E) CPA; (F) E2 0.25 mcg followed by CPA 24h later; (G) E2 2.5 mcg followed by CPA 24h later; (H) CPA followed by E2 0.25 mcg 24h later; (I) CPA followed by E2 2.5 mcg 24h later. The results indicated that: (1) castration did not significantly influence tumor growth, nor did E2 alone in castrated animals; (2) CPA was effective in castrated animals; (3) CPA followed by E2 was not different from CPA alone; (4) E2 2.5 mcg was significantly better than any other treatment.

It is thus concluded that a synergism between estrogenic recruitment and cyclophosphamide can be achieved, under particular conditions. The dose of estrogen used is important, since a near physiologic dose seems ineffective, whereas a 10 fold higher dosage is very efficient. The timing of hormone administration before chemotherapy is critical, since the extension of the delay from 24 to 48 h resulted in a total loss of the synergism.

CLINICAL STUDIES

Background

In view of the experimental results described above, and because new pharmacological means for blocking the endogenous production of oestrogens were available, a therapeutic regimen based on the concept of oestrogenic recruitment was designed. We summarize here below the final results of a pilot study, in which a hopefully synergistic hormono-chemotherapeutic combination was tested for tolerance and antitumor activity. This study was undertaken under the aegis of the EORTC Breast Cancer Cooperative Group.

Patients and methods

All patients included in this trial had advanced breast cancer, histologically proved, with evaluable and/or measurable lesions. None of them had received prior systemic anti-neoplastic therapy. Response to treatment was evaluated according to standard UICC criteria (4) and submitted to extramural review.

The endocrine part of the therapeutic regimen aimed at achieving a deep and prolonged estrogenic suppression. All patients received continuous treatment with aminoglutethimide (1.0 g/day) and hydrocortisone (40 mg/day). Since these drugs are not capable of adequately suppressing ovarian production of steroidal sex hormones, premenopausal women also underwent surgical castration. Two weeks after initiating the endocrine treatment, cyclical chemotherapy was started with a three-drug combination of 5-fluorouracil (5-FU), adriamycin (ADM), and cyclophosphamide (CPA). These drugs were given intravenously every three weeks (5-FU 500 mg/m^2; ADM 50 mg/m^2; CPA 500 mg/m^2) exactly 24 hours after the oral administration of ethinylestradiol (50 ug), the hormonal recruiting agent. After 11 cycles, ADM was replaced by methotrexate (50 mg/m^2 i.v.) in order to avoid ADM-induced cumulative cardiotoxicity, and the treatment was pursued until the disease progressed.

Results

By August 1983, 67 eligible patients registered at the EORTC Data Center by eight european institutions (Table I) had been included in the study. Ten cases were found to be inevaluable for response to therapy because of incomplete data (2 patients) or incomplete treatment (8 patients). The latter was either due to treatment refusal (2 patients) or drug withdrawal for excessive toxicity, mainly intolerance to aminoglutethimide (4 patients).

TABLE I

EORTC 10807 - PARTICIPANTS

Institut J. Bordet (R. Paridaens, J.C. Heuson)	Brussels	Belgium
Centre H. Becquerel (J.P. Julien, P. Bastit)	Rouen	France
Radiotherapeutisch Inst. (J. Blonk van der Wijst, S. The, J.G.M. Klijn)	Rotterdam	The Netherlands
Ospedale Civile (E. Ferrazzi, M. Fiorentino)	Padova	Italy
A.Z. Sint Jan (A. Clarysse)	Brugge	Belgium
Centre Hospitalier Tivoli (J. Michel, L. Debusscher)	La Louvière	Belgium
A.Z. Middelheim (D. Becquart, W. Van Bogaert)	Antwerpen	Belgium
Centre Paul Brien (C. Cauchie)	Brussels	Belgium

Among the 57 fully evaluable cases, a majority of patients (53%) had visceral metastases, mainly located in the lung and/or in the liver, which are generally deemed to share a very bad prognosis. Overall response and response according to several putative prognostic factors are detailed in table II.

TABLE II

EORTC 10807 - RESPONSE TO THERAPY

	Number of patients	Response (*)	
		CR (%)	CR+PR (%)
Dominant metastatic site			
Soft tissue	12	5 (42)	10 (83)
Bone	15	7 (47)	12 (80)
Viscera	30	8 (27)	21 (70)
Menopausal status			
Premenopausal	18	9 (50)	14 (78)
Postmenopausal	39	11 (28)	29 (74)
Estrogen receptors (**)			
> 30 fmoles/mg protein	8	3 (38)	7 (88)
< 30 fmoles/mg protein	14	5 (36)	9 (64)
unknown	35	12 (34)	27 (77)
OVERALL	57	20 (35)	43 (75)

* Median times to progression were 123 weeks (range 11-197+) for complete responders (CR) and 58 weeks (range 10-106) for partial remissions (PR).

** Assays performed according to the standardized dextran-coated charcoal method adopted by the EORTC Cancer Cooperative Group (3).

It appears that response rates were almost identical in all three categories of predominant metastatic involvement. Complete remissions (CR) (a complete disappearance of all signs and symptoms of disease according to the UICC criteria) were observed in 35 % of all the evaluable cases, representing a little less

than half of all objective (complete + partial) responses (CR + PR = 75 %). Treatment was considered as
a failure in 12 cases (21 %), and only 2 patients (4
%) were classified as having stable disease, i.e. they
had no evidence of disease progression during the
first three months of therapy. Side-effects of chemotherapy consisted mainly of transient leucopenia with
a median nadir of $2600/mm^3$ (range 1000-3800), gastro-
intestinal disturbances (88 % of patients) and alopoe-
cia (77 % of patients). Aminoglutethimide-induced
drowsiness (35 % of patients) and skin rashes (20 % of
patients) occurred mainly during the first two weeks
of treatment and were generally mild and short-lived.

DISCUSSION

The experimental studies on MXT tumors provide
evidence that estrogens, given just 24 h before chemotherapy, realize a synergistic combination. As regards therapy of hormone-dependent human breast cancer, it is premature to draw a similar conclusion.
The regimen used by the EORTC Breast Cancer Cooperative Group seems highly effective for inducing
remissions in advanced disease, and the overall and
complete remission rates obtained (75 and 35 % respectively) compare favorably with the best figures obtained by the Group with other hormonochemotherapeutic
combinations (5, 7).
    In this study, indeed, two highly effective ap-
proaches were combined, i.e. estrogens suppression
with aminoglutethimide and chemotherapy as first-line
treatment for advanced disease. The exact role of
estrogens given prior to chemotherapy is still unknown. A phase-III trial aiming to validate the concept of estrogenic recruitment has now been activated.
It is restricted to ER-positive cases and patients are
randomized to receive either ethinylestradiol or placebo, according to a double-blind design, before starting chemotherapy. So far, more than hundred patients
have been included in the study and accrual is expected to be completed within a few months.
    Two studies based on the same concept, but with
different schedules were conducted by others. In the
first, Allegra et al. (1) gave an antiestrogenic treatment (Tamoxifen 20 mg/day) for ten consecutive days,
then estrogens (premarin 0.625 mg x 2/day) days 11-14
and finally chemotherapy with methotrexate and 5
fluouracil on day 14 and leucovorin on day 15. Cycles

were repeated every 18 days. Their results were very favorable with 18 remissions, among which 14 where complete on a total of 25 evaluable patients. In the second study, Santen et al. (9) treated 37 postmenopausal women with aminoglutethimide and hydrocortisone continously; cyclic chemotherapy with the FAC regimen was repeated every 3 weeks. Patients were randomized to receive (in double blind) either a placebo (arm A) or estradiol (2 x 2 mg/d, arm B) during 3 days before the FAC injection. Among 28 evaluable cases, they observed in arm A (12 patients) 5 remissions and in arm B (16 patients) also 5 remissions. It should be noticed that, in addition to these relatively low response rates, tumor flares were observed in arm B, suggesting that chemotherapy given after 3 days of hormonal administration was unable to counteract the stimulating effects of E_2.

We conclude that appropriate hormonal manipulations and especially estrogenic recruitment represent a promising tool for enhancing the antineoplastic action of cytotoxic agents. The schedule of administration (time lapse between hormones and cytotoxic) and the dosages of hormones are critical for obtaining a true synergism. Further research is needed for improving our knowledge on cell kinetics of human breast cancer, for screening new factors modulating their growth and finally for designing synergistic combinations.

REFERENCES

1. Allegra, J.C., Woodcock, T.M., Richman, S.P., Bland, K.I. and Witliff, J.L. (1982): Breast Cancer Res. Treat., 2: 93-99.
2. Dao, T.L., Sinha, D.K., Nemoto, T. and Patel, J. (1982): Cancer Res., 42: 359-362.
3. EORTC - Breast Cancer Cooperative Group (1973): Eur. J. Cancer, 9: 379-381.
4. Hayward, J.L., Carbone, P.P., Heuson, J.C., Kumaoka, S., Segaloff, A. and Rubens, R.D. (1977): Cancer, 30: 1289-1294.
5. Heuson, J.C., Sylvester, R. and Engelsman, E. (1980): In: Breast Cancer - Experimental and Clinical Aspects, edited by H.T. Mouridsen and T. Palshof, pp. 113-117. Pergamon Press, New-York.
6. Markaverich, B.M., Medina, D. and Clark, J.H. (1983): Cancer Res., 43: 3208-3211.

7. Mouridsen, H.T. Palshof, T., Engelsman, E. and Sylvester, R. (1980): In: Breast Cancer - Experimental and Clinical Aspects, edited by H.T. Mouridsen and T. Palshof, pp. 119-123. Pergamon Press, New-York.
8. Paridaens, R.J., Danguy, A.J., Leclercq, G., Kiss, R. and Heuson, J.C. (1985): J. Natl. Cancer Inst., 74 (6): 1239-1246.
9. Santen, R.J., Harvey, H.A., Manni, A., Simonds, M.A., White, D.S., Boucher, A., Walker, B.K., Dixon, R.H., Valdivia, D.E. and Gordon, R.A. (1985): Proceedings of the ECCO meeting held in Stockholm. Abstract 615, pp. 160.
10. Stormshak, F., Leake, R., Wertz, N. and Gorski, J. (1976): Endocrinology, 99: 1501-1511.
11. Watson, C., Medina, D. and Clark, J.H. (1977): Cancer Res., 37: 3344-3348.
12. Weichselbaum, R.R., Hellman, S., Piro, A.J., Nove, J.J. and Little, J.B. (1978): Cancer Res., 38: 2339-2342.

AKNOWLEDGEMENTS

Part of this work was supported by grants of the Fonds Cancérologique de la Caisse d'Epargne et de Retraite (CGER) - Belgium.

Hormonal Manipulation of Cancer: Peptides, Growth Factors, and New (Anti) Steroidal Agents, edited by Jan G. M. Klijn et al. Raven Press, New York © 1987.

CYTOKINETIC STUDIES AND TREATMENT RESULTS OF ESTROGENS FOLLOWED BY CHEMOTHERAPY IN LOCALLY ADVANCED AND METASTATIC HUMAN BREAST CANCER

P.F. Conte, A. Rubagotti, P. Pronzato, A. Alama, D. Amadori° G. Canavese, F. Carnino* A. Catturich, M.G. Daga, R. De Micheli^ E. Di Marco, G. Gardin, P. Gentilini° A. Jacomuzzi* R. Lionetto, C. Monzeglio* C. Mossetti* A. Nicolin, R. Rosso, P. Sismondi" M. Sussio"

Istituto Nazionale per la Ricerca sul Cancro,V.le Benedetto XV,10 16132,Genova; °Ospedale G.B.Morgagni, Forlì; *Ospedale S.Anna, Torino; ^Ospedale Civile, Legnago; "Clinica Ostetrica-Ginecologica Torino, Italy

INTRODUCTION

Metastatic breast cancer is a relatively chemosensitive tumor and response rates in the order of 60-70% have been reported(3,5). Unfortunately median duration of response is usually short,the majority of these responses are not complete and very few patients remain in durable complete remission (9,15).

Undoubtedly these data suggest that mutation to drug resistance is the most important limiting factor in treatment results(12). On the other hand clinical trials aimed to overcome phenotypic resistance by combining chemo-endocrine therapy, alternating combination chemotherapies or increasing the number of drugs have failed to demonstrate any clear advantage over conventional combination chemotherapy (18). Overlapping drug-related toxicities, lack of equally active, non cross resistant regimens and the fact that the majority of patients do not have hormone-dependent tumors can partially explain the failure of therapeutic strategies aimed to overcome the phenotypic resistance. On the other side the possibility that other non genetic causes of chemoresistance are important in the clinical outcome of these patients cannot be ruled out.

In particular, a large amount of experimental data demonstrate that antiblastic drugs have a higher cell killing efficacy on proliferating in comparison to non proliferating tumor cells(10,23). Evidence that temporary chemoresistance plays a role in cancer chemotherapy comes also from clinical data: metastatic breast

cancer patients can experience an objective response to chemotherapy even if pretreated in the adjuvant setting (4),usually, response to salvage chemotherapy is as higher as longer is the progression free interval after the first remission (11)and, finally
in advanced ovarian cancer the probability of achieving a patholo
gical complete remission with chemotherapy depends upon the amount
of residual disease after primary surgery, irrespectively of tumor mass at diagnosis (13).

Human breast cancer represents the ideal situation to explore
new possibilities to overcome temporary chemoresistance by administering chemotherapy on cytokinetic basis. Many authors have de
monstrated that estrogens are able to recall into the proliferati
ve pool previously resting breast cancer cells (estrogenic recruit
ment)(1,17,24) and a few attempts to design cytokinetic regimens
based on estrogenic recruitment have been published (2,7,19,20,21)
In the present paper we present our experimental data on the effi
cacy of diethylstilbestrol (DES) as a recruiting agent in locally
advanced human breast cancer (LABC) and the results of three clinical trials based on estrogenic recruitment followed by chemothe
rapy in LABC and metastatic breast cancer.

PATIENTS AND METHODS

A. Locally advanced breast cancer

Thirty-nine consecutive patients with LABC (T_3N_1= 6 patients; T_3
N_2= 5 patients; T_4N_1= 9 patients; T_4N_2= 5 patients; inflammatory
carcinoma = 14 patients; ER+ = 13 patients; ER- = 20 patients; ER
unknwon = 6 patients) were treated with DES 1 mg/die for 3 days,
FAC (5-FU 600 mg/m^2+ Doxorubicin 50 mg/m^2+ Cytoxan 600 mg/m^2) d
4 q 21 days (DES-FAC); after 3 DES-FAC patients were submitted to
surgery + radiotherapy followed by 3 DES-FAC alternated with 3
DES-CMF.

In 23/39 patients tumor cell kinetics during therapy were evaluated on serial tumor biopsies at diagnosis (T_0),after DES (T_1),
24 hrs after the first chemotherapeutic course (T_2) and at radical surgery (T_3). Tumor kinetics were studied by thymidine labeling index (TLI = % of S-phase cells) and primer dependent DNA
polymerase (PDP-LI = % of proliferating cells). Details on the
two kinetic methods have been published elsewhere (7).

B. Metastatic breast cancer

1. CEF vs DES-CEF (I)

117 patients with metastatic breast cancer were randomized to
receive CEF (CTX 600 mg/m^2, Epi-Doxorubicin 60 mg/m^2, 5-FU 600

mg/m^2 d 1 q 21 days) or DES-CEF (CTX 600 mg/m^2_{d1} DES 1 mg on days
5,6,7; Epi-Doxorubicin 60 mg/m^2+ 5-FU 600 mg/m^2day 8) q 21 days
for 11 cycles or until progression. 47.4% of CEF patients and 45.
6% of DES-CEF patients had received previous adjuvant chemotherapy; ER status was known in a minority of patients (CEF: ER+ = 13.
6%, ER- = 16.9%; DES-CEF: ER+ = 10.5%, ER- = 24.6%). All other
possible prognostic variables(age, menopausal status, performance
status, dominant site of metastasis and number of metastatic sites) were equally distributed among the two arms. The study was
closed for accrual in October 1985.

2. CEF vs DES-CEF (II)
   In November 1985 a new trial was started in metastatic breast
cancer; patients were randomized to receive conventional CEF or
DES-CEF (II)(DES 1 mg on days 1,2,3 + CEF on day 4). The new sche
duling of DES-CEF was designed on the basis of the toxicity data
recorded in DES-CEF (I) study. So far 59 patients have entered
this ongoing trial.

RESULTS

A. L.A.B.C.
   Tumor cell kinetics during DES-FAC therapy in 23 patients are
reported in the Table below:

	T_0	T_1	T_2	T_3
TLI %	1.8+0.3	3.5+0.6	1.6+0.3	0.6+0.13
PDP-LI %	5.5+0.9	8.5+1.1	2.9+0.5	2.9+0.6

After DES TLI and PDP-LI were significantly increased in 43.5%
and 78.3% of patients respectively.
   Basal tumor proliferative activity seems to be an important
predictor of estrogenic recruitment: TLI and PDP-LI increased significantly after DES in 50% and 86.7% respectively of the patients with slowly proliferating tumors while, in the case of
spontaneously fast growing tumors, an estrogenic recruitment was
evident only in 27.3% of patients according to TLI and 50% of patients according to PDP-LI.
   Surprisingly a significant estrogenic recruitment was evident
in 85.7% of ER negative and in 55.5% of ER positive tumors.After
3 DES-FAC 15.4% of patients were in CR, 56.4% in PR, 17.9% in mi
nor response, 7.7% in stable disease and 1 patient (2.6%) had a
progressive disease (PD). After surgery + radiotherapy 52.3% of
patients was rendered disease free.
   At 30 mos actuarial survival and progression free survival are

65% and 50% respectively.

B. CEF vs DES-CEF (I)
    In metastatic breast cancer patients results by treatment were:

	CR%	PR%	SD%	PD%	Median S	Median PFS
CEF	16.1	41.1	35.7	7.1	441 days	265 days
DES-CEF	24.1	29.6	37.1	9.2	558 days	276 days

The overall differences between the two arms are not significant.

DES-CEF induced a statistically significant higher CR rate in
the subgroups of patients with dominant soft tissue metastasis
(50% vs 24. % p < 0.05) and with ER negative tumors (35.7% vs 11.1%
p < 0.025). Totally unaspected were the results by treatment in
the subgroup of patients previously treated with adjuvant chemothe
rapy:

	CR%	PR%	SD%	PD%	Median S	Median PFS
CEF	7.4	29.6	55.6	7.4	375 days	188 days
DES-CEF	20.8	16.7	54.2	8.3	> 773 days	246 days

The advantage in CR rate for DES-CEF patients is not significant while these patients experienced a significantly longer survival (p < 0.029) and progression free survival (p < 0.018) in com
parison to CEF patients.

Patients treated with DES-CEF experienced a significantly higher
bone marrow toxicity and 43.3% of DES-CEF cycles had to be delayed
because of leukopenia in comparison to 11.8% of CEF cycles (p <
0.0001).

C. CEF vs DES-CEF (II)
    Toxicity data are so far available for 40/59 randomized patients
Again, and now rather unexpectedly, the DES-CEF (II) regimen
is more myelotoxic than CEF (even if less than DES-CEF(I)): 27.5%
of DES-CEF (II) cycles have to be delayed because of leukopenia in
comparison to 10.9% of CEF cycles (p < 0.005).

DISCUSSION

Nowadays clinicians are more likely to attribute chemotherapeutic
failures to reasons which depend upon tumor biology rather than
recognize that a more rational utilization of available drugs could
improve treatment results. As a matter of fact so far treatment
strategies aimed to overcome chemoresistance due to genetic hetero
geneity have failed in human breast cancer (18). Undoubtedly soma-

tic mutation towards resistance is the ultimate cause of treatment failure, nevertheless the efforts that a few authors have per
formed in order to circumvent other, non genetic, causes of treatment failure cannot be neglected. Because of the possibility to
manipulate tumor growth by hormones, human breast cancer represents an attractive field to test the value of cytokinetic directed regimens. A few trials have been published which, while non
conclusive, suggest that tumor cell killing can be increased if
chemotherapy is administered at the time of estrogen induced kinetic recruitment (2,7,19,20,21). Our results in LABC demonstrate
that cancer cells can be recruited into the proliferative pool
by DES and that chemotherapy administered at the time of estrogenic recruitment, promptly stops the induced tumor cell proliferation. DES is able to recruit breast cancer cells irrespectively
of their ER status; while surprising these results are not completely new and other authors have outlined that estrogen receptors
do not seem to be a prerequisite to obtain an estrogenic stimulation (7,8,14). Clinical results so far achieved with DES-FAC are
promising: 71.8% of patients with locally advanced inoperable
breast cancer have obtained a major response after 3 courses and
92.3% of patients have been rendered disease free after surgery.

It is important to note that after 3 DES-FAC courses, whenever
feasible, patients have been submitted to radical mastectomy; it
is therefore likely that response rates could have been improved
with more prolonged presurgical chemotherapy. Actuarial 30 mos sur
vival and progression free survival (PFS) are 65% and 50% respectively: the advantage in PFS is significant in comparison to our
historic controls (16). Overall results from our first randomized
trial in metastatic breast cancer are not conclusive: the DES-CEF
regimen induces a higher CR rate and a slight prolongation in
survival and PFS in comparison to conventional CEF, but these dif
ferences are not significant; moreover the objective response rates (CR + PR) are identical in the two arms.

On the other hand the DES-CEF regimen induces a significantly
higher CR rate in patient with dominant soft tissue metastasis and
in patients with ER negative tumors. These results seem to indica
te that estrogenic recruitment can increase tumor cell killing by
chemotherapy in the case of chemosensitive tumors (thus transforming partial responders into complete responders) while genetically chemoresistant tumors do not show a change in response pattern
despite the more favourable kinetic situation. If this is the case
than DES-CEF should be advantageous for patients whose tumors have not been exposed to the selection pressure of chemotherapy.
In other words, if we analyze response rate, survival and PFS in

patients never treated with chemotherapy and in patients pretreated with adjuvant chemotherapy it should be reasonable to see that tumors in relapse after adjuvant chemotherapy do not modify their chemosensitivity because of estrogenic recruitment (these tumors in fact are composed by predominant genetically chemoresistant clones) while cytokinetic chemotherapy could be more effective in never treated tumors (where chemosensitive clones are still present and, hopefully, predominant).

As a matter of fact our experimental results are not so "reasonable": DES-CEF induces more CRs and a significantly prolonged survival (p < 0.029) and PFS (p < 0.018) in patients previously treated with adjuvant chemotherapy. These results are difficult to interpret but surely they cannot be explained on the basis of the predominant somatic mutation theory which postulates that failure of chemotherapy is due to the selection and emergence of pre-exsisting genetically chemoresistant clones. Better results with DES-CEF were obtained despite a higher bone marrow toxicity (44.3% of DES-CEF cycles delayed vs 11.8% of CEF cycles, p < 0.0001);this toxicity was attributed to the scheduling of antiblastic drugs: cyclophosphamide in fact was administered on day 1 while 5-FU and Epidoxorubicin were administered on day 8. This scheduling was chosen with the hope to recruit cancer cells with alkylators as demonstrated in multiple myeloma and ovarian cancer (6,22).

Surprisingly the preliminary toxicity data from the new ongoing randomized trial (CEF vs DES-CEF II) suggest that DES itself induces a more pronounced bone marrow chemosensitivity; while negative this finding further supports the view that manipulation of tissue growth can result in a larger cell killing with chemotherapy.

REFERENCES

1. Aitken, S.L., Lippman, M.E. (1982): Cancer Res., 42: 1727-1735.
2. Allegra, J.C. (1983): Sem. Oncol., 10: 23-28.
3. Bonadonna, G., Valagussa, P. (1983): Int. J. Rad. Oncol. Biol. Phys., 9: 279-297.
4. Buzdar, A.U., Legha, S.S., Hortobagyi, G.N., Yap, H.Y., Wiseman C.L., Di Stefano, A., Schell, F.C., Barnes, B.C., Campos,L.T., Blumenschein, G.R. (1981): Cancer, 47: 2798-2802.
5. Carbone, P.P., Tormey, D.C. (1977): In: Breast Cancer Advances in Research and Treatments; Edited by W.L. Mc Guire, pp 165-215 Plenum Press, New York.
6. Conte, P.F., Alama, A., Favoni, R., Trave, F., Rosso, R., Nico-

lin, A. (1984): Europ. J. Cancer Clin. Oncol., 20: 1039-1043.

7. Conte, P.F., Fraschini, G., Alama, A., Nicolin, A., Corsaro,E., Canavese,G., Rosso, R., Drewinko, B. (1985): Cancer Res., 45: 5926-5930.

8. Dao, T.L., Sinha, D.K., Nemoto, T., Patel, J. (1982): Cancer Res., 42: 359-362.

9. Decker, D.A., Ahmann, D.L., Bisel, H.F., Edmonson, H.L., Hahn, R.G., O'Fallon, J.R. (1979): JAMA, 242: 2075-2079.

10. Drewinko, B., Patchen, M., Yang, L.Y., Barlogie, B. (1981): Cancer Res., 41: 2328-2333.

11. Fisher, R.I., De Vita, V.T., Hybband, S.P., Simon, R., Young, R.C. (1979): Ann. Int. Med., 90: 761-763.

12. Goldie, J.H. (1983): Breast Cancer Res. Treat., 3: 129-136.

13. Griffits, C.T. (1975): Natl. Cancer Inst. Monogr., 42: 101-104.

14. Hug, V., Drewinko, B., Hortobagyi, G.M., Blumenschein, G.(1985): Breast Cancer Res. Treat., 6: 237-240.

15. Legha, S.S., Buzdar, A.V., Smith, T.L., Hortobagyi, G.M., Swenerton, K.D., Blumenshein, G.R., Gehan, E.A., Bidey, G.P., Freireich, E.J. (1979): Ann. Int. Med., 91: 847-852.

16. Lionetto, R., Pronzato, P., Conte, P.F., Amoroso, P., Badellino F., Bertelli, G., Canavese, G., Rosso, R. (1986): Submitted.

17. Lippman, M.E., Bolan, G., Huff, K. (1976): Cancer Res., 36: 4595-4601.

18. Lippman, M.E. (1984): Breast Cancer Res. Treat., 4: 69-77.

19. Lippman, M.E., Cassidy, J., Wesley, M., Young, R.C. (1984): J. Clin. Oncol., 2: 28-36.

20. Lippman, M.E., Sorace, R., Bagley, C., Lichter, A., Danforth, D., Wesley, M., Young, R. (1985): Proc. ASCO, 4: 65.

21. Paridaens, R., Blonk Van Der Wijst, J., Julien, J.P. (1984): Prof. ASCO, 3: 130 (abst 508).

22. Pileri, A., Conte, P.F., Hulin, M. (1976): Blood, 46: 1056-1057

23. Skipper, H.E. (1971): Prediction of Response to Chemotherapy. National Cancer Inst. Monograph. n 34.

24. Weichselbaum, R.R., Hellman, S., Piro, A.J., Nove, J.J., Little B. (1978): Cancer Res., 38: 2339-2342.

ACKNOWLEDGMENT

Supported by a Grant of the Italian National Research Council, Special Project Oncology, Contract n 85.02108.44

*Hormonal Manipulation of Cancer: Peptides,
Growth Factors, and New (Anti) Steroidal
Agents,* edited by Jan G. M. Klijn et al.
Raven Press, New York © 1987.

A PHASE II TRIAL OF TAMOXIFEN, PREMARIN
METHOTREXATE AND 5-FLUOROURACIL IN METASTATIC
BREAST CANCER. J. Allegra, T. Woodcock, J. Seeger,
D. Stevens, University of Louisville School of
Medicine, Louisville, Kentucky, U.S.A.

Breast cancer is a common disease, with approximately one
in 11-12 American women developing breast cancer. Our current
lack of success in treating breast cancer is demonstrated by the
more than 35,000 deaths attributed to this disease each year in
the United States alone.

For almost 100 years, breast tumors have been known to be
responsive to hormonal manipulation. However, in unselected
groups of patients, only 30% of women can be expected to respond
to hormonal therapy (1,2). This means that for the majority of
women, hormonal therapy alone is not adequate. Over the past
ten years, the ability to measure estrogen receptor protein has
allowed for the selection of patients with significant quantities
of this protein to receive hormonal therapy. In this select
group of women, the response rate increases to 50-60%. Perhaps
most important is the fact that tumors without a significant
amount of estrogen receptor protein have less than a 10%
objective response rate (3,5). Therefore, while the assay for
estrogen receptor has increased our ability to predict for
response to therapy by the selection of patients likely to
respond, it is not as accurate as one would like as demonstrated
by the 40% of receptor positive tumors that do not respond to
hormonal therapy. Unfortunately, the receptor is only one step
within the steroid hormone action cascade, and although
necessary for hormonal action, it is not sufficient.

Another large problem with the treatment of metastatic
breast cancer is that the response to therapy is seldom a
complete response; that is, whether one uses hormonal therapy
or even cytotoxic chemotherapy, the tumors can be made to
decrease in size but not totally disappear. This failure to
achieve a complete remission is important in any solid tumor
and, specifically, in metastatic breast cancer. Until a
significant number of patients can be made to achieve a complete
remission, cure is not a reasonable objective.

One reason for the failure to attain complete remissions in
metastatic breast cancer may lie in the concept of tumor
heterogeneity. Breast tumors have been shown to be heterogeneous for a number of characteristics, including steroid hormone
receptors. It is known that while an estrogen receptor positive
tumor contains a preponderance of cells with estrogen receptor,
it also contains some cells which do not have receptors. Likewise, estrogen receptor negative tumors contain a preponderance
of cells without receptor, but also a small fraction of cells
that do synthesize receptor proteins. This receptor heteroge-

neity may, in part, explain the failure of some estrogen
receptor positive tumors to respond to hormonal therapy and may
also explain the lack of complete remissions in metastatic breast
cancer.

The problem then becomes how to attack these divergent
subpopulations of tumor cells. One approach has been to combine
hormonal therapy which is known to be effective against hormone-
dependent cells and cytotoxic chemotherapy which is known to be
effective against rapidly dividing or hormone-independent cells.
Several regimens have been published which involve the continuous use of hormonal therapy, combined with the intermittent use
of chemotherapy. While these regimens provide slightly higher
overall response rates than either therapy alone, the rate of
complete remissions is not significantly changed, nor has
response duration or survival been altered. The clinical
implications of receptor heterogeneity and the results of
several combination chemo-hormonal regimens have recently been
reviewed (6).

The question then arises how one can achieve a higher
complete remission rate. One theory is that if a tumor is
subjected to some type of undefined growth factor prior to
exposure to the cytotoxic drugs, that a higher fraction of cells
will be killed. This undefined growth factor could potentially
make more cells susceptible to cytotoxic drugs.

Observations of breast cancer cells in tissue culture have
proven that tumor cell growth can be manipulated. Lippman et
al. (7) have shown that the anti-estrogen, tamoxifen, can
decrease the thymidine incorporation in tissue cultures of
hormone-dependent human breast cancer cells. These data show
that tamoxifen is able to arrest tumor cells in a uniform stage
of the cell cycle. Thymidine incorporation in these same cells
increases when exposed to physiological concentrations of
estrogen, and estrogen is capable of rescuing cells from the
growth inhibition effect of tamoxifen.

This chapter describes the results of a chemo-hormonal
regimen for metastatic breast cancer, based on the observations
above. Specifically, hormonal therapy is used initially to
arrest the growth of hormone-dependent cells. Then a second
hormonal therapy is used to stimulate those cells. This is
followed by cell cycle specific cytotoxic chemotherapy aimed at
the potentially increased fraction of rapidly dividing cells.
It is our hypothesis that utilizing hormones and chemotherapy in
this manner could result in a better response than either
therapy alone.

MATERIALS AND METHODS
Patients

Fifty-seven patients with histologically documented,
measurable adenocarcinoma of the breast referred to the Division
of Medical Oncology at the University of Louisville between
July, 1980 and July, 1984 were entered into this clinical trial.

Eligibility criteria for entry into this study included histologically confirmed metastatic breast cancer, measurable
disease, serum creatinine less than 1.5 mg/dl, and/or a
creatinine clearance greater than 60 mlm, an ECOG performance
status of 2 or better and an expected survival of greater than
2 months. All patients were treated without regard to their
estrogen receptor status. Patients were ineligible if they
received prior tamoxifen therapy. However, all forms of prior
chemotherapy and other forms of hormonal therapy did not make
the patient ineligible for this clinical trial, provided they
were off this therapy for 4 weeks prior to entering the study
and had fully recovered from the toxic effects of prior therapy.
Prior radiation therapy was also acceptable, provided nontreated
lesions existed for measurement. The protocol contained no age
or menopausal restrictions. All patients entered into this
trial are evaluable for response and toxicity.
    The patient characteristics are illustrated in Table I.
Their median age was 56 years, with a range of 30-80 years.
Forty-three patients were postmenopausal and 14 were premenopausal. Their median ECOG performance status was 1, with a
range of 0-2. Twenty-one patients had received no prior therapy.
Fifteen received adjuvant radiation, 11 adjuvant chemotherapy
and 1 adjuvant hormonal therapy. Ten patients had metastatic
disease irradiation, while one patient received hormonal therapy
and two patients chemotherapy for a prior recurrence.

Table I
_____

Characteristics of the Patients
_____

Number of patients	57
Median age	56 year (30-80)
Menopausal status	43 Postmenopausal
	14 Premenopausal
Median ECOG status	1 (0-2)
Disease-free interval	18 mo (0-16 yr)
Estrogen receptor status	
ER positive	30 (53%)
ER negative	20 (35%)
ER unknown	7 (12%)
Dominant site of disease	
Visceral	25%
Soft tissue	50%
Bone	25%

_____

    Thirty of the patients, or 53%, had tumors which were
estrogen receptor positive, 20 were estrogen receptor negative
and 7 had tumors of unknown estrogen receptor status. All of

the steroid hormone receptor assays were performed using a
sucrose density gradient technique or a multipoint titration
assay with dextran coated charcoal (8,9). Steroid hormone
receptor status was determined by a biopsy of metastatic tissue
prior to therapy in the majority of cases. The cutoff value for
positivity was chosen at 10 femtomoles per milligram of cytoplasmic protein.

Treatment Regimen

    Patients with metastatic breast cancer were administered
tamoxifen in a dose of 10mg orally twice a day for 10 days. The
tamoxifen was then discontinued and the patients received
premarin, a conjugated estrogen, in a dose of 0.625mg orally
twice each day for 4 days. On the fourth day of premarin
therapy, the patients received methotrexate, 200mg/m^2 intravenously, followed in 1 hour by 5-fluorouracil, 600mg/m^2
intravenously. Twenty-four hours later, the patients were
rescued with leucovorin, orally, at 10mg/m^2 every 6 hours for
6 doses. The treatment cycle repeated every 18 days. The
methotrexate dose and the 5-fluorouracil dose were altered
according to the white blood cell count and platelet count at
the time of therapy. There were no alterations in the tamoxifen
or the premarin dose. Full doses of the methotrexate and
5-fluorouracil were given if the white blood cell count was
greater than 4,000 per cubic milliliter and if the platelet
count was greater than 100,000 per cubic millileter. If the
platelet count was between 75,000 per cubic milliliter and
100,000 per cubic millimeter and the white cell count was
between 2,500 per cubic milliliter and 4,000 per cubic millimeter, 50% of the standard 5-FU and methotrexate dose was
administered. No drug was administered if the platelet count
was less than 75,000 per cubic millimeter or the white blood
cell count was less than 2,500 per cubic millimeter. In this
instance, the patients continued premarin until the white blood
cell count and platelet count increased to acceptable levels.

    In all cases, assessment of response was performed using
standardized response criteria (10). In brief, a complete
remission was defined as the clinical disappearance of all
detectable disease. This included healing of all bone lesions
and a return of the patient to premorbid performance status. A
partial remission was defined as a 50% decrease in the product
of perpendicular diameters of all measurable disease and no
evidence of new lesions. Duration of remission was calculated
from the beginning of therapy, and survival was calculated from
initiation of therapy until death.

RESULTS

    Fifty-seven patients have been entered into this Phase II
clinical trial. All are evaluable for response, survival and
toxicity.

    Thirty-eight of the patients (67%) had one site of meta-
static disease, 15 patients (26%) had two sites involved with

metastatic tumor, and only 4 patients had 3 or more sites of metastases. Approximately 25% of patients had either bone or visceral dominant disease, while 50% had soft tissue dominant disease.

Overall response rate is 62%, with 37% complete remissions, 25% partial remissions. Stable disease was achieved in 21 of the patients, and only 17% exhibited immediate progression of disease on this regimen. There were no significant differences in responses of function of estrogen receptor status (ER positive 70%, ER unknown 71%, ER negative 45%), menopausal status (pre 65%, post 50%), dominant site of disease (bone 50%, soft tissue 66%, visceral 64%) or prior therapy (none 71%, prior radiation therapy 59%, prior chemotherapy 50%, prior hormonal therapy 50%).

The median duration of remission was 14 months. If one analyzes the overall time to relapse for all patients, the median is 9 months. The median survival for the overall group was 24 months. The median survival for the responders was 28 months, and 16 months for the nonresponders. This two-fold increase in median survival was significant ($P<0.01$). Multiple subset analyses were also performed. Overall, there was no significant difference in survival between patients achieving complete remission, partial remission, or stable disease. Patients with estrogen receptor positive tumors, estrogen receptor negative tumors, and estrogen unknown tumors had similar survivals. There was no difference in survival between patients with soft tissue or visceral dominant disease, or between pre or postmenopausal patients.

Both hematologic and non-hematologic toxicities with this regimen were very tolerable. Over 750 cycles of therapy have been administered, with grade I leukopenia occurring in only 16% of the patients. Seventeen percent of the courses were associated with grade II toxicity, and 3% with grade III. No patient had a white blood cell count of less than 1,000. Only 2% of the cycles were associated with grade I thrombocytopenia and 5% with grade II. No patient ever had a platelet count of less than 50,000. With respect to non-hematologic toxicity, 42% of the cycles of therapy were associated with no toxicity whatsoever. Twelve percent of the cycles had mild nausea and 30% had vomiting easily controlled with antiemetic therapy. Only 5% of the cycles were ever associated with stomatitis.

DISCUSSION

An attempt to synchronize and stimulate tumor cell growth in order to potentially render cells more sensitive to cell cycle specific cytotoxic chemotherapy, is a concept which was clearly worthy of testing, especially in a solid tumor such as breast cancer. At the present time, almost all remissions in breast cancer are partial remissions, and this is true using either hormonal therapy or chemotherapy. Cure of metastatic breast cancer is not realistic and will not be until clinicians are able to attain complete disappearance of all measurable tumors, not just partial remissions. Standard combination chemo-hormonal therapy has not increased the curability of metastatic breast cancer, despite the appeal of attacking hormone-dependent and hormone-independent cells simultaneously.

This clinical trial was based on reproducible laboratory observations indicating that synchronization and stimulation of tumor cells is indeed possible, and also based on an elegant randomized study in patients which showed for the first time that this concept could lead to patient benefit (11). In the NCI Medicine Branch trial, patients were randomized between cytoxan, methotrexate, 5-fluorouracil and adriamycin, with or without tamoxifen and premarin, and the group receiving the anti-hormone combination had a significant longer median duration of remission. Although complete remission rates in this trial do not approach our 37% complete remission rate, the overall treatment regimens were very different, and our patient population was more favorable. In a subsequent clinical trial performed by this group in patients with locally advanced Stage III or inflammatory breast cancer, a very high complete remission rate was achieved in patients receiving the chemotherapy with anti-estrogen - estrogen synchronization - stimulation (12).

The EORTC (13) has also attempted to test this synchronization stimulation concept, using aminoglutethimide, ethinylestradiol, followed by 5-fluorouracil, adriamycin and cytoxan chemotherapy. The overall response in 41 patients was 74%, with 37% of patients achieving a complete remission. Median duration of remission and survival were not recorded, nor was estrogen receptor status of the majority of tumors, although the authors believed that the majority of patients had hormone-independent tumors since 50% of the patients had visceral dominant disease. As in our clinical trial, they found no difference in response rates as a function of dominant metastatic site, menopausal status, or estrogen receptor status.

Clearly, with multiple groups reporting promising and similar results, further large scale trials to further test these concepts and this approach to the problem of metastatic breast cancer is warranted.

REFERENCES

1. Kardinal, C.G., and Donegan, W.L. (1979). In "Cancer of the Breast" (W.L. Donegan and J.S. Spratt, eds), 2nd ed., pp. 361-404, Saunders, Philadelphia, Pennsylvania.

2. Kennedy, B.J. (1974). Semin. Oncol. 1, 119-236.

3. Legha, S.S., Davis, H.L. and Muggia, F.M. (1978). Ann Intern. Med. 88, 69-77.

4. McGuire, W.L. (1975). Cancer (Philadelphia) 36, 638-644.

5. McGuire, W.L., Horwitz, K.B., Peason, O.H., et al. (1977). Cancer 39, 2934-2947.

6. Osborne, C.K. (1985). Semin. Oncol. 12, 317-326.

7. Lippman, M., Bolan, G. and Huff, A.A. (1976). Cancer. Res. 36:4595-4691.

8. Wittliff, J.L. (1975). Methods in Cancer Res. 294-354.

9. Wittliff, J.L. and Sanlov, E.E. (1975). Estrogen Receptors in Human Breast Cancer (W.L. McGuire, P.P. Carbone and E.P. Vollmer, eds.), 73-91.

10. Breast Cancer Task Force Treatment Committee, National Cancer Institute. (1977). 11-13.

11. Sorace, R., Lippman, M., Bagley, C. et al. (1984). Proc. ASCO, Abst. #462.

12. Lippman, M.E., Cassidy, J., Eesley, M. et al. (1984). J. Clin. Onc. 28-36.

13. Aminoglutethimide and Estrogenic Recruitment for the Chemotherapy of Breast Cancer. (1983). Proc. of 13th Internal Congress of Chemotherapy. (R.J. Santen, ed.) Part 218.

Hormonal Manipulation of Cancer: Peptides, Growth Factors, and New (Anti) Steroidal Agents, edited by Jan G. M. Klijn et al. Raven Press, New York © 1987.

NEOADJUVANT CHEMOTHERAPY IN THE COMBINED MODALITY APPROACH OF LOCALLY ADVANCED NONMETASTATIC BREAST CANCER

M.E. Lippman*#, S. Swain*, C.S. Bagley*, Richard A. Sorace**, Allen S. Lichter**, David N, Danforth, Jr.***

*Medicine,** Radiation Oncology and ***Surgery Branch, National Cancer Institute, Building 10, Room 12N226 Bethesda, MD 20205.

Abstract

We treated sixty-six consecutive patients with locally advanced breast cancer, with primary induction chemotherapy including attempted hormonal synchronization, to a maximum objective clinical response before proceeding to local therapy. Patients achieving a pathologic complete response received radiation therapy while patients with residual disease received debulking surgery prior to radiation therapy; at least 6 additional months of chemotherapy were administered in all patients. Doses were escalated to targeted myelosuppression. Objective response rate to chemotherapy was 93% with 53% CR, 40% PR and 7% NC. Three patients who have already achieved a PR are still on chemotherapy with continued tumor regression. Of thirty-one patients achieving a CR to chemotherapy, twenty-nine were assessed by multiple biopsies or mastectomy. Nineteen patients (61%) were proven to be pathologic complete responders. Fortyseven patients have completed combined therapy and all have been rendered disease free (8 patients are still receiving radiation therapy and 11 patients are still on induction chemotherapy). Sixteen patients have relapsed, 5 with stage III A, 10 with stage III B and 1 with stage IV. Median survival is 33.7 months for stage III B and has not been reached for stage III A. This aggressive primary chemotherapy regimen with hormone synchronization followed by local therapy appears to provide excellent local control and encouraging early information on systemic disease control.

Introduction

Locally advanced breast cancer is difficult to control regionally and generally associated with dismal long term survival. Haagensen and Stout described the clinical features that characterize this subset of breast cancer patients;they reported that radical mastectomy failed to cure even a single patient in their series of 120 such case followed for up to 8 years (1, 2). They regarded these lesions as "categorically inoperable" and suggested that they be treated by other measures. Improved radiotherapy techniques allowed the delivery of higher doses of radiation to these patient's tumors without unacceptable local

complications, and in so doing provided increased chances of
achieving local control (3). Radiotherapy alone produces 5
year local tumor control in 28 to 74% of patients with 5 year
survival in the 12 to 38% range (4-13). The addition of surgery
to radiation has is associated 5 year survivals to 35 to 55% in
some selected series (5,14,6,7,8,10,13). However, the majority
of these patients succumbed to metastatic disease, suggesting
that disseminated micrometastases exist at the time of presentation in virtually all patients.

Retrospective data form the Harvard-Joint Center for
Radiation Therapy (7) revealed a significantly better relapse
free survival and improved local control at 4 years for patients receiving adjuvant chemotherapy with or without ablative
endocrine therapy (51% and 85% respectively) as compared to a
matched group of patients not receiving adjuvant therapy (29%
and 63% respectively). In a randomized study of patients with
operable stage III breast cancer (T_3,N_{0-2}) Grohn et al (15)
showed improved 5 year survival (57% to 73%) and freedom from
distant relapse (50% to 87.5%) when patients received 6 cycles
of cytoxan, deoxorubicin and vincristine (CAV) adjuvant chemotherapy after a modified radical mastectomy compared to those
patients who received only post-operative radiation therapy. In
Milan (16) 110 patients,were treated with preoperative chemotherapy. A 70% objective response rate was achieved with 4
cycles of doxorubicin-vincristine (AV) and an overall 3 year
survival of 53% compared to 41% for a historical control group
receiving radiation alone. Their subsequent studies comparing
surgery versus radiation after primary chemotherapy were equivalent with respect to local control, patterns of recurrence,
and overall survival (17). A similar treatment strategy of 3
cycles of 5-fluorouracil, doxorubicin and cytoxan (FAC) plus
BCG administered prior to local therapy with either radiation
alone or surgery followed by radiation was employed in 52 non
inflammatory patients at the M.D. Anderson Hospital (18). An
objective response rate to chemotherapy of 82% was achieved
with 40% actuarial 5 year survival. Hence, giving induction
chemotherapy for a fixed number of cycles prior to local therapy resulted in considerable tumor regression that enhanced
the ability to either perform a surgical resection or deliver
a tumoricidal dose of radiation in both of these institutional
experiences. The value of initial induction chemotherapy upon
the development of distant metastases is suggested by the retrospective review of Balawajder et al (5), where freedom from
distant relapse improved 2 fold when 3 cycles of cytoxan,
methotrexate and 5-fluorouracil (CMF) preceeded local therapy
with either radiation or radiation plus surgery.

We have treated woman with locally advanced breast cancer
with combination chemotherapy given to maximum objective clinical response, to reduce the tumor bulk prior to defintive

local therapy, and to destroy occult micrometastatic disease. Tamoxifen and premarin were given sequentially before the administration of cell specific agents to synchronize DNA synthesis in a proportion of these tumor cells and thus making them more susceptible to cytotoxic chemotherapy.

Materials and Methods

Sixty-four women with previously untreated locally advanced breast cancer were treated with combined modality therapy between January 1977 through February 1986). All patients were defined as stage III A or III B according to the 1983 American Joint Committee staging system. All patients were required to have a histologically documented diagnosis of mammary cancer with evidence of measurable disease. Inflammatory carcinoma was defined by the presence of dermal lymphatic invasion. All patients had a Karnofsky performance index in excess of 60 and no history of malignant neoplasms aside from curatively treated basal cell or squamous cell carcinoma of the skin or surgically cured carcinoma of the cervix in situ. Written informed consent was required before starting treatment. Two additional patients who met the above criteria, but who were found to have metastatic disease soon after starting induction chemotherapy, are included from analysis.

All patients had an initial complete history and physical examination blood cell count, urinalysis, chemistry profile, electrocardiagram, radionuclide scans of bone and liver, mammograms and radiographic examinations of the chest and skeleton. Mammograms were performed every six weeks to 3 months if lesions were present and annually when no lesion remained. Liver spleen scans and bone scans were performed every twelve weeks.

Chemotherapy Regimens

The initial 13 patients were treated as part of a large randomized protocol designed to prospectively compare two intermittent chemotherapy regimens as primary induction therapy in advanced breast cancer (19). These regimens are shown in Table 1 and termed 160B. This protocol was closed as a randomized trial in June 1983, but continued to accure subsequent patient with locally advanced breast cancer to the arm which included hormonal synchronization, with the dose adjustments shown in Table 1 and termed 160C. These dose adjustments were made in an effort to reduce bone marrow suppression and to reduce delays in treatment.

Patients were treated with induction therapy to maximum objective clinical response (20). Detailed response criteria used in these studies have been published elsewhere (21). Maximum objective clinical response was formally scored when response parameters remained stable during two consecutive determination separated by six weeks. The time to best response was taken to be the point at which the maximum objective clinical response was first observed. Dose modification for individual treatment cycles have been previously described (20).

Table 1. Treatment Regimens

160B (first 13 patients were randomly assigned)*

C	Cyclophosphamide	750 mg/m^2 iv d 1
A	Doxorubicin	30 mg/m^2 iv d 1
M	Methotrexate	40 mg/m^2 iv d 8
F	5-fluorouracil	500 mg/m^2 iv d 8

vs

C

A	T	Tamoxifen	10 mg/m^2 po d 2-6
+			
M	P	Premarin	0.652 mg/m^2 po Q12H x 3 day 7

F

160C (subsequent 53 patients received)

C	Cyclophosphamide	500 mg/m^2 i.v. day 1
A	Doxorubicin	30 mg/m^2 i.v. day 1
M	Methotrexate	300 mg/m^2 i.v. day 8
F	5-fluorouracil	500 mg/m^2 i.v. day 8
T	Tamoxifen	40 mg/m^2 p.o. days 2-6
P	Premarin	0.625 mg/m^2 p.o. Q12H x 3 day 7
L	Leucovorin	10 mg/m^2 p.o. Q6H x 6 day 9

---

*One patient received CAMF without being randomized.

Local Therapy

At the point of maximumal objective _clinical_ response to chemotherapy, patients were evaluated for local therapy. Clinical complete responders (CR) had multiple biopsies performed at the site of the original lesion in an attempt to document a pathologic complete response. Early in this study two patients received a mastectomy instead of biopsy. A 3 to 4 cm wedge biopsy was taken at the site of the original lesion with multiple biopsies taken of any surrounding suspicious areas seen at the time of the procedure. Skin was also biospied. If a pathologic

complete response was documented, patients received radical radiotherapy to the intact breast or chest wall (for the 2 mastectomy patients) and adjacent draining lymph node areas. For
patients with residual disease in their biopsy or patients
achieving only partial or no change responses, a debulking mastectomy was performed, with removal of any gross axillary disease. This was followed by radical radiotherapy. For patients
on 160B, 6 received one year of chemotherapy and 7 received six
months of chemotherapy after local therapy was completed. Complete responders to induction therapy received alternating cycles with doxourubicin. All 160C patients received six months of
chemotherapy after local therapy was completed with doxorubicin
included in every cycle. A dose of 525 mg/m^2 of doxorubicin
was not exceeded.

Pathologic complete responders received radiation to the intact breast and internal mammary nodes with opposed tangential
fields to a dose of 5000 cGy at a prescribed isodose line. The
adjacent supraclavicular nodes and axillary nodes received 5000
cGy from a single AP field at a depth of 3 cm. A posterior
axillary boost was used to bring the midplane axillary dose to
5000 cGy. The tumor bed and any sites of gross nodal disease
received a boosts of up to 1500 cGy using an AP electron beam
field. For patients undergoing debulking surgery prior to receiving radiation, the same radiation therapy technique was
used except that the chest wall and internal mammary nodes received 5000 cGy. The tumor bed and any sites of gross nodal
disease received a boost of up to 1500 cGy using an AP electron
beam field. For patients undergoing debulking surgery prior to
radiation, the same radiation therapy technique was used except
that the chest wall and internal mammary nodes received 5000
cGy total from opposed tangential fields with bolus applied
every other day. The axilla was irradiated in patient receiving a simple mastectomy. In some patients with inflammatory
breast cancer, the intact breast or chest wall received 6000
cGy with the adjacent draining modal areas receiving 5400 cGy.

Statistical Analysis

Objective standards for comparison of patient characteristics were performed using a Fisher's exact test. Survival and
time to progression distributions were estimated using the
Kaplan-Meier procedure(22).

Results

Sixty-six patients have been started on treatment and are
evaluabe for toxicity, time to progression and survival. Eight
patients are recent entrants and are too early for response
analysis. Prognostic variable information for stage III A and
IIIB patients are shown in Table 2.

Table 2. Prognostic Factors for Patients with Locally
Advanced Breast Cancer

Variable	Stage IIIA	Stage IIIB	Stage IV	All Patients
No. Pts.	31	33	2	66
Histology				
Inflammatory	0	27	0	27
Non-inflammatory	31	6	2	39
ER Status				
Positive	4	8	2	14
Negative	14	15	0	29
Unknown	13	10	0	23
Menopausal Status				
Premenopausal	14	9	0	23
Postmenopausal	17	24	2	43
Median	55	54	60	55

The overall objective response rate (CR + PR) was 93%. Thirty-one patients (53%) achieved a CR, 23 patients (40%) achieved a PR and 4 patients (7%) showed no change. Three of the patients scored as a PR remain on induction chemotherapy continued tumor regression and may achieve a complete response. Median number of chemotherapy cycles to achieve a CR, PR, or NC was 5, 3, and 4 with a range of cycles of 2 to 11, 2 to 9, and 4 to 6 respectively. No hospitalization were required as a result of toxicity. The median time for these patients to reach their best response to chemotherapy was 3 months or 4 cycles of therapy.

The distribution of various prognostic factors according to each chemotherapy response group are shown in table 3. In this relatively small sample there was no indication that estrogen receptor status, histology, nodal status, menopausal status or median age were predicive of a patient's best clinical response to induction chemotherapy. The influence of hormonal synchronization on best clinical response can only be evaluated in the 12 patients who received short course tamoxifen followed by premarin in a randomized manner on regimen 160B, since all patients on regimen 160C received hormones. By the Fisher's exact test, the addition of hormonal synchronization to cytotoxic chemotherapy was significant in achieving a CR as the best clinical response with p= 0.027.

Table 3. Prognostic Factors According to Best Chemotherapy Response

	Best	Clinical	Response
Variable	CR	PR	NC
Hormone Synchronization			
Tamoxifen + Premarin	30(5)*	19(2)	3
No Hormones	1(0)	4(4)	1(1)
Nodal Metastasis			
N_0	12	3	0
N_1	10	8	3
N_2	6	6	0
N_3	2	6	1
N_X	1	0	0
Histology			
Inflammatory	16	9	1
Noninflammatory	15	14	3
Estrogen Receptor Status			
ER Positive	7	6	1
ER Negative	13	11	3
ER Unknown	11	6	0
Menopausal Status			
Premenopausal	9	7	2
Postmenopausal	22	16	2
Median Age	55	57	46

Clinical CR status was evaluated histologically to detrmine if a pathologic CR had been attained (Table 4). Two initial clinical CR patients were evaluated with a simple mastectomy. Both of these patients had inflammatory histology. One of these patients apperared to have residual disease on gross cut section, however, only fat necrosis and fibrosis were present on microscopic analysis. No tumor was identified in any portion of the sectioned specimen. The other patient had areas of hard white gritty tissue on gross sectioning of her mastectomy specimen. These areas showed infiltrating ductal carcinoma on-microscopic analysis. No tumor was seen in the subcutaneous lymphatics. Twenty-seven patients underwent biopsy evaluation in the area of the breast previously known to be involved with tumor. Eighteen of these patients showed no evidence of residual tumor. Two biopsied patients showed residual microscopic disease only, with one of these patient's specimens showing just a few scattered tumor cells that apperared non-viable. Both of these patients proceeded to local therapy with radiation. The remaining seven biopsied patient had residual gross disease and underwent a simple mastectomy before proceeding to radiation therapy. Two patients went on to radiation therapy without histologic evaluation. This course was followed in one patient because her initial tumor was a T_2N_3 lesion that was excisionally biopsied before induction chemotherapy, hence she was felt not to have gross disease in her breast at the start of treatment. The other patient did not undergo biopsy secondary to the clinical judgement of the managing physicians. Thus, 29% of all patients recieving induction chemotherapy achieved a pathologic complete response.

Table 4.   Pathologic Evaluation of Patients Achieving
                A Clinical CR with Chemotherapy

Procedure	No. of Patients	No. of Patients Without Tumor in Specimen	No. of Patients With Tumor in Specimen	No Specimen
Mastectomy	2	1	1	0
Biopsy Only	27	18	9	0
No Biopsy	2	0	0	2
Total	31	19(61%)	10(32%)	2(7%)

Fifty-four patients have proceeded to the local therapy portion of the program (11 patients are still on chemotherapy and 1 patient left the institution). Forty-seven of these patients have completed all local therapy (8 patients are still receiving radiation therapy). All patients completing local therapy have been rendered disease free by this combined modality treatment approach. Fifteen patients have relapsed. No predictive value for eventual relapse thus far has been found for estrogen receptor status, menopausal status, age, addition of hormonal synchronization, number of cycles to best chemotherapy response. The most important predictor of relapse was the clinical TNM stage at the start of treatment. Of 15 relapsed patients, 5 were stage III A, 10 were stage IIIB and one was stage IV. Eight of the III B patients had inflammatory histolog. Patients with advanced nodal metastasis who relapsed tended to have inflammatory breast cancer. Median survival and time to progession for all patients in this series and for various subgroups are shown in Table 5. With a median follow-up of 19.8 months, the median survival for stage III B was 33.7 months and for stage III A has not been reached.

Table 5. Survival and Time to Progression

Group	No. of Patients	Median Survival (mo.)*	Median Time to Progression (mo.)*
All Patients	66	35.2	30.9
Stage III A	31	NR**	NR
Stage III B	33	33.7	27.6
Stage III B Noninflammatory	6	NR	−
Stage III B Inflammatory	27	33.4	−
Stage III A & IIIB, Noninflammatory	37	NR	−

* Median follow-up is 19.8 mo. (range 1 to 55 mo.).
** Not reached.

Discussion

We treated locally advanced breast cancer with chemotherapy for as many cycles as necessary for maximal response. This approach was used to achieve the maximum cytoreductive benefit of chemotherapy before proceeding to local therapy and to institute early systemic prophylaxis. Subsequent local therapy was guided by the patient's response to induction chemotherapy. We felt that patients achieving a pathologic CR were candidates for consolidative local therapy with definitive ra-

diation. Patients with residual gross disease received debulking surgery in an attempt to further reduce their tumor burdens
to minimal levels, ideally striving to achieve only microscopic residual disease, and then proceeded with local radiotherapy.

Patients achieving a clinical CR to chemotherapy underwent
biopsy evaluation in the area of the breast previously known to
be involved with tumor. The overall pathologic complete response rate for this induction chemotherapy regimen was 29%. In
a report from M.D. Anderson Hospital (25) of 21 patients with
inflammatory breast cancer and 69 patients with locally advanced noninflammatory breast cancer were treated with 3 cycles of
FAC chemotherapy prior to mastectomy, 15 patients (17%) had no
evidence of gross disease but only 6 patients (7%) had no evidence of microscopic disease. While great effort was made to
utilize clinical and radiologic information in guiding each
biopsy in our series, this method may be suject to sampling
errors. Nevertheless, the multiple biopsy procedure has appeared useful in identifying clinical CR patients with little
or no residual tumor. These patients are likely to do well
with consolidative local therapy with radiation alone, thereby
avoiding the need for disfiguring surgery. Twenty-one of our
patients with locally advanced breast cancer have completed
combined modality therapy and have been rendered disease free
with a cosmetically intact breast. While cosmetic issues have
not been our primary concern in the treatment of locally advanced breast cancer, the possibility of being able to maintain an
intact breast after aggressive treatment may provide an important psychologic incentive in a population of patients, some of
whom initially delayed seeking medical attention.

Hormonal synchronization was integrated into the chemotherapy regimens in all but 6 patients in this series. The
rationale for this approach is based on prior studies from our
laboratory (26,27,28) which demonstrated that antiestrogen-
induced inhibition of breast cancer cell growth could be reversed by estrogen rescue. Weichselbaum et al (29) showed
that this technique could increase the sensitivity of breast
cancer cells to cytotoxic drug treatment. Using a flow cytometry technique, Green and coworkers demonstrated that tamoxifen induced a G_1 arrest in MCF-7 human breast cancer cells in
culture (30). Our laboratory has shown that subsequent estrogen treatment could induce a synchronous wave of DNA synthesis
in human breast cancer cells (31). Hence, this strategy was
used in the present study prior to the administration of the
cell cycle specific agents methotrexate and 5-fluorouracil, in
hope of synchronizing a portion of tumor cells and making them
more susceptible to these cytotoxic drugs. Allegra et al (32)
has treated a small group of breast cancer patients with antiestrogen therapy followed by estrogen rescue plus methotrexate

and 5-fluorouracil and has reported a complete remission rate
of 56%. In a randomized study from our institution (19) using
CAMF chemotherapy with or without hormonal synchronization in
patients with metastatic breast cancer, improvement in overall
survival and time to progression was observed in objective responders in the treatment arm including tamoxifen and premarin;
however, no improvement on response rate was noticed. When the
initial patients who were randomly assigned hormonal synchronization with chemotherapy on 160B were analysed with respect to
their best response to induction chemotherapy, a significant
difference was seen favoring the achievement of a complete response when tamoxifen and premarin were included in their treatment. Therefore, all of our subsequent patients received hormonal synchronization as an integral component of their induction therapy.

Combined modality therapy as used in this series has achieved local and systemic disease free status for all those patients who completed both induction chemotherapy and local
therapy. Although the median follow-up is still short, this
aggressive regimen appears to provide excellent local control
and encouraging early information on systemic disease control
for stages III A patients. While stage III B patients have derived benefit from this combined modality approach, they still
have a high rate of relapse and an overall shorter survival.
This is most apparent in those patients with inflammmatory
breast cancer, where 7 of 8 such relapsed patients presented
with distant metastasis as a component of their initial treatment failure. This is comparable to inflammatory breast cancer
patients treated with radiation alone (33) and attests to the
aggressive nature of this form of breast cancer, even when
treated with early chemotherapy. In an effort to improve systemic control, a randomized trial is underway in which inflammatory breast cancer patients rendered disease free by this
combined modality regimen are randomized to either high dose
melphalan plus autolgous bone marrow transplant followed by
maintenance chemotherapy or maintenance chemotherapy alone.

References

1. Haagensen, C.D. Diseases of the Breast, 2nd Ed. Phila-
    delphia, Pa. W.B. Saunders, 1971, p. 629.
2. Haagensen, C.D., Stout, A.P. Carcinoma of the breast. II.
    Criteria of operability. Ann Surg 118: 859-870 and 1032-
    1051, 1943.
3. Baclesse, F. Roentgen therapy alone as the method of
    treatment of cancer of the breast. Am J Roentgenol 62:
    311-319, 1949.
4. Amalric, R., Santamaria, F., Robert, F., Seigle, J.,
    Altschuler, C., Kurtz, J.M., Spitalier, J.M., Brandone,
    H., Ayme, Y., Pollet, J.F., Burnmeister, R., Abed, R.

Radiation therapy with or without primary limited surgery for operable breast cancer. Cancer 49:30-34, 1982.

5. Balawajder, I., Antich, P.P., Boland, J. An analysis of the role of radiotherapy alone in combination with chemotherapy and surgery in the management of advanced breast carcinoma. Cancer 51:574-580, 1983.

6. Bouchard, J. Advanced cancer of the breast treated primarily by irradiation. Radiology 84:823-842, 1965.

7. Bruckman, J.E., Harris, J.R., Levene, M.B., Chaffey, J.T., Hellman, S. Results of treating stage III carcinoma of the breast by primary radiation therapy. Cancer 43: 985-993, 1979.

8. Fletcher, G.H. Local results of irradiation in the primary management of localized breast cancer. Cancer 29:545-551, 1972.

9. Langlands, A.O., Kerr, G.R., Shaw, S. The management of locally advanced breast cancer by x-ray therapy. Clinical Oncology 2:365-371, 1976.

10. Pearlman, N.W., Guerra, O., Fracchia, A.A. Primary inoperable cancer of the breast. Surg Gynecol Obstet 143: 909-913, 1976.

11. Rubens, R.D., Armitage, P., Winter, P.J., Tong, D., Hayward, J.L. Prognosis in stage III carcinoma of the breast. Eur J Cancer 13:805-811, 1977.

12. Treurniet-Donker, A.D., Hop, W.C.J., Hoed-Sijtsema, S. Radiation treatment of stage III mammary carcinoma: A review of 129 patients. Int J Radiat Oncol Biol Phys 6:1477-1482, 1980.

13. Zucali, R., Uslenghi, C., Kenda, R., Bonadonna, G. Natural history of survival of inoperable breast cancer treated with radiotherapy and radiotherapy followed by radical mastectomy. Cancer 37:1422-1431, 1976.

14. Bedwinek, J., Rao, D.V., Perez, C., Lee, J., Finberg, B. Stage III and localized stage IV breast cancer: Irradiation alone versus irradiation plus surgery. Int J Radiat Oncol Biol Phys 8:31-36, 1982.

15. Grohn, P., Heinonen, E., Klefstrom, P., Tarkkanen, J. Adjuvant PostOperative Radiotherapy, Chemotherapy and Immunotherapy in Stage III Breast Cancer. Cancer 54:670674, 1984.

16. DeLena, M., Zucali, R., Viganotti, G., Valagussa, P., Bonadonna, G. Combined chemotherapy-radiotherapy approach in locally advanced (T_{3b}-T_4) breast cancer. Cancer Chemother Pharmacol 1:53-59, 1978.

17. DeLena, M., Varini, M., Zucali, R., Rovini, D., Viganotti, G., Valagussa, P., Veronesi, U., Bonadonna, G. Multimodality treatment for locally advanced breast cancer. Cancer Clin Trials 4:229-236, 1981.

18. Hortobagyi, G.N., Blumenschein, G.R., Spanos, W., Montague, E.D., Buzdar, A.U., Yap, H.Y., Schell, F. Multimodal treatment of locoregionally advanced breast cancer. Cancer 51: 763-768, 1983.

19. Lippman, M.E., Cassidy, J., Wesley, M., Young, R.C. A randomized attempt to increase the efficacy of cytotoxic chemotherapy in metastatic breast cancer by hormonal synchronization. J Clin Oncol 2:28-36, 1984.

20. Sorace, R.A., Bagley, C.S., Lichter, A.S., Danforth, D.N., Wesley, M.W., Young, R.C., Lippman, M.E. The management of nonmetastatic locally advanced breast cancer using primary induction chemotherapy with hormonal synchronization followed by radiation therapy with or without debulking surgery. World J. Surg. 9: 775-785, 1985.

21. Breast Cancer: Suggested Protocol Guidelines for Combination Chemotherapy Trials and for Combined Modality Trials. The Breast Cancer Task Force Treatment Committee NCI National Cancer Institute. Washington, D.C. Department of Health and Human Services publication no. 77-1192.

22. Kaplan, E.L., Meier, P. Nonparametric estimation from incomplete observations. J Am Statist Assoc 53:457-481, 1958.

23. Rubens, R.D., Sexton, R., Tong, D., Winter, P.J., Knight, R.K., Hayward, J.L. Combined chemotherapy and radiotherapy for locally advanced breast cancer. Eur J Cancer 16:351-356, 1980.

24. Barker, J.L., Montague, E.D., Peters, L.J. Clinical experience with irradiation of inflammatory carcinoma of the breast with and without elective chemotherapy. Cancer 45: 625-629, 1980.

25. Feldman, L., Hortobagyi, G., Buzdar, A., Blumenschein, G. Pathologic complete remission in patients with inflammatory breast cancer and locally advanced breast cancer. Proc Am Soc Clin Oncol 25:197, 1984 (Abstr).

26. Donehower, R., Allegra, J.C., Lippman, M.E., Chabner, B. Combined effects of methotrexate and 5-fluoropyrimidine on human breast cancer cells in serum-free culture. Eur J Cancer 16:655-661, 1980.

27. Lippman, M.E., Bolan, G., Huff, K. The effects of estrogens and antiestrogens on hormone-responsive human breast cancer in long-term tissue culture. Cancer Res 36:4595-4601, 1976.

28. Nawata, H., Chong, M., Bronzert, D., Lippman, M.E. Estradiol independent growth of a subline of MCF-7 human breast cancer cell line in culture. J Biol Chem 256:6895-6902, 1981.

29. Weichselbaum, R.R., Hellman, S., Piro, A.J., Nove, J.J., Little, J.B. Proliferation kinetics of a human breast cancer cell line in vitro following treatment with 17B-estradiol and 1-B-D arabinofuranosyleytosine. Cancer Res 38: 2339-2345, 1978.

30. Green, M.D., Whybourne, A.M., Taylor, I.W., Sutherland, R.L. Effects of antiestrogens on the growth and cell cycle kinetics of cultured human mammary carcinoma cells, in Sutherland RL, Jordon VC (eds): Non-Steroidal Antiestrogens. Sydney, Academic Press 1981, p 397-413.

31. Aitken, S.C., Lippman, M.E. Hormonal regulation of net DNA synthesis in MCF-7 human breast cancer cells in tissue culture. Cancer Res 42:1727-1735, 1982.
32. Allegra, J.C., Woodcock, T.M., Richman, S.P., Bland, K.I., Wittliff, J.F. A phase II trial of tamoxifen, breast cancer premarin, methotrexate and 5-fluorouracil in metastatic breast cancer. Breast Cancer Research and Treatment 2:93-100, 1982.
33. Chu, A.M., Wood, W.C., Doucette, J.A. Inflammatory breast carcinoma treated by radical radiotherapy. Cancer 45: 2730-2737, 1980.

Hormonal Manipulation of Cancer: Peptides,
Growth Factors, and New (Anti) Steroidal
Agents, edited by Jan G. M. Klijn et al.
Raven Press, New York © 1987.

ANDROGEN PRIMING AND RESPONSE TO CHEMOTHERAPY

IN ADVANCED PROSTATE CANCER

Andrea Manni, Richard J. Santen, Alice E. Boucher, Allan Lipton,
Harold Harvey, Mary Simmonds, Debbie White-Hershey, Robert A.
Gordon, Thomas J. Rohner, *Joseph Drago, John Wettlaufer,
and Leonard M. Glode

Departments of Medicine and Surgery, The Milton S. Hershey
Medical Center, The Pennsylvania State University, P.O. Box 850,
Hershey, PA 17033; University of Colorado Health Sciences
Center, Denver, CO 80262 and *Division of Urology, The Ohio
State University, Columbus, OH 43210

INTRODUCTION

Androgen priming has been suggested as a means to increase the
sensitivity of prostate cancer cells to the effect of cytotoxic
chemotherapy (3,8). This hypothesis is based on the fact that
androgens are potent mitogens and that cytotoxic drugs may be
most effective against rapidly proliferating cells (9). We are
conducting a prospective, controlled, clinical trial in orchiectomized patients with stage D_2 prostate cancer to rigorously
test whether androgen priming potentiates the efficacy of cytotoxic chemotherapy (5). The present report provides a brief
summary of an updated analysis after a median follow-up of two
years.

MATERIALS AND METHODS

Sixty-seven patients have been entered: 33 into the control
arm and 34 into the stimulation arm. The two groups were comparable with respect to several prognostic criteria (Table 1).
Median duration of follow-up is 24 months (range, 4-47 months).
At the time of entry into the study all patients had evidence of
progressive and evaluable disease following orchiectomy. After
two patients developed spinal cord compression following androgen
administration, we initiated the routine use of pretreatment mye-
lograms in patients randomized to the stimulation arm who have
evidence of spinal metastasis on bone scan. Patients with early
spinal cord compression are excluded from the stimulation arm.
All patients receive: (a) the combination of aminoglutethimide

TABLE 1. Patient characteristics.

	Control	Stimulation
•Patient number	33	34
•Mean age, years	68	67
(range)	(52-81)	(50-82)
•Karnowski status	63.4±3.5	58.4±2.9
(mean±SEM)		
•Baseline Hct	36.8±0.9	36.7±1.0
(mean±SEM)		
•Time from castration, months	23.5±4.3	24.3±3.3
(mean±SEM)		
•Sites of metastasis		
Bone	23	22
Bone + lymph nodes	5	4
Bone + viscera	5	5
Lymph nodes	0	2
Viscera	0	1
•Elevated acid phosphatase	28	33
•Previous systemic therapy		
Orchiectomy	33	34
Estrogens	16	16
Chemotherapy	1	0

(1 gm a day) and hydrocortisone (40 mg a day) to lower adrenal androgen secretion and (b) intravenous cyclic chemotherapy every three weeks consisting initially of cytoxan (500 mg/M^2), 5-fluorouracil (500 mg/M^2), and adriamycin (50 mg/M^2). After a maximum of 400 mg/M^2 of adriamycin the chemotherapy is changed to monthly cycles of methotrexate 200 mg/M^2 followed 1 hr later by 5-fluorouracil (600 mg/M^2) and 24 hr later by citrovorum factor rescue (10 mg/M^2) four times a day for a total of . 6 doses). Patients randomized to the stimulation arm receive, in addition, the synthetic androgen fluoxymesterone (5 mg orally twice a day) for 3 days before and on the day of chemotherapy administration. Treatment is continued until there is evidence of progressive disease.

All patients were staged with established methods prior to entry into the study and at 3 monthly intervals to assess response to therapy (5). Criteria of the National Prostatic Cancer Project (6) were used for scoring responses except that a normalization of the acid phosphatase was not required for classifying a patient as an objective responder.

RESULTS

Clinical Response Rates

A significantly higher percentage of evaluable patients in the stimulation arm obtained either a remission or stabilization of disease compared to the control arm of the protocol (Table 2).

TABLE 2.   Response to treatment in the two arms of the protocol.

Response Category	Stimulation Arm			Control Arm		
	No. of pts.	Percentage of		No. of pts.	Percentage of	
		Evaluable patients (n=20)	All patients (n=34)		Evaluable patients (n=28)	All patients (n=35)
Remissions	9	45% ⎫	26% ⎫	10	36% ⎫	30% ⎫
		⎬85%[a]	⎬50%		⎬72%	⎬60%
Stable disease	8	40% ⎭	24% ⎭	10	36% ⎭	30% ⎭
Failures	3	15%	9%	8	28%	24%
Unevaluable	14	--	41%	5	--	16%

[a] $p < 0.05$ (x^2 analysis) compared to the percentage of evaluable patients in the control arm obtaining remission or disease stabilization.

However, when all randomized patients were included in the analysis, no significant difference was observed between the two groups. This was primarily due to the larger number of unevaluable patients in the stimulation arm in part as a result of fluoxymesterone toxicity (Table 3). The specific reasons which prevented adequate treatment administration in the 19 unevaluable patients are listed in Table 3.

No significant difference was observed in duration of response (remissions + disease stabilization) between the two groups. Median duration of response was 9 months both in the stimulation arm and in the control arm. No significant difference was observed in total survival between the two groups. Median survival is 13 months in the stimulation arm and 16 months in the control group. A total of 19 patients are still living, 6 in the stimulation arm and 13 in the control arm.

TABLE 3. Unevaluable patients.

Patient	Reason
	Stimulation Arm
1,2	Spinal cord compression - first therapy cycle
3,4	Pulmonary embolism during fluoxymesterone
5	Developed neurologic deficit on fluoxymesterone without clear evidence of spinal cord compression
6	Severe flare in bone pain from fluoxymesterone
7	Severe tremor and chills on aminoglutethimide
8	Died of unrelated causes before restaging
9	Death from progressive disease before chemotherapy
10	Died of disseminated intravascular coagulation 5 days after first chemotherapy
11,12	Switched to the placebo arm because of positive screening myelogram
13	Refused chemotherapy
14	Refused treatment after informed consent signed
	Control Arm
1,2	Poor compliance/multiple unrelated medical problems
3	Died within a few days of subdural hematoma
4	Disseminated Herpes Zoster
5	Died within 3 weeks of progressive disease

Drug Toxicity

Two episodes of reversible spinal cord compression were observed during the first cycle of therapy prior to the introduction of the routine screening myelogram (see Methods). Since then only one patient has developed reversible neurological deficit on fluoxymesterone which, however, on repeat myelogram was not due to spinal cord compression. The specific etiology of the neurological deficit during androgen priming in this patient remains undetermined. Most patients experienced exacerbation of bone pain during fluoxymesterone administration. In two patients this was sufficient severity to require discontinuation of treatment. The exacerbation of bone pain with fluoxymesterone declined and in some cases totally disappeared after a few cycles of therapy. Other androgen and chemotherapy-related toxicities are recorded in Table 3.

DISCUSSION

Advanced prostate cancer which has become refractory to orchiectomy is associated with poor prognosis and a 6 month survival of only 50% (2,4). Under these circumstances, the administration of cytotoxic chemotherapy has usually met with limited success (10). Transient stimulation of tumor growth with androgen administration offers a potential new tool to enhance the efficacy of cytotoxic chemotherapy in advanced prostate cancer. The hypothetical concept underlying this strategy is that androgens increase the growth fraction of the tumor and enhance its susceptibility to the action of chemotherpy. Preliminary experimental evidence exists to indicate that androgen-induced stimulation of growth potentiates the effects of chemotherapy on normal prostatic tissue (7) as well as on experimental prostatic cancer (1). Two other clinical trials have employed a strategy of hormonal stimulation plus chemotherapy in the treatment of advanced prostate cancer in humans. While one study reported an encouraging response rate of 85% in a group of 30 men with stage D prostate cancer (3), the other demonstrated only a 43% respone rate in a similar group of 21 men (8). Since, however, neither study was controlled, no conclusion can be drawn on the potential superiority of this treatment strategy over administration of chemotherapy alone.

Our data indicate that the benefit from androgen priming may be partially offset by its greater toxicity in patients with markedly advanced disease. This possibility is suggested by the increased frequency of toxicity and greater percentage of unevaluable patients in the stimulation arm compared to the control arm (41% versus 16%, Table 2). Considerations of tumor biology suggest that risk benefit ratios for this strategy would be more favorable in patients with less advanced disease. Since all of our study patients had evidence of progressive disease following orchiectomy, it is likely that a significant fraction of their tumor cells had become androgen insensitive and, thus, not likely to be influenced by hormonal priming. If this hypothesis is correct, the androgen priming strategy would be more beneficial if instituted earlier in the patient's course. At the time of initial castration, a larger fraction of hormone-responsive cells are present and androgen priming should be more efficacious. We conclude that the present study provides experimental support for the concept of androgen priming which now should be tested in a more favorable group of patients.

REFERENCES

1. Grossman, H.B., Kleinert, E.L., Lesser, M.L., Herr, H.W., and Whitmore, W.F. (1981): Urol. Res., 9:237-240.

2. Johnson, D.E., Scott, W.W., Gibbons, R.P., Prout, G.R., Schmidt, J.D., Chu, T.M., Gaeta, J., Saroff, J., Murphy, G.P. (1977): Cancer Treat. Rep., 61:317-323.

3. Kedia, K.R., Kellermeyer, R.W., and Persky, L. (1981): In: Proc. Amer. Urol. Assoc., pp. 191A.

4. Klein, L.A. (1979): N. Engl. J. Med., 300:824-833.

5. Manni, A., Santen, R.J., Boucher, A., Harvey, H., Simmonds, M., White, D., Gordone, R., Rohner, T., Drago, J., Wettlaufer, J., and Glode, M. (1985): Anticancer Res., 5:161-165.

6. Murphy, G.P. and Slack, N.H. (1980): Prostate, 1:375-382.

7. Sloan, W.R., Heston, W.D.W., and Coffey, D.S. (1975): Cancer Chemother. Rep., 59:185-194.

8. Suarez, A.J., Lamm, D.L., Radvin, H.M., Sarosdy, M., Clark, G., and Osborne, C.K. (1982): Cancer Chemother. Pharmacol., 8:261-265.

9. Sulkes, A., Livingston, R.B., and Murphy, W.K. (1979): J. Natl. Cancer Inst., 62:513-515.

10. Torti, II, F.M. and Carter, S.K. (1980): Ann. Int. Med., 92:681-689.

Subject Index